A Primer on Stroke Prevention Treatment:
An Overview Based on AHA/ASA Guidelines

A Primer on Stroke Prevention Treatment: An Overview Based on AHA/ASA Guidelines

Edited by

Larry B. Goldstein
Professor of Medicine
Duke University Medical Center
Durham, North Carolina
USA

WILEY-BLACKWELL
A John Wiley & Sons, Ltd., Publication

This edition first published 2009, © 2009 American Heart Association
American Heart Association National Center, 7272 Greenville Avenue, Dallas, TX 75231, USA
For further information on the American Heart Association:
www.americanheart.org

Blackwell Publishing was acquired by John Wiley & Sons in February 2007. Blackwell's publishing program has been merged with Wiley's global Scientific, Technical and Medical business to form Wiley-Blackwell.

Registered office: John Wiley & Sons Ltd, The Atrium, Southern Gate, Chichester, West Sussex, PO19 8SQ, UK
Editorial offices: 9600 Garsington Road, Oxford, OX4 2DQ, UK
      The Atrium, Southern Gate, Chichester, West Sussex, PO19 8SQ, UK
      111 River Street, Hoboken, NJ 07030-5774, USA

For details of our global editorial offices, for customer services and for information about how to apply for permission to reuse the copyright material in this book please see our website at www.wiley.com/wiley-blackwell

Library of Congress Cataloging-in-Publication Data

A primer on stroke prevention and treatment : an overview based on AHA/ASA
guidelines / edited by Larry B. Goldstein.
    p. ; cm.
  Includes bibliographical references.
  ISBN 978-1-4051-8651-3
  1. Cerebrovascular disease. I. Goldstein, Larry B. II. American Heart Association.
III. American Stroke Association.
  [DNLM: 1. Stroke–prevention & control–Practice Guideline. 2. Stroke–therapy–Practice
Guideline. WL 355 P9537 2009]
  RC388.5.P6785 2009
  616.8'105–dc22

                            2008051435

ISBN: 9781405186513

A catalogue record for this book is available from the British Library.

Set in 9.25 on 12 Minion by SNP Best-set Typesetter Ltd., Hong Kong
Printed & bound in Singapore by Fabulous Printers Pte Ltd
1   2009

Contents

A companion website:

www.wiley.com/go/strokeguidelines,

will keep you informed of new and updated guidelines.

Contributors

Harold P. Adams, Jr., MD
Director of the Division of Cerebrovascular
Diseases
Department of Neurology
Carver College of Medicine
University of Iowa
Iowa City, IA, USA

Robert J. Adams, MS, MD
Stroke Center
Medical University of South Carolina
Charleston, SC, USA

Opeolu Adeoye, MD
Assistant Professor
Departments of Emergency Medicine and
Neurosurgery
University of Cincinnati
Cincinnati, OH, USA

Richard C. Becker, MD
Professor of Medicine
Divisions of Cardiology and Hematology
Duke University School of Medicine
Duke Clinical Research Institute
Durham, NC, USA

Danielle Blankenship
Doctor of Physical Therapy Division
Department of Community and Family Medicine
Duke University
Durham, NC, USA

Jonathan L. Brisman, MD
Director, Cerebrovascular and Endovascular
Neurosurgery
Winthrop University Hospital
Long Island, NY, USA

Cheryl D. Bushnell, MD, MHS
Associate Professor, Department of Neurology
Wake Forest University Health Sciences
Medical Center Boulevard
Winston-Salem, NC, USA

Joseph P. Broderick, MD
Professor and Chair
Department of Neurology
UC Neuroscience Institute
University of Cincinnati
Cincinnati, OH, USA

Mark Chan, MD
Research Fellow
Duke Clinical Research Institute
Durham, NC, USA

Seemant Chaturvedi, MD, FAHA, FAAN
Professor of Neurology
Stroke Program and Department of Neurology
Wayne State University
Detroit, MI, USA

Burhan Z. Chaudhry, MD
Zeenat Qureshi Stroke Research Center
Department of Neurology
University of Minnesota
Minneapolis, MN, USA

Gabrielle A. deVeber, MD
Director, Children's Stroke Program
Division of Neurology
Hospital for Sick Children
Toronto, Ontario, Canada

Pamela Woods Duncan PhD, PT, FAPTA, FAHA
Professor and Bette Busch Maniscalco Research
Fellow
Doctor of Physical Therapy Division
Department of Community and Family Medicine
Duke University
Senior Fellow
Duke Center for Clinical Health Policy Research
Durham, NC, USA

Philip B. Gorelick, MD, MPH
John S. Garvin Professor and Head
Director, Center for Stroke Research
Department of Neurology and Rehabilitation
Section of Cerebrovascular Disease and
Neurological Critical Care
University of Illinois College of Medicine at
Chicago
Chicago, IL, USA

Vladimir Hachinski, MD, DSc, FRCP (C)
Distinguished University Professor and Professor
of Neurology
University of Western Ontario
London, ON, Canada

Shunichi Homma, MD
Margaret Milliken Hatch Professor of Medicine
Division of Cardiology
Columbia University
New York, NY, USA

George Howard, DrPH
Professor and Chair
Department of Biostatistics
School of Public Health
University of Alabama at Birmingham
1665 University Boulevard
Birmingham, AL, USA

Virginia J. Howard, PhD
Research Assistant Professor
Department of Epidemiology
School of Public Health
University of Alabama at Birmingham
Birmingham, AL, USA

Nicol Korner-Bitensky, PhD, OT
McGill University
Faculty of Medicine, School of Physical and
Occupational Therapy
Centre de recherche interdisciplinaire en
réadaptation du Montréal métropolitain
Canadian
Stroke Network (Theme – Rehabilitation)
CanDRIVE – Keeping Safe Older Drivers Driving
Montreal, QC, Canada

Steven R. Levine, MD
Professor of Neurology
Director, Cerebrovascular Education Program
Stroke Center
The Mount Sinai School of Medicine
New York, NY, USA

Marc R. Mayberg, MD
Director, Seattle Neuroscience Institute
Swedish Medical Center
Seattle, WA, USA

José G. Merino, MD, MPhil
Medical Director
Suburban Hospital Stroke Program
Bethesda, MD, USA

Nikolaos I.H. Papamitsakis, MD
Director, Stroke Service
Assistant Professor of Neurology
Medical University of South Carolina
Charleston, SC, USA

Soojin Park, MD
Massachusetts General Hospital
Boston, MA, USA

Adnan I. Qureshi, MD
Zeenat Qureshi Stroke Research Center
Department of Neurology
University of Minnesota
Minneapolis, MN, USA

Kumar Rajamani, MD
Stroke Program and Department of Neurology
Wayne State University
Detroit, MI, USA

Jose G. Romano, MD
Associate Professor of Neurology
Director, Cerebrovascular Division
University of Miami Miller School of Medicine
Miami, FL, USA

Jonathan Rosand, MD, MSc
Department of Neurology and Center for Human
Genetic Research
Massachusetts General Hospital
Program in Medical and Population Genetics
Broad Institute of MIT and Harvard
Boston, MA, USA

Natalia Rost, MD
Massachusetts General Hospital and Center for
Human Genetic Research
Program in Medical and Population Genetics
Broad Institute of MIT and Harvard
Boston, MA, USA

Ralph L. Sacco, MD, MS, FAAN, FAHA
Chairman of Neurology
Olemberg Family Chair in Neurological Disorders
Miller Professor of Neurology, Epidemiology, and
Human Genetics
Neurologist-in-Chief, Jackson Memorial Hospital
University of Miami Miller School of Medicine
Miami, FL, USA

Lee H. Schwamm, MD
Massachusetts General Hospital
Boston, MA, USA

Svati H. Shah, MD
Assistant Professor of Medicine
Division of Cardiology
Duke Center for Human Genetics
Duke University School of Medicine
Durham, NC, USA

Farhan Siddiq, MD
Zeenat Qureshi Stroke Research Center
Department of Neurology
University of Minnesota
Minneapolis, MN, USA

Fernando D. Testai, MD, PhD
Neurology Clinical Instructor
Department of Neurology and Rehabilitation
Section of Cerebrovascular Disease and
Neurological Critical Care
University of Illinois College of Medicine at
Chicago
Chicago, IL, USA

Marco R. Di Tullio, MD
Professor of Medicine
Division of Cardiology
Columbia University
New York, NY, USA

Linda Williams, MD
Chief of Neurology, Roudebush VAMC
Research Coordinator, VA Stroke QUERI
Associate Professor, Neurology
Indiana University
Bloomington, IN, USA

Preface

The American Stroke Association/American Heart Association Guidelines are intended to distill a vast amount of information to support the practice of evidence-based medicine. Yet clinical guideline statements can be a challenge to use and apply in routine practice. In addition, patients are often encountered for whom the available guidelines do not seem to apply directly.

The development of practice guidelines is only one step in the process of improving clinical care. The American Stroke Association/American Heart Association is dedicated not only to increasing knowledge related to stroke and cardiovascular diseases but also to translating the best available science in a way that informs and improves the health and outcomes of both patients and the general public. This book is intended to help bridge the gap between guidelines and practice.

The book is divided into two sections. Chapters in the first section deal with general issues, and those in the second section with focused topics. Each chapter's major points are highlighted in a bullet point table. To provide clinical context, each chapter begins with a patient example that is referred to in the subsequent discussion. Some chapters use several illustrative cases. The ASA/AHA guidelines are referenced wherever applicable; however, clinical issues not covered in available guidelines are also reviewed. Although taking a clinical perspective, each chapter is thoroughly referenced, providing helpful content for both generalists and stroke specialists.

Clinicians think in terms of people, not guidelines. By example, the approach taken in this book should serve to help providers integrate the information provided in the ASA/AHA guidelines into their practices to the betterment of their patients.

Larry B. Goldstein, MD, FAAN, FAHA
Professor of Medicine Duke University
Medical Center
Durham, NC

Classification of Recommendations and Level of Evidence

Reference is made throughout this book to ASA/AHA Guideline recommendations. The scheme is summarized in the table and serves as a reference for the reader's interpretation of both estimates of certainty of treatment effects (i.e., Level A, B, or C) and the magnitude of that effect (Class I, IIa, IIb, and III). It should be noted that in this scheme, Class III reflects a treatment for which the risk generally outweighs its benefit. The table also provides phrases that are generally used to reflect the strength of a recommendation.

Applying Classification of Recommendations and Level of Evidence

	SIZE OF TREATMENT EFFECT			
	CLASS I *Benefit >>> Risk* Procedure/Treatment **SHOULD** be performed/administered	**CLASS IIa** *Benefit >> Risk* *Additional studies with focused objectives needed* **IT IS REASONABLE** to perform procedure/administer treatment	**CLASS IIb** *Benefit ≥ Risk* *Additional studies with broad objectives needed; additional registry data would be helpful* Procedure/Treatment **MAY BE CONSIDERED**	**CLASS III** *Risk ≥ Benefit* Procedure/Treatment should **NOT** be performed/administered **SINCE IT IS NOT HELPFUL AND MAY BE HARMFUL**
LEVEL A Multiple populations evaluated* Data derived from multiple randomized clinical trials or meta-analyses	■ Recommendation that procedure or treatment is useful/effective ■ Sufficient evidence from multiple randomized trials or meta-analyses	■ Recommendation in favor of treatment or procedure being useful/effective ■ Some conflicting evidence from multiple randomized trials or meta-analyses	■ Recommendation's usefulness/efficacy less well established ■ Greater conflicting evidence from multiple randomized trials or meta-analyses	■ Recommendation that procedure or treatment is not useful/effective and may be harmful ■ Sufficient evidence from multiple randomized trials or meta-analyses
LEVEL B Limited populations evaluated* Data derived from a single randomized trial or nonrandomized studies	■ Recommendation that procedure or treatment is useful/effective ■ Evidence from single randomized trial or nonrandomized studies	■ Recommendation in favor of treatment or procedure being useful/effective ■ Some conflicting evidence from single randomized trial or nonrandomized studies	■ Recommendation's usefulness/efficacy less well established ■ Greater conflicting evidence from single randomized trial or nonrandomized studies	■ Recommendation that procedure or treatment is not useful/effective and may be harmful ■ Evidence from single randomized trial or nonrandomized studies
LEVEL C Very limited populations evaluated* Only consensus opinion of experts, case studies, or standard of care	■ Recommendation that procedure or treatment is useful/effective ■ Only expert opinion, case studies, or standard of care	■ Recommendation in favor of treatment or procedure being useful/effective ■ Only diverging expert opinion, case studies, or standard of care	■ Recommendation's usefulness/efficacy less well established ■ Only diverging expert opinion, case studies, or standard of care	■ Recommendation that procedure or treatment is not useful/effective and may be harmful ■ Only expert opinion, case studies, or standard of care
Suggested phrases for writing recommendations[†]	should is recommended is indicated is useful/effective/beneficial	is reasonable can be useful/effective/beneficial is probably recommended or indicated	may/might be considered may/might be reasonable usefulness/effectiveness is unknown/unclear/uncertain or not well established	is not recommended is not indicated should not is not useful/effective/beneficial may be harmful

ESTIMATE OF CERTAINTY (PRECISION) OF TREATMENT EFFECT

*Data available from clinical trials or registries about the usefulness/efficacy in different subpopulations, such as gender, age, history of diabetes, history of prior myocardial infarction, history of heart failure, and prior aspirin use. A recommendation with Level of Evidence B or C does not imply that the recommendation is weak. Many important clinical questions addressed in the guidelines do not lend themselves to clinical trials. Even though randomized trials are not available, there may be a very clear clinical consensus that a particular test or therapy is useful or effective.

†In 2003, the ACC/AHA Task Force on Practice Guidelines developed a list of suggested phrases to use when writing recommendations. All guideline recommendations have been written in full sentences that express a complete thought, such that a recommendation, even if separated and presented apart from the rest of the document (including headings above sets of recommendations), would still convey the full intent of the recommendation. It is hoped that this will increase readers' comprehension of the guidelines and will allow queries at the individual recommendation level.

Part I

Overview Topics

Stroke Epidemiology

George Howard and Virginia J. Howard

EXAMPLE CASE

A 45-year-old right-handed African-American man residing in central North Carolina has a history of hypertension and presents with right-sided weakness without a language impairment and visual or sensory deficits. He also has a 50-pack-year history of cigarette smoking. His examination revels a body mass index (BMI) of 35, a blood pressure of 180/95 mm Hg, a regular pulse, no cervical bruits, and no cardiac murmur. His neurological examination is notable only for a right upper-motor neuron pattern facial paresis and 3/5 strength in his right arm and leg with depressed right-sided deep tendon reflexes and a right plantar-extensor response. A brain CT scan obtained 4 hours after symptom onset was normal. An EKG followed by a transthoracic echocardiogram showed left ventricular hypertrophy (LVH).

MAJOR POINTS

- Although overall stroke mortality rates have been rapidly declining, consistently higher rates remain among African-Americans (particularly between ages 45 and 65) and Southerners.
- Risk factors influencing stroke incidence can be stratified into two tiers:
  - Tier 1. Risk factors consistently identified as playing a major role
    - The "big three" risk factors contributing over half of the population attributable risk: hypertension, diabetes, and smoking
    - Others: left ventricular hypertrophy, atrial fibrillation, and heart disease
  - Tier 2. Risk factors likely playing a role
    - Risk factors for risk factors: obesity, fat distribution, and physical activities may have minor direct impact but play a major role by increasing the risk for hypertension and diabetes (tier 1 factors)
    - Risk factors important to control regardless of direct stroke risk: dyslipidemia and metabolic syndrome
    - Risk factors playing an important role in special populations: asymptomatic carotid stenosis, postmenopausal hormone therapy, and sickle-cell disease
    - Risk factors likely playing a smaller or questionable role.
- The "graying of America" is likely to have a major impact on the absolute number of stroke events in the next half-century, with an anticipated dramatic increase in the number of stroke events particularly among elderly women.

A Primer on Stroke Prevention Treatment: An Overview Based on AHA/ASA Guidelines, 1st Edition. Edited by L Goldstein.
© 2009 American Heart Association, ISBN: 9781405186513

Stroke mortality and its disparities

There are few US national data describing stroke incidence, and as a result, most of what is known about stroke epidemiology focuses on mortality rates. The age–sex-adjusted stroke mortality rates by race-ethnic group for the United States between 1979 and 2005 are shown in Figure 1.1. This figure reflects the remarkable successes and failures in stroke. During this brief 26-year period, stroke mortality has declined by 48.4% for African-Americans, by 52.9% for whites, and by 45.5% for other races [1] – a decline in a chronic disease that is simply striking. Along with similar reductions in heart disease mortality, this decline was acknowledged as one of the "Ten Great Public Health Achievements" of the 20th century (the only two achievements that were listed for a specific disease) [2].

This same figure, however, underscores one of the great failures in the 20th century – striking disparities by race. Using the year 2000 age standard, in 1979, African-Americans had an age-adjusted stroke mortality rate that was 30.8% higher than whites, whereas other races had a rate that was 26.7% below whites. This is in contrast to 2005, when African-Americans had stroke mortality rates 43.0% higher than whites, a relative *increase* of 39.6% ([43.0–30.8]/30.8) in the magnitude of the racial disparity in stroke deaths. This increase in stroke mortality

among African-Americans persists despite the Healthy Persons 2010 goals (one of the guiding documents for the entire Department of Health and Human Services) having as one of its two primary aims "to eliminate health disparities among segments of the population, including differences that occur by gender, race or ethnicity, education or income, disability, geographic location, or sexual orientation" [3].

This figure obscures another disturbing pattern. The African-American–white differences in stroke mortality rates are three to four times (300–400%) higher between the ages of 40 and 60. These are attenuated with increasing age to become approximately equivalent above age 85 (see Figure 1.2) [4]. Data from the Greater Cincinnati/Northern Kentucky Stroke Study suggest that this excess burden of stroke mortality is primarily attributable to higher stroke incidence rates in African-Americans (rather than case fatality), and is uniformly shared between first and recurrent stroke, as well as between ischemic and hemorrhagic (both intracerebral and subarachnoid) stroke subtypes; all have incidence race ratios between 1.8 and 2.0 [5,6].

Another great disparity in stroke mortality is the "stroke belt" – a region in the southeastern United States with high stroke mortality that has persisted since at least 1940 (see Figure 1.3 [7]). Whereas the overall magnitude of geographic disparity is between

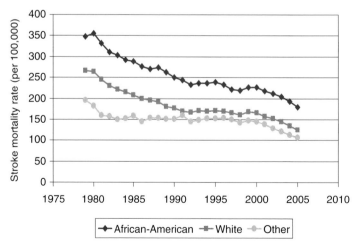

Fig. 1.1 Age-adjusted (2000 standard) stroke mortality rates for ages 45 and older, shown for African-American, white, and all other races. Data were retrieved from the Centers for Disease Control Wonder System [1], with ICD-9 codes 430–438 for years 1979–1998, and ICD-10 codes I60 to I69 for years 1999–2005.

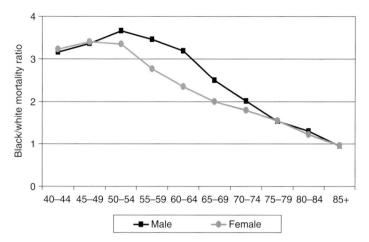

Fig. 1.2 African-American-to-white age-specific stroke mortality ratio for 2005 for the United States [4].

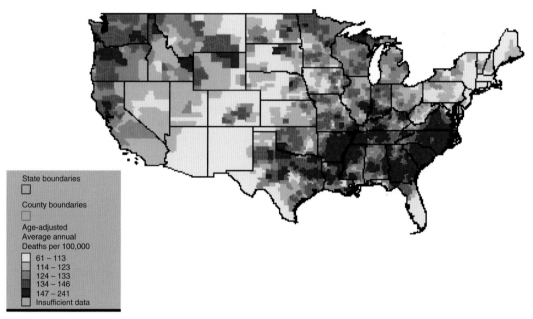

Fig. 1.3 Geographic pattern of stroke mortality rates between 1991 and 1998 for US residents aged 35 and older. Centers for Disease Control and Prevention, Stroke Atlas. www.cdc.gov/DHDSP/library/maps/strokeatlas/index.htm.

30% and 50%, this map shows that specific regions (such as the "buckle" region of the stroke belt along the coastal plain of North Carolina, South Carolina, and Georgia) have stroke mortality rates well over twice those of other regions. There are as many as 10 published hypothesized causes of this geographic disparity [8,9], but the reason for its existence remains uncertain. Finally, depending on sex and age strata, the magnitude of the southern excess stroke mortality is between 6% and 21% greater for African-Americans than for whites [10]. The example patient is at a higher risk of stroke and stroke mortality compared with Americans of other race-ethnic groups because he is an African-American and because he resides within the stroke-belt region of the country.

Stroke risk factors

The current American Heart Association/American Stroke Association Primary Stroke Prevention Guidelines provides a comprehensive review of potential stroke risk factors with an extensive listing of references (offering a total of 572) [11]. A list of more than 30 separate risk factors and conditions reviewed in these guidelines is summarized in Table 1.1, along with classifications on the support for treatment and the level of evidence regarding the role of the factor in modifying stroke risk. Although the table is comprehensive, the goal of this section is to provide a more focused discussion within a framework that may be quickly considered by practicing clinicians. Any attempt to reorganize the listing provided in the guidelines should not be interpreted as minimizing the importance of any factor in an individual patient, but rather as helping to set priorities in a resource-limited environment.

The foundation of the approach to organize risk factors is to consider efforts to establish "risk functions" for stroke in which the factors are considered as independent predictors of stroke risk taken from the more comprehensive list. Although reported over 15 years ago, the most well known of these risk assessments is from the Framingham Study cohort in which independent stroke predictors included age, systolic blood pressure, use of antihypertensive medications, diabetes mellitus, current smoking, established coronary disease (any one of myocardial

Table 1.1 Summary of recommendations from the American Heart Association Guidelines for primary stroke prevention

Nonmodifiable	**11** Physical inactivity (I, B)
1 Age	**12** Obesity and body fat distribution (I, A)
2 Sex	
3 Low birth weight	Less well-documented or potentially modifiable risk factors
4 Race ethnicity	**1** Metabolic syndrome (see individual components)
5 Genetic factors (IIb, C)	**2** Alcohol abuse (IIb, B)
	3 Drug abuse (IIb, C)
Well-documented and modifiable risk factors	**4** Oral contraceptive use (III, B/C)
1 Hypertension (I, A)	**5** Sleep-disordered breathing (IIb, C)
2 Cigarette smoking (I, B)	**6** Migraine (ratings not provided, but considered "insufficient" to
3 Diabetes (I, A)	recommend a treatment approach)
4 Atrial fibrillation (I, A)	**7** Hyperhomocysteinemia (IIb, C)
5 Other cardiac conditions	**8** Elevated lipoprotein (a) (IIb, C)
• Left ventricular hypertrophy (IIa, A)	**9** Elevated lipoprotein-associated phospholipase A_2 (absence of
• Heart failure (IIb, C)	evidence)
6 Dyslipidemia (I, A)	**10** Hypercoagulability (absence of evidence)
7 Asymptomatic carotid stenosis (I, C)	**11** Inflammation (IIa, B)
8 Sickle-cell disease (I, B)	**12** Infection (absence of evidence)
9 Postmenopausal hormone therapy (III, A)	**13** Aspirin for primary stroke prevention (III, A)
10 Diet and nutrition	
• Sodium intake (I, A)	
• Healthy diet (DASH) (I, A)	
• Fruit and vegetable diet (IIb, C)	

DASH, Dietary Approaches to Stop Hypertension

Attempts were made to classify each potential risk factor on two scales (shown in the table as Roman numerals and letters). First, each was classified by the strength of evidence for a treatment approach into strata: I) conditions for which there is evidence for and/or general agreement that the procedure or treatment is useful and effective; IIa) conditions for which there is conflicting evidence and/or a divergence of opinion about the usefulness/efficacy of a procedure or treatment, but the weight of evidence or opinion is in favor of the procedure or treatment; IIb) conditions for which there is conflicting evidence and/or a divergence of opinion about the usefulness/efficacy of a procedure or treatment, and the usefulness/efficacy is less well established by evidence or opinion; and III) conditions for which there is evidence and/or general agreement that the procedure or treatment is not useful/effective and in some cases may be harmful. The second classification was on the level of evidence into strata: A) data derived from multiple randomized clinical trials; B) data derived from a single randomized trial or nonrandomized studies; or C) consensus opinion of experts.

infarction [MI], angina or coronary insufficiency, congestive heart failure, or intermittent claudication), atrial fibrillation, and LVH [12]. It is striking that this list of independent predictors was confirmed by perhaps the second best known of these risk functions, produced from the Cardiovascular Health Study, which included precisely the same list of risk factors (plus additional measures of frailty) [13]. Not accounting for age as a disease risk factor and considering systolic blood pressure and use of antihypertensive medications as one factor, that these two risk functions were concordant with the independent risk factors for stroke strongly suggests these six factors as "first-tier" risk factors for stroke (see Table 1.2). The example patient has a history of hypertension, an additional, modifiable, "first-tier" stroke risk factor.

The "population attributable risk" (the proportion of stroke events attributable to specific risk factors) is a product of both the magnitude of the impact of a risk factor and its prevalence in the at-risk population, and provides important insights to the contributions of these first-tier risk factors. The population attributable risk for major stroke types was recently reported from the Atherosclerosis Risk in Communities Study (Figure 1.4) [14] showing that the combination of hypertension, diabetes, and cigarette smoking contributes the great majority of

Table 1.2 A proposed structure for consideration for modifiable stroke risk factors

1 First-tier factors
- The "big three" factors (based on population attributable risk)
  a. Hypertension
  b. Diabetes
  c. Cigarette smoking
- Other first-tier factors
  a. Heart diseases
  b. Atrial fibrillation
  c. Left ventricular hypertrophy

2 Second-tier factors
- Risk factors for risk factors. Examples:
  a. Obesity and body fat distribution
  b. Physical inactivity
- Risk factors important to control (regardless of stroke risk). Examples:
  a. Dyslipidemia
  b. Metabolic syndrome
- Risk factors important in special populations
  a. Asymptomatic carotid stenosis
  b. Postmenopausal hormone therapy
  c. Sickle-cell condition
- Risk factors with a smaller effect or questionable effect (others)

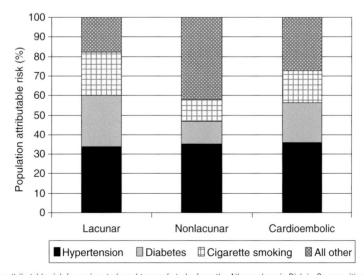

Fig. 1.4 Population attributable risk for major stroke subtypes of stroke from the Atherosclerosis Risk in Communities study for the "big three" risk factors and all others (including second-tier risk factors). Adapted from data available in Ohira *et al.* [14].

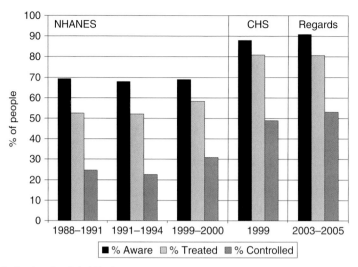

Fig. 1.5 Awareness, treatment, and control of blood pressure.
CHS, Cardiovascular Health Study; NHANES, National Health and Nutrition Examination Survey; REGARDS, Reasons for Geographic and Racial Differences in Stroke.

risk for lacunar (82%), nonlacunar (58%), and cardioembolic (73%) stroke. The substantial contribution of these three risk factors to stroke risk is underscored by the population attributable risk in the American Heart Association (AHA)/American Stroke Association (ASA) guidelines paper [11], which, while based on different studies, sums to more than 100% (i.e., more than 100% of the risk of stroke is attributed to different causes). The guidelines statement suggests that hypertension alone contributed between 30% and 40% of stroke risk, cigarette smoking between 12% and 18%, and diabetes between 5% and 27% [11]. Clearly, these three risk factors could be called "the big three" of the first tier. In addition to being an African-American residing in the stroke belt with a history of hypertension, the example patient smokes cigarettes, further increasing his stroke risk. His clinical syndrome is consistent with a "lacunar" syndrome.

As a clinician, it is not only important to treat specific risk factors in individual patients, but it is also important to think at the level of a group of patients (e.g., a practice) and allocate resources where they can have the greatest impact. Importantly, treatment approaches that will lead to substantial reductions in the overall burden of stroke would need to particularly target this "big three" cluster of risk factors. Although there have been some improvements in their management over

time, the control of these risk factors remains suboptimal. For example, awareness, treatment, and control of high blood pressure in the National Health and Nutrition Examination Survey (NHANES) Study over the period 1988–1991 to 1999–2000, and from the Reasons for Geographic and Racial Differences in Stroke Study through 2003–2005, are shown in Figure 1.5 [15]. These data suggest that while there may have been an increase in awareness of hypertension from 70% to 90%, an increase in treatment from 52% to 80%, and an increase in control (to systolic blood pressure < 140 and diastolic blood pressure < 90) from 25% to 52%, approximately 50% of hypertensive individuals still fail to achieve control of their condition. Likewise, while there were substantial decreases in the prevalence of cigarette smoking from 1965 (with a prevalence of 51.2% in men and 33.7% in women) to 1990 (with a prevalence of 28.0% in men and 22.9% in women), the rate of decline substantially slowed in the 16 years between 1990 and 2005. The prevalence only decreased to 23.4% in men and to 18.3% in women – with one in every five adults remaining as active smokers [16]. We are also largely failing at adequate control of diabetes, for which between 35% and 50% of type 2 diabetics in the NHANES study had hemoglobin A1c values at or above 8% [17]. Although we know that impacting these "big three" risk factors would reduce stroke incidence by more than 50%, interventions to manage these risk factors are not being optimally employed.

The other three "first-tier" risk factors – history of heart diseases, atrial fibrillation, and LVH – are as important (or perhaps even more important) in individual patients with these prevalent conditions [12,13]. The population prevalence of each of these conditions is lower, thereby making their overall contributions smaller. Also, it is clear that effective treatments exist for high-risk patients with atrial fibrillation using warfarin [18–20], although the standard treatments for LVH and previous heart disease are more complex. Hence, it could be suggested that a primary care physician could have the largest impact intervening on the "big three," but the awareness and treatment of individual patients who have these "other first-tier" risk factors remain important. The example patient also had LVH, possibly related to his history of hypertension.

Although non-first-tier risk factors should not be thought of as being unimportant, it is useful to use a different framework for their consideration. This framework includes thinking about these "other" risk factors in three classes.

There are several risk factors that do not directly impact stroke risk, but rather act as risk factors for one or more of the first-tier risk factors. For example, obesity is largely absent or has a relatively minor role in multivariable stroke risk models. In the Framingham and other studies, obesity is a potent risk factor for diabetes and carries an odds ratio 2.5 times greater for incident diabetes among participants with a BMI of 30 or greater [21]. In the Incidence of Hypertension in a French Working Population (IHPAF) study, obesity was the single greatest predictor of incident hypertension; individuals with a BMI above 30 had an odds ratio for incident hypertension 5.5 times greater for men and 2.8 times greater for women [22]. With obesity playing such a major role on the risk for two of the three "first-tier" stroke risk factors (and also having a relationship with atrial fibrillation and LVH), its absence in the major risk models should not be interpreted as reflecting a lack of importance, but rather as identifying obesity prevention and treatment as a point of intervention to reduce the major risk factors for stroke. A similar argument could be made for other non-first-tier stroke risk factors, most notably physical inactivity. The example patient had a BMI in the obese range – a factor that increased his chances of developing hypertension.

There are other non-first-tier risk factors for which treatment is critical for reasons that extend quite beyond protection from stroke. Examples of this class include treatments for dyslipidemia. With statin treatment, patients with coronary heart disease or additional risk factors such as hypertension or diabetes not only have a reduction in their risk of coronary heart events, but also a reduction in the risk of a first stroke [11]. In the Stroke Prevention by Aggressive Reduction in Cholesterol Levels (SPARCL) trial that assessed statin treatment for secondary stroke prevention among stroke/transient ischemic attack patients with a low-density lipoprotein level between 100 and 190 mg/dL, there was a 48% reduction (hazard ratio [HR] of 0.58) for subsequent coronary events in addition to a 16% reduction (HR of 0.84) in stroke events [23]. While in SPARCL there were more stroke than MI events, in most populations, the incidence of MI overwhelms that of stroke, and the impact of statin treatment is more powerful for coronary event prevention – suggesting that individuals with elevated lipid levels should be treated with statins almost regardless of their stroke risk. The interpretation of the role of the metabolic syndrome, a clustering of other well-documented cardiovascular risk factors, may also fall to this consideration.

There are also risk factors in special populations. For example, it is clear that surgical treatment of individuals with asymptomatic carotid disease will reduce stroke risk if the operation is performed safely; however, it is not clear whether (a) this is a risk factor for stroke or part of the causal pathway (i.e., hypertension and diabetes cause advancement of atherosclerosis that in turn causes stroke) and (b) treatment is warranted given the relatively small absolute risk reduction [24]. This is reviewed in the chapter on carotid surgery. A similar "special population" is the use of postmenopausal hormone therapy, which has been shown in three randomized trials to be associated with higher cardiovascular risk (including stroke) [25–27]. In all three of these studies, however, the risk of placing women on hormone therapy appeared to be associated with an early higher risk of thrombotic events, raising the question of the optimal treatment for women already on such treatment (who have already passed this high-risk period).

A number of other risk factors discussed in the AHA/ASA Primary Prevention Guideline have been documented in individual studies as potentially related to increased stroke risk [11]. Although their role in increasing stroke risk may be relatively smaller, and additional information may be needed to better understand their roles, the treating physician should be aware of each and consider them for treatment.

The projected future burden of stroke on the healthcare system

As noted earlier, the decline in stroke mortality, presumed to be at least partially attributable to declines in stroke incidence, has been a striking success [2]. Even assuming a continued decline in stroke incidence (perhaps a bold assumption), these declines are likely to be overwhelmed by the "graying of America" as reflected in the population pyramids shown in Figure 1.6. The year 2000 pyramid makes the "baby-boomer" bulge at approximately 45 years apparent – and it is noteworthy that this bulge is at the age when stroke risk is frequently considered to increase. Between 2000 and 2050, it is anticipated that the overall US population will grow by approximately 48% [28]. This "baby-boomer" bulge suggests that there will be a 109% growth among individuals aged 60–69, a

100% growth for individuals aged 70–79, a 196% growth for individuals aged 80–89, and a remarkable 569% growth for individuals over 90 [29]. With the risk of stroke approximately doubling with each increasing decade of age, these increases in the elderly population are likely to lead to more than a doubling in the number of stroke events before 2050 [30]. This increase in the number of persons having strokes, particularly among Hispanic and African-American populations, has been estimated to be associated with public health costs in excess of $2.2 trillion dollars over this period – $1.52 trillion for non-Hispanic whites, $313 billion for Hispanics, and $379 billion for African-Americans [30]. Unfortunately, the graying of America makes it likely that the absolute numbers of Americans having and being disabled by stroke will be increasing.

The example patient's stroke may have largely been preventable. Although he was an African-American residing in the stroke belt, lifestyle changes such as smoking cessation and weight loss would have lowered his risk. Effective control of his blood pressure would also be important as the stroke that occurred can be attributed to occlusion of a small intracranial artery, which is particularly sensitive to the effects of hypertension.

References available online at www.wiley.com/go/ strokeguidelines.

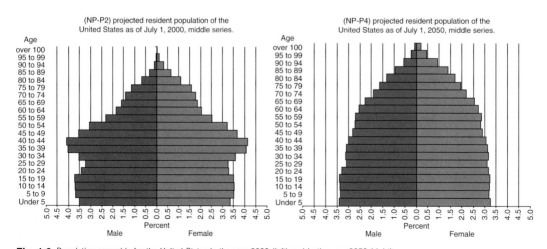

Fig. 1.6 Population pyramids for the United States in the year 2000 (left) and in the year 2050 (right).

Stroke Systems

Soojin Park and Lee H. Schwamm

EXAMPLE CASES

Case 1

A 61-year-old white male arrived at a 120-bed community and regional teaching hospital at 11:30 PM, with left-sided weakness and right-gaze preference. His family insisted he was completely normal at 10:30 PM (1 hour earlier) when, as they were finishing dinner, they witnessed him develop these symptoms. Emergency medical services (EMS) were called and the patient was brought by ambulance to this hospital, which was the nearest one with an emergency department (ED). He was examined by the ED physician who estimated his National Institutes of Health Stroke Scale (NIHSS) score to be 23; he had occasional respiratory pauses and was subsequently intubated for an unenhanced computed tomography (CT) scan of the brain. The

MAJOR POINTS

- A systems-based approach to stroke care delivery is needed to increase access to limited stroke resources and eliminate geographic and financial disparities.
- Telemedicine technology and air medical transport can help collapse the barriers of time and distance between patients and stroke expertise to facilitate rapid delivery of thrombolytic therapy or other advanced interventions.
- Systematic implementation of guideline-based care is essential, and providers should focus on delivering these interventions in each domain of the stroke care continuum.
- Stroke care systems should strive to address the consensus recommendations contained in the Stroke Systems of Care framework, and should focus not just on the individual domains but also on the linkages between the discrete domains of care.

- Lessons can be learned from other successful disease-centered systems of care delivery such as the trauma and acute cardiac systems of care.
- Whenever possible, objective and verifiable criteria should be used to establish hospitals' acute stroke capability and stroke center status, and this information should be made publicly available.
- Continuous quality improvement activities and evaluation should occur within each domain and the stroke system of care model itself should be subject to evaluation and modification over time.
- Gaps in knowledge exist and further research is needed to identify the best methods to measure the effectiveness of systems of care implementation, and to refine the elements necessary within each domain. Legislation efforts and strong financial incentives will likely be needed to make significant improvements.

A Primer on Stroke Prevention Treatment: An Overview Based on AHA/ASA Guidelines, 1st Edition. Edited by L Goldstein.
© 2009 American Heart Association, ISBN: 9781405186513

radiologist's dictation read "dense middle cerebral artery (MCA) sign on the right and subtle ischemic changes."

The neurologist on call for the ED was contacted by telephone and was apprised of the following additional history. The patient had atrial fibrillation and had been on warfarin for stroke prevention until a month ago, when he had a gastrointestinal hemorrhage requiring admission but no blood transfusions. A colonoscopy during that admission revealed two polyps, which were felt to be the cause of bleeding, and were removed. Three days after the colonoscopy, he restarted warfarin. Two weeks after restarting warfarin, when a little blood was noted in his stool, he was instructed to discontinue warfarin until a follow-up appointment could be arranged. After learning the additional history, the neurologist recommended admission and advised against IV thrombolysis (IV tissue-type plasminogen activator [tPA]) because of the bleeding risk and because he felt that the NIHSS score was "too high." The neurologist planned to see the patient in the morning because he was not an IV tPA candidate.

The ED physician phoned the acute stroke service at a nearby tertiary care hospital for a second opinion at 11:55 PM. After reviewing the elements of the ED physician's examination in detail, the acute stroke physician estimated the NIHSS at 18. Without being able to view the CT images that were described over the telephone as having "subtle ischemic changes," the stroke physician felt uncomfortable recommending IV tPA. The patient's family was concerned and requested transfer to the tertiary care hospital in order to have the opportunity to be enrolled in an acute care clinical trial or be screened for endovascular treatment. Because the NIHSS by itself was not considered to be a contraindication for IV or intra-arterial (IA) therapy, the patient was transported by helicopter. On arrival, he was intubated with persistent chemical paralysis and sedation required for the helicopter transport. CT angiogram was performed as soon as the patient arrived at 4:30 AM, 5 hours after the onset of symptoms. The CT angiography revealed an occlusion of the right internal carotid artery and an evolving infarction in the entire MCA and anterior cerebral artery distributions with no visible collaterals. Due to the presence of completed infarct on CT, no endovascular therapy was recommended. Of note, bilateral aspiration pneumonia was visualized on CT.

Early hemicraniectomy was considered and discussed with the family, emphasizing the possibility of reduced mortality without any expected early improvement in the stroke symptoms, but the family declined the intervention. The patient was transferred to the neurointensive care unit, where he was closely monitored overnight. Within 36 hours, despite aggressive medical measures to treat malignant cerebral edema, the patient died as a result of transtentorial herniation.

Case 2

A 51-year-old woman with a history of hypothyroidism and tobacco dependence described the onset of language difficulty and right-sided weakness at 9:45 PM after getting out of the bath. She had no symptoms at 9:00 PM when her boyfriend last saw her, but when she called a friend at 10:00 PM, she was difficult to understand on the telephone. EMS was called, and the ambulance was routed past a nearby hospital to be brought to the nearest state-designated stroke center at 10:45 PM. Because of the prearrival notification by EMS, the CT scan technologist was alerted and was holding open a CT scanner for the patient when she arrived. On examination at the hospital's ED, she was noted to have right-sided weakness and aphasia. Her blood pressure was 150/80 mm Hg, and her pulse was regular at 80 bpm. There was no evidence of acute aortic dissection, myocardial ischemia, hypoglycemia, or comorbid terminal illness. She was not taking any aspirin or prescription medications.

An unenhanced head CT was interpreted as showing no mass lesion, bleeding, or clearly visible new infarction. The ED physician's assessment was that this patient might be a potential IV tPA candidate. Rather than trying to transfer the patient prior to treatment to the nearest comprehensive stroke center (40 miles away), they contacted the stroke center for a telemedicine-enabled stroke (telestroke) consultation at 11:00 PM, 2 hours after she was last known to be well.

The telestroke consultation was initiated, and the diagnosis was felt to be acute ischemic stroke, with ischemia likely in the left MCA territory. An NIHSS score performed over interactive videoconferencing was 9. After the patient's history and CT images were reviewed by the telestroke consultant, it was agreed that the patient should receive IV tPA, and together, they reviewed with her family the risks and benefits, calculated the dose, and supervised its administration. The IV tPA bolus was given at 11:30 PM, 2.5 hours after she was last seen well. She was then transferred to the regional stroke center.

Her neurological condition improved en route, and by the time she arrived, she had only a mild right pronator drift and right facial weakness. She had an magnetic resonance imaging (MRI) with magnetic resonance angiography (MRA) of the head and neck and magnetic resonance perfusion imaging. There were several cortical foci of restricted diffusion-weighted imaging in the left MCA territory, one in the left middle frontal gyrus, one in the frontal operculum, one in the precentral gyrus, and one in the postcentral gyrus, consistent with acute ischemia. A region of abnormality on perfusion-weighted MRI with prolonged relative mean tissue transit time and reduced relative cerebral blood flow was centered in the left frontal operculum, considerably larger in size than the patient's focal area of restricted diffusion in this location. MRA identified a dissection in the left cervical internal carotid artery. She was discharged on a 3-month course of warfarin anticoagulation. The patient recovered fully and returned home after 4 days in the hospital.

Discussion

Acute care demands on general neurologists are rising as geography, practice environments, and reimbursement issues contribute to disparities in acute stroke coverage (Figure 2.1). These two cases demonstrate how access to stroke expertise and treatment options can differ based on different practice environments, financial incentives, and manpower constraints. In the absence of an organized stroke system of care, centers of excellence can be surrounded by other centers struggling to provide even rudimentary stroke services. The advent of organized networks of prehospital care coupled with stroke centers, as well as the utilization of new technology such as telemedicine, increases access to specialty acute care for those who would not have otherwise received opportunities for thrombolytic therapy or other advanced interventions. The old paradigm of preliminary evaluation over several hours in a small community hospital ED, followed by transfer to a tertiary center after the window for intervention had expired (a "drift and shift" approach), is being gradually replaced by rapid evaluation and initial administration of therapeutics in consultation with expert centers prior to transfer (the "drip and ship" approach).

A stroke system strives to ensure a more equitable distribution of scarce resources. Within any one community, there are often too many urgent needs, and not enough qualified healthcare providers to meet them. Not all hospitals need to possess all capabilities. Because patients arriving at hospitals with acute stroke within the 3-hour time window (generally within 2 hours of symptom onset) is a low-frequency, high-impact event, and because half of all strokes result in minimal disability (NIHSS score <4), which generally does not require thrombolytic intervention, acute stroke expertise on-site may not be practical. Strategies such as telemedicine or air medical transport that can bring patients and providers together rapidly and efficiently may help reduce disparities in access to acute stroke care. Coordinated approaches to addressing the acute stroke needs of an entire state or region are best pursued in the context of a stroke systems of care framework that engages key stakeholders and forges links between the different critical components of care delivery.

Florida - stroke deate rates
Total population, ages 35+, 1991–1998

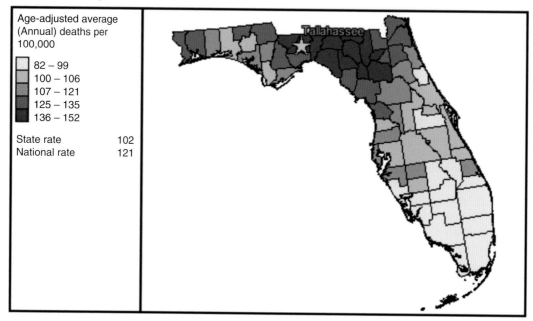

Florida - neurologists per 10,000 population, ages 65+

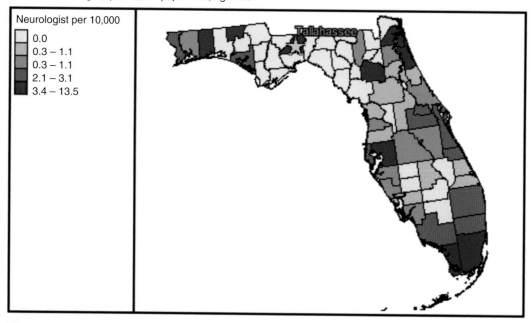

Fig. 2.1 Relationship between stroke mortality and distribution of neurologists based on the Centers for Disease Control and Prevention's Online Atlas of Stroke Mortality (http://apps.nccd.cdc.gov/giscvh2/Select2Maps.aspx).

New York- stroke deate rates
Total population, ages 35+, 1991–1998

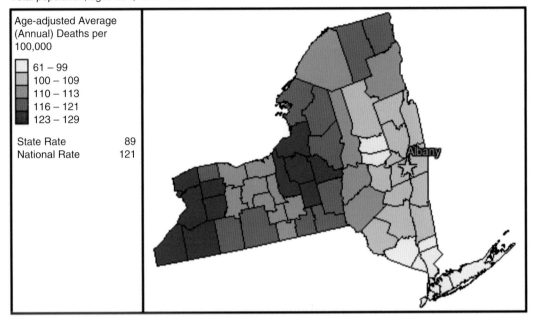

New York - neurologists per 10,000 population, ages 65+

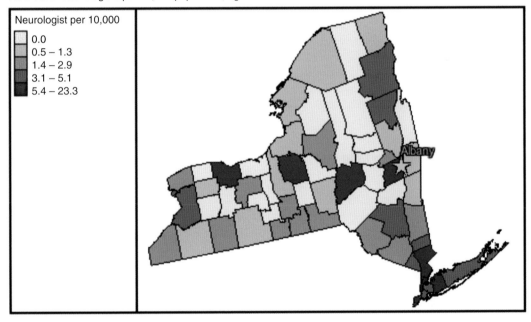

Fig. 2.1 *Continued*

A model for stroke systems

The trauma system is a successful model from which useful parallels for stroke care may be drawn. A trauma system is a network involving all phases of patient care – starting from injury prevention, to the scene of injury, through the trauma center, recovery, and rehabilitation. Putting in place a trauma system, or improvements in an aspect of a trauma system, is associated with improved hospital survival among the seriously injured [1]. Within a region, there is a hierarchy of centers based on demonstrated need in the community, the capability to provide care to the seriously injured, and a predetermined expectation of proper coordination and rapid transportation of the most seriously injured from less capable to tertiary care centers. Trauma systems strive to provide similar coverage between urban and rural communities within a region.

The potential to improve stroke outcomes by focusing on building infrastructure and systems of care was recognized early in the stroke center movement. While a standardized approach to hospital-based stroke care had been evolving, innovative programs in prehospital EMS, community education, and rehabilitation were being developed in isolation. There was a clear need for a more integrated approach to address the disparities in care delivery and access observed throughout the United States and within smaller regions (e.g., cities, counties, states).

Defining the components of the ideal stroke system

The American Stroke Association's (ASA) Task Force on the Development of Stroke Systems examined ongoing stroke initiatives in the United States (publications from 1994 to 2003) and drafted the Recommendations for the Establishment of Stroke Systems of Care in 2005 [2]. The recommendations were organized by the *seven components* that an ideal stroke system would address (Table 2.1), elaborating on the prior concept of the chain of stroke survival, which was organized based on the temporal sequence of acute stroke care. The Task Force recommendations offered a set of guiding principles for state and regional collaboratives that were developing their own stroke systems of care, with an emphasis on

Table 2.1 Seven components that an ideal stroke system should address (adapted from the American Stroke Association's Recommendations for the establishment of Stroke Systems of Care 2005) [2]

1 Primordial and primary prevention
2 Community education
3 Notification and response of emergency medical services
4 Acute stroke treatment
5 Subacute stroke treatment and secondary prevention
6 Rehabilitation
7 Continuous quality improvement activities within each domain and across the system itself

providing maximal access to care to the greatest number of individuals, rather than carving out special or unique populations of patients based on corporate affiliations or hospital financial interests. The Task Force provided strategies to overcome barriers and acknowledge key shared goals.

Seven stroke system components

Primordial and primary prevention

Improving systems to detect and treat disease earlier will help decrease death, disability, and costs associated with untreated disease. Primordial prevention refers to strategies designed to prevent or minimize the development of the intermediate disease states that are themselves risk factors for stroke (e.g., smoking, obesity prevention, and control). It is, essentially, primary prevention of the diseases or risk factors that increase the risk of stroke. Primary prevention of stroke refers to treatment of already established diseases in the population (e.g., hypertension, atherosclerosis, diabetes) to reduce the risk of stroke. This topic will be covered in more detail in Chapter 3.

Heart disease and stroke share many common risk factors; partnering with other stakeholders improves the chances of adequate funding for prevention programs and research. The American Cancer Society, the American Diabetes Association, and the American Heart Association (AHA) published a joint scientific statement pledging their common goals in 2004 [3]. The Center for Disease Control set Healthy People goals for 2010, which included a reduction of death from heart disease and stroke by 25% (these goals were met earlier than expected in 2008) [4].

Community education

Within a stroke system, it is important to develop initiatives to enhance public knowledge and awareness in collaboration with key community partners so as to maximize the cultural appropriateness and effectiveness of the message. Shared goals include education regarding the signs and symptoms of stroke and stroke risk factors, and reinforcing the appropriate use of EMS for patients or bystanders who note the onset of stroke symptoms. The general public's knowledge of stroke symptoms has been dangerously inadequate [5–10]. While traumatic injury is readily apparent, stroke symptoms and their significance can be more difficult to appreciate and do not consistently trigger notification of EMS.

Historically, the public's knowledge of stroke has lagged behind the knowledge of heart disease [6,11]. The AHA/ASA views public education as a vital component of its mission.

Notification and response of EMS

A multidisciplinary expert panel convened by the ASA addressed the role of EMS systems in the wider stroke system of care (Table 2.2) [12]. Key goals, barriers, potential solutions, and appropriate measurement parameters were identified.

Among the recommendations were universal access and coverage for enhanced 911 (land and wireless) services for all callers in all geographic areas covered by the relevant stroke system of care.

Table 2.2 Adapted from the American Stroke Association (ASA) Panel on emergency medical service systems (EMSS) role in the wider stroke system of care [12]

1 Universal access and coverage for enhanced 911 services
2 Pivotal role of EMSS communicators
3 Prioritization of acute stroke in dispatch guidelines
4 American Heart Association/ASA-approved caller interrogation tools
5 Statewide emergency stroke system protocols
6 Measure and share key process measures for continuous quality improvement

They emphasize the pivotal role played by EMS communicators, as they are the first point of contact for the patient, family, and EMS responder. EMS communicators, by recognizing stroke symptoms and triaging appropriately, hold the power to prime the stroke system to efficiently and expertly care for an acute stroke patient. Therefore, it is critical to provide accurate and frequent education on the recognition of stroke symptoms. The challenges inherent in this task vary distinctly with geography (e.g., rural, urban, proportion of population with limited English-language skills) and are hampered by a lack of national standards for the equitable coordination and delivery of emergency medical care [13].

EMS dispatch guidelines should be reorganized to require that acute stroke patients be assigned to the highest priority response. The use of AHA/ASA-approved caller interrogation tools is recommended to help EMS communicators to identify suspected stroke patients accurately and to err on the side of "over-triage" so as to minimize the risk of false-negative assessments.

Until statewide emergency stroke system protocols are universal, regions should be responsible for coordinating local transport protocols and emphasizing transport to the nearest designated stroke center, even if efforts are sometimes at odds with geopolitical forces. Issues of ambulance ownership and scarcity of resources in certain communities offer a special challenge for stroke systems to provide adequate coverage and opportunities for acute care.

For the purposes of continuous quality improvement (CQI), it is vital that data reflecting key process measures are recorded and shared in a useful way. Data should be collected and analyzed both at an individual EMS transactional level as well as a regional aggregate to influence behavior and improve quality. Analysis of the time intervals between contact with an EMS dispatcher, EMS dispatch, scene arrival, and hospital arrival may help develop strategies to reduce delays and direct patients' triage appropriately.

Air transport may be more efficient than ground transport if it is initiated quickly [14–17]. At the same time, in the face of the rising costs of health care, specific indications for initiating air transport should be analyzed on a regional basis. Geospatial characteristics of the region should be taken into account [18] as well as the realistic likelihood of arrival at destination within a treatable time window. Given the complex nature of air transport, most patients transported by helicopter or fixed wing aircraft would not arrive at a stroke center in time to receive IV tPA, unless the helicopter were to be dispatched directly to the scene, as is done in some communities for acute trauma. In most cases, the rationale for air medical transport is access to advanced therapeutics such as catheter-based therapies beyond 3 hours after symptom onset.

Through the use of telemedicine and other strategies to facilitate access to acute stroke expertise, it is feasible to create an environment in which many hospitals can function as "acute stroke capable" centers in which patients can be initially triaged and rapidly assessed. If acute stroke expertise is not consistently available at a given institution, every effort should be made to establish referral relationships with nearby stroke centers, so that patients can be transferred to an appropriate facility for admission after stabilization and possible treatment with IV thrombolysis.

Finally, there will always be hospitals without the infrastructure to care for acute stroke patients, and some patients will still arrive via private car, or be transported by EMS to these facilities when stroke may not be rapidly diagnosed or patients are hemodynamically unstable. These hospitals must still be considered when creating a stroke system of care and EMS triage algorithm, even if they have opted out of the role of being "acute stroke capable" or even providing the basic components of inpatient stroke care. Small size, rural location, or limited resources may compel certain hospitals to routinely transfer their complex stroke patients, or all their stroke patients, to larger, better-resourced facilities. These relationships should be built into the fabric of the system of care, so that the process of rapid evaluation and delivery of care is as seamless as possible for all patients, regardless of their geographic or economic circumstance.

Acute stroke treatment

As recently as 12 years ago, ischemic stroke was a syndrome without an acute treatment option, for which management was largely focused on rehabilitation and avoidance of adverse outcomes in the subacute setting. Despite the landmark approval of IV tPA as an acute treatment for ischemic stroke in 1996, administration rates were low. According to regional and nationwide studies (United States and Canada) from 1996 to 2002, only 0.6–8.5% of patients presenting with nonhemorrhagic stroke were being treated with IV tPA [19–23].

The reasons for the low rate of IV tPA administration were probably multifactorial [23,24] (Table 2.3). These included the lack of painful symptoms, impaired communication that often accompanies stroke, the wide variety of possible symptoms, the frequent delays in activating EMS, and the public's lack of knowledge of stroke symptoms. Studies that have evaluated arrival times suggest that only 17–35% of stroke patients arrive within the time that allows treatment in the 3-hour window [19,20,22,23]. The lack of an organized infrastructure to rapidly triage and evaluate patients compounds the problem and reduces the likelihood of timely treatment, even where treatment is available. In the presence of these obstacles, and the concerns over malpractice litigation if complications should occur, rates of IV tPA administration have remained low. In studies that delineated reasons for nontreatment of patients arriving within 3 hours, physician-determined contraindications to IV tPA accounted for only 27–52% [19,23].

Interestingly, one center that had participated in the original National Institute of Neurological Disorder and Stroke IV tPA clinical trial [25] achieved a postmarketing administration rate of up to 15% of all ischemic strokes admitted to its hospital [26] (compared with the 0.6–8.5% national rates in the

Table 2.3 Possible reasons for low administration rates of IV tissue-type plasminogen activator (tPA), 1996–1999

1 Clinicians' concerns about the efficacy of tPA
2 Clinicians' fear of complications of tPA, especially bleeding
3 Inability to rapidly transport patients from remote regions to hospitals
4 Lack of infrastructure to rapidly evaluate stroke patients
5 Patients rarely presented within 3 hours (due to lack of awareness or knowledge, infrequent activation of emergency medical systems)

same time period). This center had an established program for prearrival notification of its experienced acute stroke team by EMS. This is one example of how an integrated stroke system of care can contribute to higher rates of acute stroke treatment by linking together different components within the continuum of providers.

It is imperative that organizations within a stroke system of care work together to formulate a pre-specified care plan for any potential stroke patient arriving at any hospital. As discussed in the previous section, prearrival notification and mobilization of internal hospital resources in preparation for a stroke patient's arrival increases the likelihood of IV tPA administration [27].

In many academic or comprehensive stroke centers, acute ischemic stroke patients are evaluated rapidly up to 8 hours after the onset of stroke symptoms. The options available include catheter-based therapy and various acute clinical trials. Although the Food and Drug Administration has approved the use of two devices as tools for *clot removal* in acute ischemic stroke, there are no data from randomized controlled trials demonstrating that treatment with these devices is associated with improved clinical outcome. Ironically, because many stroke physicians believe that rapid reperfusion in selected cases will be associated with improved clinical outcomes, it has been difficult to fund and complete the necessary trials to evaluate the efficacy of these therapies in a randomized, placebo-controlled fashion. Two NIH-sponsored trials (Magnetic Resonance and Recanalization of Stroke Clots Using Embolectomy [28] and Interventional Management of Stroke [29]) that will address these strategies are under way.

Further discussion on the merits or limitations of catheter-based therapy is provided in Chapter 15. In any event, a plan should exist for the management of patients who have a significant nonfluctuating neurological deficit (expected to result in long-term disability) but are either ineligible for IV tPA or unable to receive it within 3 hours of onset. Consideration should be given to identifying these patients in a consistent manner and providing them with the option of alternative treatments, utilizing predetermined protocols for triggering rapid transport to an appropriate center.

Subacute stroke treatment and secondary prevention

Between 1980 and 1995, the results of multiple randomized controlled trials indicated that care of the stroke patient in a dedicated unit was related to a reduction in dependency and death, as well as a decreased length of hospital stay [30]. The Brain Attack Coalition (BAC), a multidisciplinary group of the major professional organizations dedicated to stroke care, performed a review of the English-language literature published from 1966 to 2000, with special attention to logistical issues regarding delivery of acute stroke care and cost-effectiveness. Their published recommendations subsequently formed the basis for a certification program for the establishment of primary stroke centers nationwide, a level that was felt to be obtainable by many US hospitals (Table 2.4) [31]. The BAC has also recommended the recognition and certification of a more advanced type of center, known as a comprehensive stroke center, to deliver more complex and challenging therapies for a broader array of cerebrovascular conditions. These centers, like Level 1 trauma centers, require significant resources and personnel. In contrast to primary stroke centers, it is not

Table 2.4 Major elements of a primary stroke center [31]

Patient care areas
1 Acute stroke teams
2 Written care protocols
3 Emergency medical services
4 Emergency department
5 Stroke unit (only required for centers that will provide ongoing in-hospital care for patients with stroke)
6 Neurosurgical services

Support services
1 Commitment and support of medical organization; a stroke center director
2 Neuroimaging services 24 hours a day
3 Laboratory services 24 hours a day
4 Outcome- and quality-improvement activities
5 Continuing medical education

Reproduced from the Brain Attack Coalition Recommendations for Primary Stroke Centers; used with permission.

expected that most hospitals can achieve this level of designation.

Rehabilitation

In a secondary review of their own trials, the Stroke Unit Trialists' Collaboration sought the features of an organized stroke unit care that seemed most likely to predict improved outcome. Compared with general medical wards, the typical stroke unit was more multidisciplinary and its staff had more interest, training, and expertise in stroke and rehabilitation [30]. Decreased lengths of stay and reduced hospitalization costs translated into substantial financial benefits for hospitals [32].

The AHA endorses the Veterans Affairs/Department of Defense (VA/DoD) clinical guidelines for the management of post-stroke rehabilitation care (Table 2.5; see Chapter 8) [33]. Standardized approaches to assess the rehabilitation needs of all stroke inpatients are a critical step in providing appropriate access to rehabilitation care and in improving patient outcomes. They are also a recognized measure of high-quality stroke care by the Joint Commission, the Centers for Disease Control (CDC), and the AHA.

Patients must be referred to suitable levels of rehabilitation. The VA/DoD recommendation indicates that "as much appropriate therapy" should be delivered as the patient can "tolerate" as early as medically possible [33]. Patients who are discharged home should be matched with the correct follow-up and primary care.

CQI activities within each domain and across the system

To track the quality of acute stroke care nationally, Congress charged the CDC to establish the Paul Coverdell National Acute Stroke Registry (PCNASR) in 2001 [34,35]. Recognizing the importance of also optimizing in-hospital subacute stroke care and secondary prevention measures, the ASA expanded its pilot quality improvement program for coronary artery disease "Get With The Guidelines-CAD" (GWTG-CAD) by adding a stroke quality improvement module entitled GWTG-Stroke. GWTG-Stroke uses a quality improvement model that incorporates sharing of best practices, collaborative learning sessions, and an online patient management tool for data collection and performance measurement to improve stroke care delivery within hospitals [36]. This highly successful program has already led to significant improvements in acute stroke care and secondary prevention in its initial phase, and promises to help drive the agenda for stroke quality improvement in the coming years [37]. In collaboration with the ASA, the Joint Commission started its primary stroke center certification program in 2003 [38], becoming the first nationwide program to monitor and certify hospitals for meeting established standards for hospital-based stroke care in the United States (Table 2.6). In 2008, the AHA, CDC, and the Joint Commission

Table 2.5 Recommended elements of post-stroke rehabilitation care (adapted from [American Heart Association/American Stroke Association adapted] Veterans Affairs/Department of Defense clinical guidelines for post-stroke rehabilitation care) [33]

1 Interdisciplinary teams including rehabilitation
2 Rehabilitation should be provided – as much and as early as medically tolerable
3 Maintain current databases and referral information on community and national resources for families and caregivers

Table 2.6 Summary of major national quality improvement programs in stroke

Acute Stroke Treatment Program (American Stroke Association [ASA])
   Provided resources to hospitals developing primary stroke centers, based on ASA 2000 consensus guidelines.

Paul Coverdell National Acute Stroke Registry (Centers for Disease Control) [34,35]
   Established in 2001, tracks the quality of acute stroke care nationally. Seeking permanent funding through the Stop Stroke Act.

Get With The Guidelines-Stroke (ASA) [37]
   QI model focusing on optimal in-hospital subacute stroke care and secondary prevention measures by sharing best practices, collaborative learning sessions, and online patient management tool for data collection and performance measurement.

Primary Stroke Center Certification (the Joint Commission) [38]
   Starting in 2003, in collaboration with the ASA, the Joint Commission launches the first nationwide program to certify and monitor hospital-based stroke care in the United States.

completed a year-long effort to harmonize their quality-improvement performance metrics, and a consolidated set of 10 measures was adopted [39]. Eight of these measures were recently endorsed by the National Quality Forum, and the Centers for Medicare and Medicaid Services (CMS) has announced its intention to include them in the 2011 update to the core measure set for hospital quality reporting.

Examples of regional stroke systems and state legislative efforts

The New York State Stroke Center Designation Project is an example of a successful collaborative effort between a state department of health and EMS that allowed triage of acute stroke patients to self-designated primary stroke centers. It was shown to significantly improve the quality of emergency care and acute case management in the two urban city boroughs in which the effort occurred (Brooklyn and Queens) [40].

In Massachusetts, statewide EMS protocols have been implemented to ensure rapid triage of acute stroke patients to more than 60 Department of Public Health–licensed "primary stroke service" hospitals [41]. Each of these hospitals underwent rigorous on-site inspections to achieve designation, and state regulations require that EMS transport all eligible acute stroke patients to the nearest primary stroke facility.

Several states have passed legislation defining stroke systems; examples of regulatory language from these statutes are available online (Table 2.7) [42–44]. They are mainly structured along the seven domains identified by the ASA Stroke Systems of Care Task Force. The area with the most need for improvement remains the organized linkage between acute and post-acute care, emphasizing the challenges to continuity of care posed by the transition to rehabilitation and ensuring that adequate resources exist within stroke systems to provide comprehensive rehabilitation coverage. Examples of innovative ways in which stroke systems of care are being implemented regionally are listed in Table 2.8.

Conclusion

In the United States, there persists an inequitable distribution of acute stroke care and a patchwork of stroke care delivery systems across a variably dispersed population. The development of stroke systems of care is critical to address this disparity. Broad implementation of stroke systems of care

Table 2.7 State legislative guidelines for development of stroke centers/systems (Maryland example) [44]

1 Stroke Fellowship Trained Director of Stroke Center
2 24-hour availability of neurosurgical operating rooms
3 Emergency Department Clinical Staff Assessment within 10 minutes
4 Acute stroke team assessment within 15 minutes
5 Laboratory and diagnostical services within 45 minutes
6 Neuroimaging services within 25 minutes
7 Inpatient stroke unit available for treatment beyond the acute period
8 Continuing education requirement for staff exposed to stroke patients
9 Secondary and primary prevention for stroke patients and their families
10 Accreditation by the Joint Commission
11 Participation in a stroke registry through Centers for Medicare and Medicaid Services or a Centers for Disease Control Paul Coverdell National Acute Stroke State Registry

Table 2.8 Innovation in development of stroke systems

1 King County Medic One (Seattle, WA) [47] – tiered emergency medical service system; link in the public health system including enhanced 911 and public disclosure of continuous quality improvement measures.
2 Birmingham Regional Emergency Medical Services System [48] – multidisciplinary stroke system encompassing seven counties in central Alabama; real-time matching of patients with resources.
3 Remote Evaluation of Acute Ischemic Stroke [49,50] – telestroke program linking nine rural hospital emergency rooms to the Medical College of Georgia neurologists.
4 Partners TeleStroke Program – telestroke program linking 21 hospitals in New England to Massachusetts General Hospital and the Brigham and Women's Hospital, with affiliated hub and spoke networks in Washington, Virginia, Oklahoma, and Connecticut [51].
5 Multidisciplinary Rounds [52] – Berkshire Medical Center's (Massachusetts) collaborative approach; consistently surpasses goals of continuous QI in heart disease and stroke.

would have significant financial implications, since it might lead to concentrating resources and patients at a smaller number of better staffed and better resourced facilities. As efforts to improve hospital reimbursement for ischemic stroke have led to more favorable financial profiles for stroke admissions, especially after thrombolytic administration, rerouting of patients may meet increased resistance from community hospitals.

While regional development of stroke systems is vital, efforts on a national level to reduce death and disability from stroke through systems of care are also important. The Stroke Treatment and Ongoing Prevention (STOP) Stroke Coalition, a group of over 25 major health organizations, was formed to support the STOP Stroke Act, a piece of legislation first introduced in the 107th Congress in 2002 and reintroduced every year since. STOP Stroke aims to maintain a national stroke registry and clearinghouse of information and best practices, to promote telehealth solutions to reduce stroke care disparity, to standardize EMS triage and response, and to support regional consortiums and stroke systems development through block grants. On March 27, 2007, STOP Stroke was passed by the US House of Representatives of the 110th Congress [45]. It was later integrated into a package of bills, called the Advancing America's Priorities Act, and considered by the Senate on July 28, 2008. Unfortunately, the package did not obtain the 60 votes needed to advance to consideration by the full Senate, so the bill has not yet been enacted [46]. However, momentum continues to grow, and with the endorsement of stroke performance measures by the National Quality Forum and probable incorporation into the CMS core measures, it is likely that improvements in acute stroke care delivery and the stroke systems of care model will continue to develop and mature.

The good news is that hospitals continue to voluntarily improve the quality of stroke care they provide, and increasing numbers are pursuing opportunities for quality improvement through programs like GWTG-Stroke, PCNASR, and the Joint Commission's Primary Stroke Center certification. The data suggest that more care opportunities are being fulfilled in the inpatient hospital setting every year, but further efforts are needed to link together the disparate elements of prehospital and post-acute care into a seamless system of care delivery.

Gaps in current knowledge

Little is currently known about the quantifiable impact of stroke systems of care on quality of care and about the most appropriate means to measure this improvement. It is also difficult to estimate the costs of implementation of such systems throughout the continuum of care to permit a cost-effectiveness analysis to be performed. Although much is known about the merits of individual interventions within some of the components, significant gaps in understanding still exist in the prehospital and post-acute domains, in which substantial resource investments are likely to be needed. Stroke quality improvement science is still in its infancy, and new models of implementation and evaluation are currently being refined and tested.

Further research is needed to identify the best methods to measure the effectiveness of systems of care implementation, and to refine the elements necessary within each domain. Additional financial investment is needed to match care delivery system capabilities to the needs of the population, and legislative efforts will probably be necessary to promote the integration of delivery across the continuum of care and the diverse array of providers involved.

References available online at www.wiley.com/go/ strokeguidelines.

3 Primordial and Primary Prevention of Stroke

Nikolaos I.H. Papamitsakis and Robert J. Adams

EXAMPLE CASE

A 49-year-old man without a significant medical history except for cigarette smoking presented for a neurology clinic visit because of chronic headaches. His blood pressure (BP) on two occasions in the office was 155/95 mm Hg. Brain magnetic resonance imaging (MRI) was performed as part of the headache evaluation and was normal.

Primary stroke prevention: a primer

Every patient encounter is an opportunity for preventive interventions, and the scenario illustrated during this patient visit is not uncommon. It is imperative to advise patients and the population in general on the importance of treating vascular risk factors with the goal of preventing a first stroke. Stroke is the third leading cause of death in the United States, with an estimated total annual cost of $65.5 billion, and is a leading cause of disability and functional impairment [1]. This chapter will focus on the available evidence for the evaluation and treatment of such patients.

Primordial prevention

The Centers for Disease Control (CDC) defines primordial cardiovascular and stroke prevention as a set of interventions targeting people without risk factors or overt cardiovascular disease, which includes the maintenance or restoration of favorable social and environmental conditions and the promotion of healthy behavioral patterns to prevent the development of risk factors (http://www.cdc.gov/DHDSP/library/action_plan/full_appendix_a.htm). As such, this approach directly corresponds to the goals of the Healthy People 2010 Heart and Stroke Partnership. While this approach was originally tar-

MAJOR POINTS

- Interventions to decrease the risk of a first stroke should be considered at every patient encounter.
- Patients should know their stroke risk.
- Lifestyle modifications can decrease stroke risk.
- Hypertension is the most important treatable stroke risk factor.
- Smoking cessation decreases stroke risk to baseline after 5 years.

- Treatment of hypertension, hyperlipidemia, diabetes, and smoking cessation are the cornerstones of cardiovascular and cerebrovascular disease prevention.
- Aspirin can be beneficial for primary stroke prevention in high-risk women, without cardiac disease, but not in men.

A Primer on Stroke Prevention Treatment: An Overview Based on AHA/ASA Guidelines, 1st Edition. Edited by L Goldstein.
© 2009 American Heart Association, ISBN: 9781405186513

geted at the societal or community level, it is often used to refer to efforts to keep individuals without risk factors from developing them. The term has acquired more common usage to refer to both the promotion of physical fitness and healthy behaviors in individuals and strategies for improving cardiovascular health at the community level [2].

What is the risk of a first stroke?

It is beneficial for both the public and healthcare providers to estimate a person's risk of a first stroke as a first step in attempting to lower the risk with the appropriate interventions. In the example earlier, the patient being evaluated does not have a history of stroke or transient ischemic attack (TIA), and his obvious stroke risk factors include tobacco use and probable hypertension. There is solid evidence for many stroke risk factors. For others, the evidence is not as strong, and clear data supporting specific treatments are sometimes lacking. There are several risk assessment tools evaluating the impact of a series of factors on stroke risk. One example, recommended in the American Stroke Association Primary Stroke Prevention Guidelines, is the Framingham Stroke Profile (FSP) [3,4]. The FSP includes as predictors age, presence of hypertension, systolic BP, diabetes mellitus (DM), smoking, cardiovascular disease, angina, atrial fibrillation (AF), and left ventricular hypertrophy on ECG.

Stroke risk factors

Several factors contribute to a person's stroke risk, even if no previous history of brain ischemia (stroke or TIA) is present. They can be broadly divided into nonmodifiable and modifiable factors.

Nonmodifiable risk factors

These can identify the persons who are at the highest stroke risk and benefit from the aggressive treatment of modifiable risk factors, and include age, sex, race, low birth weight, and genetic factors (Table 3.1).

Table 3.1 Nonmodifiable stroke risk factors

Age
Race
Sex
Family history of stroke/transient ischemic attack

Age

Although stroke can impact persons of any age, it is a disease mainly affecting the older population: the risk of stroke doubles for each decade after age 55 [5].

Sex

As with cardiovascular disease, the prevalence of stroke is higher in men than in women, and this holds true for most age groups, with the exception of the 35- to 44-year-olds and individuals older than 85. In these age groups, women have a higher age-specific stroke incidence [6]. Women's use of oral contraceptives (OCs) and pregnancy contribute to the higher incidence. Men die earlier from cardiovascular disease, and this explains the higher risk of stroke in older women; women account for the majority of stroke deaths in the United States (61.5%) [1].

Race–ethnic group

African-Americans and Hispanics have a higher incidence of stroke compared with Americans of the European ancestry [6,7]. They have a higher prevalence of hypertension, diabetes, and obesity.

Low birth weight

It has been estimated that the stroke risk more than doubles in persons with birth weight <2.5 kg compared with >4 kg [8]. The reasons for this association are uncertain but may explain regional differences in stroke-related mortality.

Genetics

Increased risk in patients with paternal and, to a lesser degree, maternal histories of stroke has been established [9]. This could be due to the genetic inheritance of established modifiable stroke risk factors and environmental risk factors, such as similarities in diet and lifestyle between parents and their offspring. Certain hypercoagulable states (protein C and S deficiency, factor V Leiden mutation) are inherited as autosomal dominant disorders. Conditions that can lead to arterial dissections, such as fibromuscular dysplasia, also have a genetic component. Cerebral autosomal dominant arteriopathy with subcortical infarcts and leukoencephalopathy is caused by mutations in the *NOTCH3* gene on chromosome 19 [10]; Fabry's disease is an X-linked disorder caused by lysosomal α-galactosidase A deficiency, leading to the deposits of glycosphingolipids in small vessels in the brain and other organs. A recent study from Germany reported that up to 2% of all cryptogenic strokes are caused by Fabry's [11]. Finally, the evaluation of large genetic databases, as the one from Iceland (DeCode group), found mutations of phosphodiesterase 4D associated with ischemic stroke [12], although this has not been found in studies in other populations. Specific gene therapies have not yet been established, but in some conditions, such as Fabry's disease, enzyme replacement therapies have been tried.

Modifiable risk factors

These include well-documented, modifiable factors such as hypertension, DM, tobacco use, hyperlipidemia, asymptomatic carotid stenosis, AF, sickle-cell disease (SCD), hormone replacement therapies, physical inactivity, obesity, poor dietary habits, and others that are potentially modifiable, including alcohol and drug use, obstructive sleep apnea (OSA), OC use, elevated homocysteine, migraine, metabolic syndrome, elevated lipoprotein (a), and elevated lipoprotein-associated phospholipase A2 (Lp-PLA2), as well as underlying hypercoagulability and infec-tion/inflammation (Table 3.2) [4]. It should also be emphasized that patients with cardiovascular or peripheral vascular disease have an increased risk of a first stroke. The management of those conditions and their risk factors, which overlap with the ones pertaining to stroke, should also reduce the risk of stroke for such patients.

Hypertension

This is arguably the most important of the modifiable risk factors, responsible overall for approximately 50% of all strokes, and especially for intracerebral hemorrhages [13]. Although there is a continuous relationship between BP and cardiovascular risk, hypertension is defined as a BP greater than 140/90 mm Hg in the guidelines (7th Report) by the Joint National Committee on Prevention, Detection, Evaluation and Treatment of High Blood Pressure (JNC 7) [14], which are endorsed in the American Heart Association (AHA) Primary Prevention Guidelines [4]. The risk of developing hypertension increases with age: over 90% of persons who are normotensive at age 55 will become hypertensive by their ninth decade [15]. There is also solid evidence that adequate treatment of elevated BP prevents stroke, as well as renal failure, congestive

Table 3.2 Modifiable stroke risk factors, well-documented [4]

Factor	Prevalence	Relative risk	Risk reduction with treatment
Cardiovascular disease	8.4% (men)	1.73 (men)	
	5.6% (women)	1.55 (women)	
Hypertension	30% in age 60	4.0	38%
	60% in age 90	1.0	
Smoking	25%	1.8	50% within 1 year
Diabetes	7.3%	1.8–6	blood pressure control
Asymptomatic carotid stenosis	2–8%	2.0	~50% with carotid endarterectomy after 5 years
Atrial fibrillation	0.5% (50–59 years)	4.0	45% with warfarin (vs. aspirin)
	8.8% (80–89 years)	4.5	
Sickle-cell disease	0.25% in African-Americans	200–400	91% with transfusion therapy
Dyslipidemia	25%	2.0	27–32% with statins in high-risk patients
Dietary factors; Na intake >2,300 mg	75–90%	?	8% decrease in mortality after 3 mm Hg blood pressure decrease
Obesity	17.9%	1.75–2.37	?
Physical inactivity	25%	2.7	?
Hormone therapy (postmenopausal)	20% in women 50–74 years	1.4	Unclear

heart failure (CHF), and other conditions arising from end-organ damage. Antihypertensive treatment is associated with approximately 40% stroke risk reduction [16]. BP targets of 140/90 mm Hg or less, and 130/80 mm Hg or less in diabetics have been recommended, along with the use of two or more antihypertensive agents for better BP control [14]. There is no clear relationship between specific types of antihypertensive medications and improved stroke outcomes attributed to other characteristics than BP-lowering effects. AHA guidelines recommend treatment with any of the commonly available antihypertensives, as long as the BP is adequately controlled [4]. The Losartan Intervention for Endpoint Reduction in Hypertension (LIFE) Study showed that in patients with hypertension and left ventricular hypertrophy on ECG, an angiotensin II receptor blocker had an increased effect compared with a beta adrenergic receptor blocker in cardiovascular and, in particular, stroke risk reduction [17]. However, a recent ON TARGET study (Telmisartan, ramipril, or both in patients at high risk for vascular events) showed comparable stroke prevention with either drug and no benefit with the combination [18]. Benefits have also been documented in the control of isolated systolic hypertension and diastolic BP. In the JNC 7 recommendations, treatment of BP, less than 140/90 mm Hg and greater than 120/80 mm Hg is recommended if there is underlying CHF, myocardial infarction (MI), DM, chronic renal failure, or recent stroke. In our patient, lifestyle modifications could be attempted first before starting with antihypertensives, with a target BP of <140/90 mm Hg and probably close to 120/80 mm Hg.

Diabetes mellitus

DM conveys an increased risk for ischemic stroke of up to six times [19]. Multifaceted intensive interventions in patients with DM (including the use of statins, angiotensin receptor blockers [ARB], angiotensin-converting enzyme inhibitors [ACE-I], antiplatelet drugs, and behavioral modifications) decrease the risk of stroke, as well as cardiovascular events. Particular focus in the tight management of BP in patients with DM was shown to be beneficial in the prevention of stroke and cardiovascular complications (United Kingdom Prospective Diabetes Study) [20]. There is, at present, no evidence that tight glycemic control leads to reduced stroke risk, although it has been shown that it reduces microvascular complications of diabetes. In the Heart Outcomes Prevention Evaluation (HOPE) and LIFE studies, there was a significant benefit in stroke risk reduction in patients with DM and history of cardiovascular events or hypertension, who were treated with an ACE-I or an ARB, respectively [17,21]. In the Health Protection Study (HPS), the use of a statin in patients with DM led to a significant reduction in stroke risk and major vascular events [22].

A recent meta-analysis on the effect of rosiglitazone, which has been extensively used to lower blood glucose levels in patients with type 2 DM, on cardiovascular morbidity and mortality showed increased risk of MI and death from cardiovascular causes [23]. This emphasizes the importance of well-designed trials and registries in order to monitor the potential side effects of medications used in the management of vascular risk factors.

Smoking

Smoking is associated with a 2-fold increased risk of ischemic stroke, and it is estimated to contribute to 12–14% of all stroke deaths [24]. There is also a synergistic effect between smoking and OC use: over three times higher risk compared with nonsmoking OC users [25]. Passive smoking is also associated with an increased risk for heart disease and stroke. Physiological effects of smoking include increase of heart rate and mean arterial pressure and decrease in arterial distensibility. Quitting smoking is associated with a decreased risk for stroke, which approaches baseline after approximately 5 years from quitting [26,27]. In our patient, smoking cessation would be a major intervention aiming at primary stroke and cardiovascular disease prevention.

Hyperlipidemia

Several studies have found an increased risk for ischemic stroke in patients with elevated total cholesterol. For example, the Asia Pacific Cohort Studies Collaboration found a 25% increase in ischemic stroke rates for every 1 mmol/L increase in total cholesterol [28]. The data on the relationship between low-density lipoprotein (LDL) cholesterol and ischemic stroke are weaker, whereas several studies have shown increased prevalence of ischemic stroke in persons with low high-density lipoprotein

(HDL) cholesterol (especially less than 30 mg/dL) [29]. Elevated triglycerides are also associated with higher rates of cerebral ischemia. Statin use is associated with decreased stroke rate of approximately 30% in patients with coronary artery disease (CAD) (i.e., HPS, Anglo-Scandinavian Cardiac Outcomes Trial) [30,31].

A recent trial evaluated the use of an inhibitor of cholesteryl esterase transfer protein, torcetrapib, which has been shown to increase HDL cholesterol, in reducing major cardiovascular events. The results were surprising: although HDL levels increased by 72.1% and LDL cholesterol decreased by 24.9%, major cardiovascular events increased by 40%, and death rate increased by 25% in the treatment group. Potential explanations include altered immune and inflammatory functions of HDL [32].

Asymptomatic carotid stenosis

Approximately 5–10% of men and women older than 65 years have an asymptomatic carotid stenosis of more than 50%, with an annual stroke risk rate between 1% and 3.4% [33,34]. In the North American Carotid Endarterectomy Trial (NACET), the annual risk of stroke in the territory of an asymptomatic carotid artery stenosis was 3.2% (over 5 years); however, it should be emphasized that 45% of the strokes ipsilateral to an asymptomatic stenosis (contralateral to a symptomatic vessel) can be attributed to other mechanisms [35]. Overall, the stroke rate ipsilateral to a hemodynamically significant internal carotid artery stenosis is estimated between 1% and 2% per year. Several large trials have evaluated the benefit of carotid endarterectomy [36–38] and angioplasty and stenting [39] in patients with asymptomatic stenosis [36–38]. Please refer to Chapter 14 for a detailed discussion of management issues.

Atrial fibrillation

AF is responsible for approximately 60,000 strokes per year in the United States, or in 2–4% of persons with AF without previous history of cerebral ischemia. It is prevalent in older patients, affecting 5% of persons older than 70 years. It is responsible for almost 25% of all strokes in patients older than 80 years [40]. Treatment with antithrombotics reduces the odds of stroke. Warfarin is more efficacious than aspirin, leading to 45% stroke risk reduction compared with aspirin in persons with AF [41]. Patients

with AF who have other vascular risks are at a higher risk of stroke. The American College of Cardiology recommends anticoagulation with warfarin in patients with AF who are over 60 years of age and have a history of hypertension, diabetes, CAD, heart failure, history of prior thromboembolism, and for all persons with AF who are over 75 years of age. The so-called CHADS2 score assigns 1 point each for CHF, hypertension, age ≥75, and DM, and 2 points for prior stroke or TIA, stratifying patients for future stroke risk [42]. Patients with a low CHADS2 score (0–1) have a low risk for stroke (~1% per year); patients with a score of 2 have a moderate risk (~2.5% per year); and patients with high scores (3 or greater) have a high risk (~5% per year). The exceptions in this stratification scheme are the few patients with a history of stroke or TIA and no vascular risk factors (score of 2), who were found in the Stroke Prevention in Atrial Fibrillation (SPAF) trials to have a stroke rate of 5.9% per year, and who should be considered at high risk for recurrence [43]. Patients with a yearly stroke risk of 4% or more should be treated with warfarin, whereas for patients with low stroke rates (1% per year), aspirin should be sufficient. The recommended anticoagulation target is an international normalization ratio (INR) of 2.0–3.0. The importance of controlling vascular risk factors in patients with AF cannot be overemphasized [44]. Only approximately half of eligible patients are treated with anticoagulation with warfarin, and this is more pronounced in elderly patients. The elderly have a higher risk of bleeding complications when anticoagulated, but they also benefit more, especially when they have a high risk for ischemic stroke (as patients with a previous history of central nervous system ischemia).

Several other cardiac conditions have been associated with significant or moderate stroke risk, including prosthetic cardiac valves, endocarditis, MI, congenital defects such as patent foramen ovale (PFO), and cardiomyopathy. Patients with ST-elevation MI and significant wall motion abnormalities can be treated with warfarin for several months. For patients with a decreased ejection fraction (EF < 29%), the relative stroke risk compared with patients with EF > 35% is 1.86 [45]. There is, however, no strong evidence at present that treatment with warfarin is superior to antiplatelet drugs in such patients, and a large trial is evaluating primary and secondary stroke prevention strategies in these patients (Warfarin versus Aspirin in Reduced Cardiac Ejection Fraction [WARCEF]).

SCD

SCD is an autosomal recessive disease in which the genetic mutation leads to abnormal hemoglobin synthesis, usually manifesting with painful episodes involving the extremities ("sickle-cell/vaso-occlusive crises") and organ infarctions/strokes, due to severe hemolysis [46]. A substantial number of patients with homozygous SCD have silent strokes, noted on brain imaging. The identification of patients with higher stroke risk has been made possible by the use of transcranial Doppler (TCD) testing. Patients with maximum mean flow velocities in the middle cerebral artery of greater than 200 cm/s have a yearly stroke rate of ~10% versus 1% in patients with SCD in general [47,48]. The Stroke Prevention Trial in Sickle Cell Anemia (STOP) evaluated blood transfusions compared with standard care in children with SCD and high stroke risk, having as a target reducing hemoglobin S to <30% of total, a treatment that reduced stroke rates to a baseline of 1% [49]. A follow-up randomized trial (STOP-II) evaluated whether transfusions could be safely discontinued after at least 30 months of treatment in children without a stroke and decreased TCD velocities after transfusion therapy (<170 cm/s). The study showed poorer outcomes in patients who discontinued their transfusions despite frequent TCD surveillance [50]. Other approaches, such as the use of hydroxyurea or bone marrow transplantation, are currently being investigated.

Postmenopausal hormone therapy

Several prospective trials have evaluated the effects of hormone therapy on the incidence of vascular events. The Women's Estrogen for Stroke Trial (WEST) showed that in patients with stroke, hormone therapy with estradiol was associated with higher risk of recurrent stroke and death [51]. In the Heart and Estrogen/Progesterone Replacement Study (HERS), hormone therapy did not have an effect on the risk of stroke in postmenopausal women who had an MI [52]. Finally, in the Women's Health Initiative study, hormone therapy was evaluated for the primary prevention of cardiovascular disease in postmenopausal women. There was,

instead, an increase in vascular events, including strokes, in women with an intact uterus treated with estrogen and progesterone, as well as in women with hysterectomy who were treated with estrogen [53].

Diet and nutrition

Several studies have documented that increased consumption of fruits and vegetables is associated with a decreased risk of stroke. For every increase of one serving per day, the stroke risk is decreased by 6% [54]. Higher sodium and lower potassium levels are associated with increased stroke risk in prospective studies, probably partially mediated through elevations in BP, as well as through other mechanisms [55,56].

Physical inactivity and sedentary lifestyle

The beneficial effects of physical activity have been documented for the prevention of cardiovascular disease and stroke in numerous prospective studies (Framingham Heart Study, Honolulu Heart Program, Oslo Study, Nurses' Health Study, National Health and Nutrition Examination Survey [NHANES I], and the Northern Manhattan Stroke Study [NOMASS]) [57–59]. This protective effect might be mediated through BP reduction and control of weight and diabetes. The National Institutes of Health and CDC recommend moderate exercise for ≥30 minutes almost daily [4,60].

Obesity and body fat distribution

A body mass index of ≥30 kg/m^2 is classified as being obese; abdominal obesity is defined by a waist circumference of >102 cm (40 inches) in men and 88 cm (35 inches) in women. In the United States, 65.7% of adults are overweight or obese, and 30.4% are obese, with the prevalence of obesity being particularly high in black and Hispanic children. Large studies have documented an association between increased weight and increased risk for ischemic and hemorrhagic stroke, even after controlling for other cardiovascular risk factors (although then there is a reduction in the strength of association) [61,62]. Weight reduction is associated with BP reduction, although not directly shown to reduce stroke risk.

Potentially modifiable stroke risk factors

These include metabolic syndrome, alcohol and drug use, OSA, OC use, elevated homocysteine, migraine, metabolic syndrome, elevated Lp(a), and elevated Lp-PLA2, as well as underlying hypercoagulability and infection/inflammation (Table 3.3) [4].

Metabolic syndrome

Metabolic syndrome is defined by the presence of three or more of the following: abdominal obesity determined by a waist circumference of more than 40 inches for men and more than 35 inches in women; triglycerides greater than 150 mg/dL; HDL cholesterol less than 40 mg/dL in men and less than 50 mg/dL in women; BP greater than 130/85 mm Hg; and fasting glucose greater than 110 mg/dL. Hyperinsulinemia is also present [63]. The fat deposition in metabolic syndrome is associated with insulin resistance, diabetes, and other metabolic changes, promoting hyperlipidemia, hypertension, and renal damage. Hyperinsulinemia and insulin resistance appear to be associated with increased stroke risk [64]. Approximately 47 million Americans are estimated to have metabolic syndrome, with its preva-

lence being higher in Mexican-Americans and in African-American women. Overall, however, the specific stroke risk in patients with metabolic syndrome is uncertain. Lifestyle modifications are recommended, as well as pharmacotherapy for BP, lipid, and glycemic control as appropriate.

Alcohol abuse

Alcohol abuse can lead to medical complications and stroke. A J-shaped relationship between alcohol consumption and ischemic stroke risk is reported in several studies, indicating a protective effect of alcohol in light and moderate drinkers (≤1 drink per day in women and ≤2 drinks per day in men). Its benefits are quickly eliminated in persons with higher alcohol consumption [65,66]. Consumers of more than five alcoholic drinks per day have a 69% increased stroke risk compared with abstainers. Light alcohol use can increase HDL cholesterol, reduce platelet aggregation, and lower plasma fibrinogen, whereas heavy alcohol consumption can lead to hypertension, hypercoagulability, reduced

Table 3.3 Potentially modifiable stroke risk factors (less documented) [4]

Factor	Prevalence	RR	Risk reduction with treatment
Metabolic syndrome	23.7%	N/A	
Alcohol abuse	5–7%	1.6	?
≥5 drinks per day			
Hyperhomocysteinemia	43% (men)	1.3–2.3	?
In persons >60 years	47% (women)		
Drug abuse	3–14%	6.5	?
Hypercoagulability	19.7% (men)	1.3	0.99 with warfarin
Anticardiolipin antibodies	17.6% (women)	1.9	
Oral contraceptive (OC) use	13%	2.8	No protection with OC use
In women 25–44 years			
Inflammatory processes	16.8%	2.11	?
Periodontal disease			
Elevated high-sensitivity CRP in women ≥45 years	28.13%	3.0	?
Migraine	12%	2.1	?
High Lp(a)	20% in men ≥65 years	2.92	?
High Lp-PLA2	N/A	1.97 (highest vs. lowest quartile)	?
Sleep-disordered breathing	4%	1.2%/year	?

CRP, C-reactive protein; Lp(a), lipoprotein (a); Lp-PLA2, lipoprotein-associated phospoholipase A2.

cerebral blood flow, and greater likelihood of AF. Reducing alcohol consumption in heavy drinkers is recommended, and for persons who do consume alcohol, moderation is recommended. It is not recommended for nondrinkers to start consuming alcohol.

Drug abuse

Cocaine, heroin, and amphetamine use are associated with increased stroke risk, causing BP changes, vasculitic and vasoconstrictive changes, and infective endocarditis, and inducing hematological abnormalities resulting in increased blood viscosity and platelet aggregation [67,68]. The treatment of drug addiction can be challenging, and referral to counseling should always be attempted.

Oral contraceptive use

Increased risk of stroke was found in women using "first generation" OCs, containing >50 mcg of estradiol. There may also be an increased risk of stroke in women using second and third generation OCs [69]. Meta-analyses have been conflicting [70]. There is an association between sinus venous thrombosis and OC use, especially in women with underlying hypercoagulability states such as factor V Leiden or prothrombin gene mutations. Women who are older than 35 years, are current cigarette smokers, have hypertension or diabetes, have migraines, or have had previous thromboembolic events (especially while on OCs) are at a higher stroke risk when they use OCs, although the issue is not settled for low-dose OCs [71]. Even with the higher estimates of stroke risk, the risk of stroke associated with OC use remains lower than the mortality rate of pregnancy in the United States.

Obstructive sleep apnea or sleep-disordered breathing (SDB)

Habitual snoring is a risk factor for ischemic stroke. Excessive daytime sleepiness due to OSA has been found to be associated with stroke risk [72]. A large study of men with severe OSA (apnea–hypopnea index >30 per hour of sleep) found increased risk of fatal and nonfatal cardiovascular events (MI, acute coronary insufficiency requiring intervention, and stroke) [73]. The outcomes of those treated with continuous positive airway pressure (CPAP) did not differ from controls. Snoring and SDB can increase stroke risk by leading to hypertension and heart disease, and possibly by causing reduction in cerebral blood flow, altered autoregulation, impaired endothelial function, hypercoagulability, inflammation, and paradoxical embolism in patients with PFO [74]. In one study, each additional apneic event per hour of sleep increased the odds of hypertension by 1%, and each 10% decrease in nocturnal oxygen saturation increased the stroke risk by 13% [75]. Cardiac arrhythmias and AF may occur in patients with advanced SDB in which the oxyhemoglobin saturation falls to less than 65%. The treatment of SDB includes the use of CPAP, as well as a variety of prosthetic oral devices and surgical interventions.

Migraine

Migraine has been associated with increased stroke risk mainly in young women and not in those older than 60. The odds ratio (OR) for stroke was 2.08 in a meta-analysis of case-control studies in patients with migraine and stroke [76]. Patients with additional risk factors can have a further increase in stroke risk. In a population-based study from the Netherlands, there was a 7-fold increased odds of silent brain infarction on MRI in the posterior circulation in migraine patients [77]. Additional risk factors such as hypertension, smoking, and OC use did not modify the effects of migraine, and there is no evidence that preventing migraine attacks can decrease that risk. Potential mechanisms that could explain the association of migraine headaches with increased stroke risk include reduced blood flow, blood volume, posterior circulation oligemia, increased platelet activation, and platelet–leukocyte aggregation, as well as paradoxical embolism through PFO, with microemboli through PFO causing brain ischemia and triggering migraine with aura [78–80].

Hyperhomocysteinemia

Several studies have reported an association between elevated homocysteine levels and atherosclerotic disease. The OR for stroke was 2.3 in subjects in the highest quartile for serum homocysteine in the NHANES Follow-up Study III [81]. In the Framingham Study, the baseline total homocysteine levels were an independent risk factor for stroke in the elderly [82]. In the same study, the OR for stroke comparing the higher with the lower quartile of homocysteine levels was 1.82. Homocysteine is an amino acid derived from dietary methionine. Methylene-tetrahydrofolate reductase (MTHFR) is the enzyme that metabolizes homocysteine, and a single mutation in its gene at base position 677 in which cytosine (C) is replaced by thymidine (T) results in elevated homocysteine concentration. The TT genotype is found in ~10–12% of the population and is associated with a 25% higher homocysteine levels than the CC genotype. In recent meta-analyses of *MTHFR* gene prevalence studies in vascular disease and serum homocysteine in disease risk, an increase of serum homocysteine by 5 µmol/L was associated with a 1.42 OR for ischemic heart disease and 1.59 OR for stroke. A 3 µmol/L decrease in homocysteine levels was associated with a 16% decrease in ischemic CAD and 24% decrease in stroke [83]. High homocysteine was defined as >11.4 µmol/L for men and >10.4 µmol/L in NHANES III and >16.4 µmol/L in the Framingham Heart Study. Although treatment with B-complex vitamins reduces homocysteine levels, as well as atherosclerotic plaque progression, no randomized studies have yet shown that lowering elevated homocysteine reduces the risk of a first stroke, including the Vitamin Intervention for Stroke Prevention Study (VISP) [84]. The benefit of treatment cannot be excluded, and until further data are available, the use of folic acid and B vitamins in patients with elevated homocysteine levels may be considered.

Elevated lipoprotein (a)

Lp(a) is a lipid–protein complex that has emerged as a risk factor for CAD. It consists of apolipoprotein B-100 that is linked by a disulfide bridge to apolipoprotein (a). It enhances cholesterol deposition and increases the risk of thrombosis through the inhibition of plasminogen activation. A meta-analysis of several studies found that patients with baseline Lp(a) levels in the top third of the concentration distribution, have ~60% increased risk as compared with those with Lp(a) in the bottom third [85]. There are no consistent findings demonstrating that Lp(a) levels promote ischemic stroke, although they have been associated with ischemic stroke in childhood. High Lp(a) levels have also been associated with intracranial large artery occlusive disease.

Treatment with niacin can reduce elevated levels of Lp(a) by ~25% [86], but studies showing that this decreases stroke risk have not been carried out.

Elevated lipoprotein-associated phospholipase A2

Lp-PLA2 is a calcium-independent serine lipase that is associated with LDL. Elevated levels of Lp-PLA2 are associated with an increased risk of cardiovascular events; in a population-based study, the persons in the highest versus the lowest quartile of Lp-PLA2 levels had a 2-fold increased risk of ischemic stroke, even after adjusting for other stroke risk factors [87,88]. Although levels of Lp-PLA2 can be reduced by statins, fenofibrate, and beta-blockers, there are, as yet, no studies showing that reducing Lp-PLA2 leads to reduction in ischemic stroke risk.

Hypercoagulability

Hypercoagulable states are usually associated with venous thrombosis rather than cerebral infarction. Antiphospholipid antibodies, including anticardiolipin antibodies (ACLs) and lupus anticoagulants can be associated with arterial thrombosis and infarctions. Several studies, including the Antiphospholipid Antibody and Stroke Study (APASS), did not find increased risk for subsequent vascular events in patients with ischemic stroke and ACLs [89]. Furthermore, in the APASS trial, even if elevated ACL titers were found in a stroke patient, treatment with aspirin was not different than treatment with warfarin in the prevention of recurrent events [89]. The examination for anti-beta 2 glycoprotein 1 antibodies, a cofactor for antiphospholipid binding, is specific for thrombosis [90]. Young women with antiphospholipid syndrome, who have a history of thrombotic events, might benefit from primary prevention strategies including warfarin with a target INR of 2.0–3.0. Hypercoagulable states may be more frequent in stroke patients with a PFO compared with those without a PFO.

Inflammation

Atherosclerosis is a chronic inflammatory condition initiated by several agents injuring the endothelial surface. C-reactive protein (CRP) is an acute phase reactant increasing responses to inflammatory stimuli and is a known mediator of complement activity and thrombogenic factor release. Several

Table 3.4 Summary of recommendations [4]

Factor	Recommendations
Assessing risk of first stroke	Use a risk assessment tool, such as the Framingham Stroke Profile, to assess individuals who could benefit from interventions.
Genetic causes of stroke	Genetic counseling in patients with rare genetic stroke causes.
Cardiovascular and peripheral vascular disease	Management of underlying disease, including antiplatelets.
Hypertension	Regular screening (at least every 2 years in adults) and appropriate management including JNC 7 recommended pharmacotherapy.
Cigarette smoking	Abstinence is recommended. Counseling and nicotine products and oral-smoking cessation medications can be used.
Diabetes	Tight control of hypertension with BP target <130/80; use of ACE-I or ARB; use of statin.
Atrial fibrillation	Anticoagulation with warfarin (target 2.0–3.0) is recommended for high (>4% annual stroke risk) and moderate risk patients with nonvalvular AFib.
Other cardiac conditions	Warfarin for patients with MI and ST-elevation syndrome, as well as for patients with MI and LV dysfunction.
Dyslipidemia	Patients with known heart disease or high-risk hypertensive patients should be treated with lifestyle measures and a statin or with niacin versus gemfibrozil if they have low HDL.
Asymptomatic carotid stenosis	Therapy of all identified stroke risk factors, use of aspirin. Prophylactic endarterectomy recommended on selected patients with high-grade stenosis (>60%) to be performed by surgeons with <3% morbidity/mortality. Unclear at present if carotid angioplasty and stenting should be considered in such patients.
Sickle-cell disease	Children with SCD should be screened with TCD from age 2 and transfusion therapy should be considered for those with increased risk. Transfusions should be continued in those whose TCD velocities return to normal. Children with velocities in the conditional range should be screened more frequently. In adults with SCD, management of stroke risk factors is recommended.
Postmenopausal hormone therapy	Estrogen +/− progesterone should not be used for primary stroke prevention.
Diet and nutrition	Reduced intake of sodium (<2.3 g/d) and increased intake of potassium (>4.7 g/d) is recommended in patients with hypertension. Fruits, vegetables, and low-fat diary products recommended, including ≥5 servings of fruits and vegetables.
Physical inactivity	≥30 minutes of moderate intensity activity daily is recommended by CDC and NIH.
Obesity	Weight reduction is recommended due to its effect in lowering BP.
Metabolic syndrome	Exercise, weight loss, and proper diet recommended. Antihypertensive, lipid-lowering and hypoglycemic agents should be considered in appropriate patients.
Alcohol abuse	For alcohol consumers, ≤2 drinks/d for men and ≤1 drink/d for nonpregnant women is recommended.
Drug abuse	Referral for counseling.
Oral contraceptives (OC)	OC should not be used by women with additional vascular risk factors.
Sleep-disordered breathing	Referral to a sleep specialist along with appropriate testing (sleep study) is recommended.
Migraine	No clear data exist on the best treatment approach.
Hyperhomocysteinemia	Follow guidelines on daily intake of folate, B6, and B12 by consumption of vegetables, fruits, legumes, meats, fish, and fortified cereals. Unclear if treatment with folic acid and vitamin B complex reduces risk of first stroke in patients with hyperhomocysteinemia, but given their safety and low cost, they could be given for such patients.
Elevated lipoprotein (a)	Consider treatment with niacin (up to a total dose of 2,000 mg/d), which reduces Lp(a) levels by ~25%. Prospective trials results are pending.

Table 3.4 *Continued*

Factor	Recommendations
Elevated lipoprotein-associated phospholipase A2	No data exist on clinical benefit with reduction in blood levels.
Hypercoagulability	No specific recommendations for primary stroke prevention exist.
Inflammation	Use of hs-CRP level can be helpful in considering the intensity of risk factor modification in those at moderate general cardiovascular risk.
Infection	Insufficient data are available to recommend antibiotic therapy for primary stroke prevention in patients with seropositivity for certain pathogenic organisms.
Aspirin	Not recommended for primary stroke prevention in men.
	Can be useful for primary stroke prevention in women with sufficiently high cardiovascular risk.

ACE-I, angiotensin-converting enzyme inhibitor; AFib, atrial fibrillation; ARB, angiotensin receptor blocker; BP, blood pressure; CDC, Centers for Disease Control; HDL, high-density lipoprotein; hs-CRP, high-sensitivity C-reactive protein; JNC 7, Joint National Committee on Prevention, Detection, Evaluation and Treatment of High Blood Pressure; LV, left ventricle; MI, myocardial infarction; NIH, National Institutes of Health; SCD, sickle-cell disease; TCD, transcranial Doppler.

studies have shown a strong correlation between CRP levels and cardiovascular/cerebrovascular events with a 2- to 3-fold increase in stroke risk. The OR for the first ischemic stroke and TIA between the highest and lowest quartile of CRP levels in men was 2.0 in some of the studies performed [91]. Treatment with statins shows reduction in coronary atherosclerotic plaque progression and reduction of CRP levels. Lower CRP levels after statin therapy were associated with better clinical outcomes in patients with acute coronary syndromes [92]. It is unclear if asymptomatic patients with increased CRP levels reduce their risk of stroke with the use of statins [93]. The vascular response to injury prompts the migration of inflammatory cells and the release of pro-inflammatory cytokines that convert the endothelial surface over a plaque to a prothrombotic state [94]. These inflammatory cells mediate the release of matrix metalloproteinases, including MMP-9, MMP-3, and MMP-2, leading to instability of the fibrous cap and plaque rupture. The CD40/CD40 ligand system (CD40/CD40L) plays a role in the activation of inflammatory mediators in atherogenesis. In the Women's Health Study, CD40L concentrations above 95th percentile had a relative risk of MI, stroke, and cardiac death of 3.3 [95]. Other pro-inflammatory cytokines as IL-18 have been associated with cardiovascular events. Prospective trials are needed for further understanding of the inflammatory profile in atherosclerosis. There is no evidence that widespread screening of a general adult population with the high-sensitivity CRP is indicated, although it can be reserved for patients with moderate general risk [4].

Infection

Recent infections have been associated with acute stroke, possibly due to generalized activation of circulating leukocytes at the atherosclerotic plaque. *Chlamydia pneumoniae* has been identified in atherosclerotic plaques, and in the NOMASS trial elevated immunoglobulin titers of *C. pneumoniae* were associated with increased stroke risk [96]. No clear benefit of treatment with antibiotics was documented in seropositive patients. Periodontal disease has been associated with carotid atherosclerosis and stroke risk, probably related to the continuous seeding of the bloodstream with Gram-negative organisms. Cytomegalovirus has been associated with increased carotid atherosclerosis and all vascular events risk. *Helicobacter pylori* has been found in atherosclerotic plaque. No single organism accounts for all cases of atherosclerosis, although an "infectious burden" (of several seropositivities) has been associated with atherosclerotic plaque progression [97]. A single anti-infectious regimen will likely not be effective in stroke prevention in such patients.

Aspirin for primary stroke prevention

Aspirin at a dose of 75 mg/d has been recommended for cardiac prophylaxis in persons with high coronary risk, defined as ≥10% risk per 10 years [98]. Until the recent Women's Health Study, there was no evidence that aspirin would be beneficial for primary stroke prevention. In that trial, almost 40,000 women older than 45 years of age, who were asymptomatic at the onset of the trial, were randomized to receive aspirin 100 mg every other day versus placebo, and were followed for 10 years for a first major vascular event [99]. In contrast to previous studies that included mostly men, this study found a nonsignificant reduction (9%) in the primary end point, but a significant (17%) reduction in the risk of stroke, with an absolute risk reduction of 0.02% per year. The most consistent benefit was for women ≥65 years at study entry, who had 26% reduction in cardiovascular events and 30% reduction in ischemic stroke rates, especially in women with a history of hypertension, hyperlipidemia, and diabetes. Aspirin is not recommended for the prevention of a first stroke in men, but it can be helpful for the prevention of a first stroke in women whose risk is sufficiently high [4].

Summary of recommendations is shown in Table 3.4.

References available online at www.wiley.com/go/ strokeguidelines.

4 Treatment of Patients with Acute Ischemic Stroke

Harold P. Adams, Jr.

EXAMPLE CASE

A 77-year-old woman was at home with her husband. At approximately 7:30 PM, her husband heard a noise and found her slumped against a chair in the living room. She denied that she had a problem. However, he noticed that her speech was slurred. She had sagging on the left side of the face, and she was not moving her left arm.

Introduction

Annually, approximately 780,000 Americans have a first or recurrent stroke; approximately 80% of these events are secondary to a thromboembolic occlusion of an artery perfusing the brain [1]. Ischemic stroke is the third leading cause of death in the United States, a leading cause of long-term disability, and the second most common cause of dementia (vascular dementia). The management of patients with ischemic cerebrovascular disease includes measures to control risk factors, antithrombotic medications, and medical or surgical interventions, particularly among persons who have had warning symptoms of stroke (transient ischemic attack [TIA] or previous stroke). Unfortunately, these therapies only reduce the likelihood of ischemic stroke; they do not eliminate the risk. In addition, many persons do not have warning symptoms of stroke, and their first manifestation of the vascular disease is an ischemic stroke. Thus, acute treatment remains a key aspect of management of patients with ischemic cerebrovascular disease.

This chapter outlines the components of the evaluation and treatment of persons with an acute or

MAJOR POINTS

- Stroke is a medical emergency.
- Patients should seek medical attention immediately.
- 911 and emergency medical services should respond quickly.
- The receiving hospital should have a code stroke protocol for emergency evaluation and treatment.
- Evaluation is aimed at confirming stroke and eliminating alternative diagnoses.
- Management includes measures to treat acute complications such as hypertension.
- Patients should be screened for treatment with intravenous rt-PA.
- Intravenous thrombolysis is recommended for eligible patients that can be treated within 3 hours of onset of stroke.
- Admission to the hospital for subsequent treatment is recommended.
- Measures to prevent or control complications of stroke should be instituted.

A Primer on Stroke Prevention Treatment: An Overview Based on AHA/ASA Guidelines, 1st Edition. Edited by L Goldstein.
© 2009 American Heart Association, ISBN: 9781405186513

recent stroke. Such management is complex with treatment priorities influenced by the interval from the onset of the ischemic symptoms, the severity of the stroke, and the development of medical or neurological complications (Table 4.1). Most of the initial evaluation and treatment occurs in the hospital emergency department. The elements of subsequent inpatient treatment are determined on the basis of the patient's neurological status and the presence of comorbid diseases. The recommendations included in this chapter are based on the current American Heart Association/American Stroke Association guidelines [2,3]. Although primarily intended for physicians, this chapter also includes suggestions for treatment by emergency medical services (EMS) personnel and other healthcare professionals. The chapter is divided into two major components: emergency treatment within the first hours after stroke and treatment after admission to an acute care hospital. Although rehabilitation and institution of measures to prevent recurrent stroke are critical components of treatment in the hospital, these aspects of management are covered in other chapters in this book.

An integrated approach to treatment of acute ischemic stroke

The awareness of the symptoms of stroke among the public is distressingly low, especially among high-risk groups such as the elderly [4–7]. Public educational programs emphasizing the recognition of stroke and the correct response (to seek medical attention immediately) are fundamental to the success of treatment [7]. The most common reason that patients with ischemic stroke cannot be treated with IV thrombolysis, the only treatment currently approved by the Food and Drug Administration (FDA), is that they arrive well after the required 3-hour treatment window [8,9]. The clinical features of stroke, which may be taught to the public, are listed in Table 4.2. Because stroke affects the brain, the patient may not be aware of the symptoms, or their thinking may be impaired; as a result, education of family members, neighbors, coworkers or acquaintances of persons at risk for stroke is crucial. Lags in seeking treatment are most likely to occur if the patient is alone or in a nonpublic location, such as the patient's home. In addition, the public needs to know the correct response – to activate the EMS system by calling 911.

Table 4.1 Components of management of a patient with an acute or recent ischemic stroke

Public (including persons at higher risk)
    Recognize the symptoms of ischemic stroke
    Immediately seek medical attention

Emergency medical services
    Early dispatch and rapid evaluation in the field
    Prompt transportation to closest appropriate hospital
    Initiate general emergency treatment

Emergency department
    General emergency treatment
    Evaluate for ischemic stroke
    Treat acute ischemic stroke
    Prevent or treat medical and neurological complications
    Admit to the hospital

Hospital
    Continue measures to treat the ischemic stroke
    Prevent or treat medical and neurological complications
    Evaluate for cause of ischemic stroke
    Initiate treatment to prevent recurrent stroke
    Start rehabilitation and plans for discharge

Table 4.2 Public educational stroke programs

The clinical features of stroke
    Sudden onset of:
        Weakness or paralysis – face, arm, hand, leg
        Numbness – face, arm, hand, leg
        Inability to speak or understand others
        Speech that is slurred or difficult to understand
        Dizziness (vertigo) or imbalance with walking
        Loss of vision in one or both eyes
        Unusually severe headache
    Symptoms can occur at any time, usually not with pain
    Symptoms usually occur in combination – area of brain injury

The correct response to suspected stroke
    Call 911 – seek emergency medical treatment
    Go to an emergency department (ride with someone else)
    Do not call the doctor's office
    Do not stay home waiting for the symptoms to clear

Example Case, cont'd.

The husband calls 911, and the local paramedics arrived at 7:50 PM. Her blood pressure was 175/95 mm Hg. Her pulse was 88 and irregularly irregular. They noted slurred speech with weakness on the left side of the face, left arm, and left leg. She had a high probability of stroke based on the Cincinnati Prehospital Stroke Scale.

They obtained additional history. She had hypertension and diabetes mellitus. She had been diagnosed as having atrial fibrillation 2 years earlier. She had been taking warfarin, but her dosage was reduced 2 weeks earlier because her international normalization ratio (INR) had been 3.3. She had been scheduled to have a follow-up INR in 2 days. She had had no recent serious illnesses or trauma. Her other medications included losartan, hydrochlorothiazide, metformin, and atorvastatin. They also asked her husband when was the last time he knew that she was not having problems; it had been at approximately 7:15 PM.

Emergency stroke care is based on a multidisciplinary, community-wide, and institutional program that involves the collaboration of EMS, hospitals, physicians, and other healthcare providers [10,11]. Much of the management of stroke mimics that for the treatment of patients with acute myocardial ischemia (Table 4.3). The mantra for emergency stroke care is "time is brain" [12]. The development of integrated stroke systems including the organization of EMS, creation of hospital stroke protocols, and the designation of stroke centers are outlined in Chapter 2. All potential sources of delay in treatment should be addressed [7].

Example Case, cont'd.

En route to the hospital, the paramedics informed the emergency department that they were transporting a patient with a suspected stroke and to activate the local stroke emergency team. They checked her blood glucose level; it was at 125 mg/dL. She arrived at the hospital at 8:25 PM.

Table 4.3 Similarities and differences in emergency treatment of ischemic stroke and myocardial infarction

Similarities
  Two most common acute medical emergencies
    Stroke common among persons with heart disease
      Stroke complicates myocardial infarction
    Heart disease common among persons with stroke
      Cardiac complications of stroke
  Two leading causes of death and disability
  Both accompanied by life-threatening complications
  Both usually due to a thromboembolic arterial occlusion
  Early reperfusion is a key to successful treatment
    Pharmacological or mechanical thrombolysis

Differences
  Pain is the primary symptom of myocardial infarction
    People respond quickly to severe pain
    Pain is not a prominent symptom in most strokes
  The symptoms of myocardial infarction are relatively stereotyped
  The symptoms of stroke are diverse – depending on brain location
  The brain is healthy in most patients with myocardial infarction
    Thinking is clear, should be able to respond
  The brain is affected in stroke
    Impaired thinking, lack of awareness

Patients should be transported to hospitals that have the expertise and resources to promptly evaluate and treat persons with suspected stroke. In many parts of the United States, these hospitals have been designated as primary stroke centers by either the Joint Commission or state public health authorities [13,14]. Protocols that include the required components of evaluation and treatment should be developed with the goal of meeting national guidelines [3]. If the patient cannot be treated with IV tissue-type plasminogen activator (tPA) at a community hospital, protocols should be in place to facilitate possible transfer to a stroke center. The components of such a stroke center include a full range of diagnostic studies, surgical procedures, and endovascular services [15]. Specific quality markers for the treatment of patients, based primarily on the American Heart Association guidelines, have been developed by the Joint Commission [3,16] (Table 4.4).

Stroke units, which provide comprehensive treatment of patients with acute stroke, are associated

Table 4.4 Quality indicators for hospitals ischemic stroke

Emergency treatment
    Thrombolytic therapy administered (or considered)
After admission to the hospital
    Prophylaxis against deep vein thrombosis prescribed
        (ambulation, antithrombotic medications, devices)
    Screening for dysphagia before receiving food or water by mouth
    Antithrombotic agents to prevent recurrent stroke started
        Started within 48 hours of stroke
        Patients with atrial fibrillation receive anticoagulants (unless a
        specific contraindication)
    Cholesterol-lowering medication started if low-density
        lipoprotein cholesterol is >100 mg/dL
    Assessed for rehabilitation prior to discharge
    Stroke education provided to patient and family
    Smoking cessation services should be offered

---

with improved outcomes [17–19]. The magnitude of the benefit of stroke unit care is similar to that achieved by early treatment with tPA. These benefits occur in a broad population of patients, including those who are not treated with tPA [20]. A stroke unit is usually a geographically defined facility that includes monitored beds and is staffed by medical, nursing, and rehabilitation personnel who have special expertise in treating patients with acute stroke.

Example Case, cont'd.

Upon arrival, her blood pressure was 190/105 mm Hg. She was upset with her husband and everyone else because she believed there was no reason for her to be at the hospital. She denied headache or chest pain. The history obtained from the paramedics was confirmed. She had no history of bleeding or intracranial hemorrhage. Diagnostic studies were ordered. Her weight was 80 kg. At approximately 8:40 PM, her husband arrived at the hospital, and he reconfirmed the relevant history.

Clinical presentations of acute ischemic stroke

The history of the onset and evolution of the symptoms is a crucial component of the initial evaluation. Many patients with stroke may be unable to provide a history because of impairments of language or consciousness, and historical information may need to be obtained from observers. Alternative diagnoses are relatively few; the most important is hemorrhagic stroke (Table 4.5). Differentiating hemorrhagic from ischemic stroke based only on clinical findings is difficult, and brain imaging is required [21,22].

Patients have the loss of neurological function (neurological impairments) reflecting the area of the brain injury. The most common symptoms are weakness, sensory loss, visual complaints, or difficulty with speech or language. Symptoms may occur in isolation or in combination. Some patients may have nausea or vomiting. Approximately 20% of patients have headache, particularly when vascular events are in the vertebrobasilar circulation. A severe headache or neck pain also may be prominent among patients with stroke related to an intracranial or extracranial arterial dissection [23,24]. Loss of consciousness or confusion (delirium) is rare. Seizures may occur with embolic events that affect the cerebral cortex. In general, the symptoms are of sudden onset, but the findings may evolve (worsen) or wax and wane during the first hours after stroke.

Another important component of the history is defining the time of symptom onset (taken as the time the patient was last at his or her baseline status). For patients who awaken with neurological symptoms, the time of onset is considered to be the time the patients were last awake and known to be symptom free. Some patients may have warning symptoms that resolve (i.e., TIA) prior to the new neurological findings. In these circumstances, the time of onset that is used to determine emergency interventions begins anew. For a patient that had mild neurological impairments and subsequent neurological worsening, the time of stroke onset is calculated as the time when the first symptoms were present. Information about the presence of risk factors for atherosclerosis or heart disease, migraine, seizures, trauma, drug abuse, infection, or pregnancy should also be sought. The use of medications, especially anticoagulants, should be queried.

The physical examination includes an assessment of vital signs and the status of the airway and pulse oximetry. Cardiac examination may point to the cause of the stroke or acute cardiovascular complications. The neurological examination focuses on

Table 4.5 Differential diagnosis of acute ischemic stroke

Diagnosis	Findings supportive of alternative diagnosis
Intracerebral hemorrhage	Prominent headache Nausea and vomiting Early decreased consciousness Very sudden and severe onset
Hypertensive encephalopathy	Headache Decreased consciousness Delirium Elevated blood pressure Visual loss Seizures
Migraine	History of prior events Positive phenomena (aura) Prominent headache Nausea and vomiting Younger age (especially women)
Seizure (with post-ictal signs)	History of seizures Witnessed seizure activity Confusion Lateral tongue bites March of symptoms Onset/resolution
Mass lesion (subdural hematoma/tumor)	Evolution of signs Headache Personality changes History of trauma
Encephalitis	Evolution of signs Decreased consciousness Seizures Fever Malaise and other constitutional symptoms
Hypoglycemia	History of diabetes/insulin use Decreased consciousness Confusion/delirium Autonomic signs – clammy
Conversion disorder	Lack of cranial nerve findings Findings – nonvascular pattern Inconsistent examination Unusual emotional reaction for the situation

the pattern and extent of the impairments, which reflect the location and severity of the stroke. The general rules of localization are included in Table 4.6. Patients with occlusion of the basilar artery may have the sudden onset of decreased consciousness [25].

Example Case, cont'd.
On neurological examination, which was performed at 8:30 PM, she was alert and oriented. She denied there was a problem, and she did not recognize her left arm as her own. She preferred to look to the right and ignored threats in the left visual field. She had mild dysarthria and left-sided facial weakness. She was unable to move her left arm and left leg. She did not respond to painful stimuli on the left. Her total National Institutes of Health Stroke Scale (NIHSS) score was calculated as 17.

The neurological assessment is enhanced by the use of standardized stroke scales such as the NIHSS [26,27] (Table 4.7). This clinical rating instrument, which is extensively used in clinical trials, is a standard way to measure the severity and types of neurological impairments following ischemic stroke. The scale facilitates communications among healthcare providers. It can be completed rapidly and accurately by a broad spectrum of healthcare professionals [28]. The pattern of impairments helps identify the location of the brain injury and the arterial occlusion. The total NIHSS score provides important prognostic information, including the potential for neurological complications, and assists in the identification of patients who may be eligible for emergency stroke therapies including tPA [3,29].

Example Case, cont'd.
Her complete blood count, platelet count, cardiac enzymes, and renal studies were normal. Her blood glucose level was 130 mg/dL. Her activated partial thromboplastin time was normal, and her INR was 1.7. The electrocardiogram showed atrial fibrillation. The CT scan was completed at 8:45 PM. It did not show bleeding or ischemic changes in the brain. A dense artery sign was seen in the right middle cerebral artery.

Table 4.6 Patterns of neurological impairment subtypes of ischemic stroke

Multilobar hemisphere infarction
  Consciousness – alert to drowsy (subsequently stupor/coma)
  Behavioral or cognitive signs are prominent
    Right (nondominant) hemisphere – neglect, aprosodia
    Left (dominant) hemisphere – aphasia, apraxia
  Contralateral visual field defect
  Conjugate eye deviation toward the lesion
  Dysarthria
  Contralateral hemiparesis and sensory loss
    Motor and sensory impairments usually similar
    Affect face, arm, and leg

Branch cortical hemisphere infarction
  Alert
  Behavioral cognitive signs are prominent
    Right (nondominant) hemisphere – neglect, aprosodia
    Left (dominant) hemisphere – aphasia, apraxia
  Contralateral visual field defect found with posterior infarctions
  Conjugate eye deviation toward the lesion often mild or absent
  Dysarthria is uncommon
  Contralateral hemiparesis and sensory loss
    May not affect face, arm, and leg equally
    Motor and sensory impairments may not be equal

Subcortical (lacunar) hemisphere infarction
  Alert
  Behavioral and cognitive signs less prominent or subtle
    Right (nondominant) hemisphere – neglect, aprosodia
    Left (dominant) hemisphere – aphasia, ataxia
  Contralateral visual field defects are uncommon
  Dysarthria is common
  Contralateral hemiparesis and sensory loss are common
    Generally affects face, arm, and leg equally
    May involve motor or sensory loss in isolation

Brain stem – cerebellar infarction
  Consciousness ranges from alert to coma
  Behavioral and cognitive signs are absent
  Visual field defects are absent
  Cranial nerve palsies present, ipsilateral to side of lesion
  Oculorotatory disturbances are prominent
  Dysarthria is often severe
  Paralysis may be contralateral, bilateral, or crossed
  Sensory loss may be contralateral, dissociated, or crossed
  Motor and sensory loss may occur in isolation
  Prominent ataxia ipsilateral to side of lesion

Evaluation of a patient with ischemic stroke

The diagnostic studies complement the clinical assessment. The initial (emergency) evaluation is performed when a patient with a suspected stroke is first seen. The goals of testing are to establish ischemia as the cause of the neurological symptoms (and to exclude alternative diagnoses), to screen for acute neurological or medical complications, and to determine the patient's eligibility for emergency treatment with reperfusion therapy. The guidelines delineate the diagnostic tests that need to be available in most community hospitals on a 24-hour per day and 7-day per week basis [3]. The goal is to complete the evaluation within 1 hour of the patient's arrival in the emergency department (Table 4.8). The additional (optional) tests listed in Table 4.8 may be performed as indicated by the patient's history, clinical findings, or comorbidities.

Brain imaging is the cornerstone of the evaluation; potential findings include the size, location, and vascular territory of the infarction, the presence of intracranial bleeding, or the presence of acute complications such as hydrocephalus or a mass. The tests also provide information about the possible degree of reversible brain ischemia, the status of intracranial arteries, and the hemodynamic status [30]. Brain imaging tests help select patients who might be treated with reperfusion therapies, including IV tPA, the risk for hemorrhagic complications of treatment, and the presence of arterial occlusions that may be treated with intra-arterial interventions. The most commonly performed tests are CT and magnetic resonance imaging (MRI). While MRI provides more information on stroke than CT, the treatment of a patient with a suspected ischemic stroke should not be delayed in order to perform an MRI when CT is readily available.

Nonenhanced CT of the brain is recommended for the initial evaluation of most patients [3,31]. CT is noninvasive, and it does provide important information; the yield in detecting intracerebral hemorrhage or subarachnoid hemorrhage is very high [32,33]. CT can also detect an intracranial mass such as a tumor or subdural hematoma. In most cases, CT will not demonstrate the acute effects of brain ischemia. The assumption is that acute ischemia is the explanation of a patient's focal neurological

Table 4.7 Components of the National Institutes of Health Stroke Scale

Level of consciousness			Orientation questions (2)	
Alert	0		Answers both correctly	0
Drowsy	1		Answers one correctly	1
Stupor	2		Answers neither correctly	2
Coma	3			
Response to commands (2)			Lateral eye movements	
Both tasks correct	0		Normal movements	0
One task performed	1		Partial gaze paresis	1
Performs neither task	2		Complete gaze paresis	2
Visual fields			Facial movement	
No visual field defect	0		Normal facial movement	0
Partial hemianopia	1		Minor facial weakness	1
Complete hemianopia	2		Partial facial weakness	2
Bilateral hemianopia	3		Complete facial palsy	3
Motor function (arm)			Motor function (leg)	
Both right and left rated independently				
No drift	0		No drift	0
Drift before 5 seconds	1		Drift before 5 seconds	1
Falls before 10 seconds	2		Falls before 10 seconds	2
No effort against gravity	3		No effort against gravity	3
No movement	4		No movement	4
Limb ataxia			Sensory examination	
No ataxia	0		No sensory loss	0
Ataxia in one limb	1		Mild sensory loss	1
Ataxia in two limbs	2		Severe sensory loss	2
Language			Articulation	
Normal language	0		Normal speech	0
Mild aphasia	1		Mild dysarthria	1
Severe aphasia	2		Severe dysarthria	2
Global aphasia or mute	3			
Extinction or inattention (two modalities tested)				
Absent	0			
Mild loss (one sensory)	1			
Severe loss (two sensory)	2			

symptoms of sudden and recent onset when a CT is normal and other causes are excluded. Physicians may recognize the subtle early abnormalities that can be demonstrated on CT [34–36]. The findings evolve over the first hours after stroke and include the development of lenticular hypodensity, loss of the gray-white matter differentiation, particularly in the lateral margins of the insula, and sulcal efface-ment. CT may also demonstrate an acute arterial occlusion, most commonly found in the middle cerebral artery or its branches (dense artery sign and dot sign) (Figure 4.1a and 4.1b). A thrombus may also be found in the basilar artery. These findings are most likely among patients with major multilobar infarctions, and they are associated with poorer out-comes [37]. Focal areas of cortical swelling have

Table 4.8 Emergency evaluation of a patient with suspected ischemic stroke

---

Baseline evaluation

   Noncontrast enhanced CT or magnetic resonance imaging of the brain

   Complete blood count, platelet count

   Coagulation tests (prothrombin time/international normalization ratio and activated partial thromboplastin time)

   Blood glucose

   Serum electrolytes/renal function tests

   Electrocardiogram

   Markers of myocardial ischemia (troponin)

   Oxygen (pulse oximetry)

Evaluation in selected patients

   Arterial blood gas tests (if hypoxia is suspected)

   Chest radiogram (if acute heart, aorta, or lung disease is suspected)

   Pregnancy test (women of childbearing potential)

   Toxicology screen and blood alcohol (if intoxication is suspected)

   Hepatic function tests (if metabolic disorder is suspected)

   Cerebrospinal fluid examination (if subarachnoid hemorrhage is suspected and brain imaging is negative for blood, or if an inflammatory vasculopathy, i.e., infection or vasculitis, is suspected)

   Electroencephalogram (if seizures are suspected)

---

been detected on CT, but this finding is not specific for cerebral ischemia [38]. There are insufficient data to state that any specific CT finding, other than hemorrhage, disqualifies a patient for treatment with tPA within 3 hours of stroke onset [3]. Sequential CT studies can be used to monitor for secondary hemorrhagic changes or prior to starting antithrombotic agents [39].

Dynamic CT perfusion and CT angiography may provide information about cerebral blood flow, mean transient time, cerebral blood volume, and vascular status [40,41]. The changes on perfusion CT may be compared with unenhanced CT to identify hypoperfused, but potentially salvageable ischemic brain (i.e., the ischemic penumbra) [42]. CT angiography is accurate in detecting lesions of major intracranial or extracranial arteries [41,43]. These tests can be done on an emergency basis with the contrast-enhanced studies performed immediately following the traditional unenhanced scan. However, the equipment and professional expertise to perform these tests are not widely available, especially in a community setting. The patient should be screened for renal dysfunction. Some patients are allergic to the contrast agent. In addition, the volume of contrast is considerable, and it may affect decisions about intra-arterial treatment, which require additional injections of contrast. While the role of

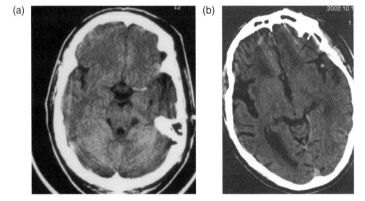

(a)   (b)

Fig. 4.1 (a and b) Axial views of a computed tomographic scan of a patient with an occlusion of the left middle cerebral artery. The scan demonstrates a thrombus in the artery (dense artery sign) (a) and the higher image also demonstrates a thrombus in a distal branch of the middle cerebral artery (dot sign). Images courtesy of Patricia Davis, MD, University of Iowa, Iowa City, IA.

contrast-enhanced CT is likely to increase in the future, current guidelines recommend that treatment with tPA should not be delayed in order to obtain these tests [3].

MRI is also useful for the emergency evaluation of patients with suspected stroke. It has several advantages, including the detection of acute, small, and posterior fossa infarctions; differentiation of acute from older infarction; excellent spatial resolution; and detection of arterial occlusions. It also avoids exposure to ionizing radiation. A suggested sequences of studies would include diffusion-weighted imaging (DWI), FLAIR, and gradient-echo sequences done without contrast (Figure 4.2). Subsequently, the patient could undergo MRI perfusion imaging that can be obtained with gadolinium contrast. The perfusion sequences can assess the time to peak, mean transient time, cerebral blood flow, and cerebral blood volume. Magnetic resonance angiography (MRA) of the intracranial and extracranial vasculature may follow; this can include a contrast-enhanced time of flight study. MRI can rapidly visualize the acute ischemic lesion (particularly with DWI sequences) and occlusions of major intracranial arteries [44,45]. A contrast-enhanced study can be performed to assess perfusion to the brain. It does provide some measures of the cerebral hemodynamic status. A comparison of the volume of the lesions found between DWI and perfusion sequences has been used to help define the ischemic penumbra (i.e., diffusion–perfusion mismatch; Figure 4.3a and 4.3b). MRA can demonstrate severe stenosis or occlusion of the major intracranial or extracranial vasculature [46] (Figure 4.4). Limitations of MRI

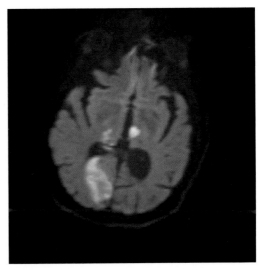

Fig. 4.2 Axial diffusion-weighted magnetic resonance image of a patient with an acute ischemic stroke. The scan shows bilateral thalamic and right occipital infarctions.

(a) (b)

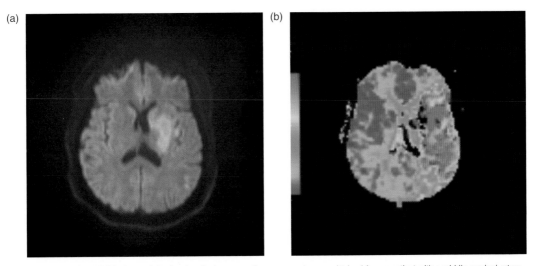

Fig. 4.3 (a and b) Axial diffusion-weighted and perfusion magnetic resonance images obtained from a patient with a middle cerebral artery occlusion. The area of ischemia (diffusion-weighted image) is smaller than the area of decreased perfusion (diffusion/perfusion mismatch).

include its cost, relatively limited availability, and contraindications including claustrophobia, cardiac pacemakers, and metal implants. Nephrogenic systemic fibrosis has been associated with gadolinium used for enhanced MRI studies, and patients' renal function should be screened before the agent is given. Current guidelines indicate that multimodal MRI studies may be considered for the evaluation of some patients with acute stroke, but are not required [3].

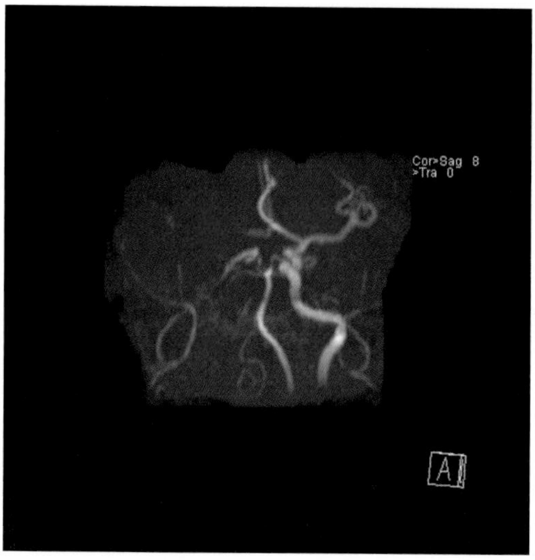

CT angiography, MRA, transcranial Doppler ultrasonography, carotid duplex, and catheter-based angiography can be used to assess the intracranial and extracranial vasculatures. The latter is often used as part of a procedure that includes intra-arterial administration of a thrombolytic agent or use of a mechanical intervention (Figure 4.5a and 4.5b). These tests are also performed after the patient has been admitted to the hospital, and the results are used in making decisions about the prevention of recurrent stroke.

Electrocardiography, which is a component of the emergency evaluation, is performed to screen for concomitant heart disease including myocardial ischemia and arrhythmias. Besides affecting acute management, the results also influence decisions about the prevention of recurrent stroke. Transthoracic echocardiography or transesophageal echocardiography is a component of evaluation of a patient with stroke because the results influence decisions about long-term prophylaxis against recurrent stroke. The other diagnostic studies outlined in Table 4.9 include assessments for risk factors for premature atherosclerosis and screening for hypercoagulable disorders or autoimmune diseases.

Fig. 4.4 Anterior-posterior view of a magnetic resonance angiographic study shows occlusions of the right internal carotid and middle cerebral arteries.

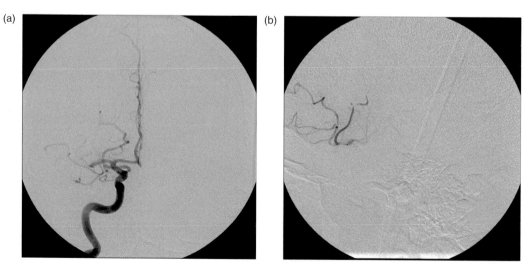

(a) (b)

Fig. 4.5 Anterior-posterior view of a cerebral arteriogram demonstrates an occlusion of the middle cerebral artery (a). The second image visualizes distal vasculature after a microcatheter has been passed through the thrombus (b). An embolus is seen in a distal branch artery. These films were obtained prior to local intra-arterial administration of a thrombolytic agent.

Table 4.9 Additional diagnostic tests for evaluation of a patient with an ischemic stroke

Vascular imaging
    Magnetic resonance angiography
    CT angiography
    Carotid duplex ultrasonography
    Transcranial Doppler ultrasonography
    Catheter-based arteriography

Cardiac imaging
    Transthoracic echocardiography
    Transesophageal echocardiography
    Cardiac CT
    Cardiac magnetic resonance imaging

Risk factor evaluation
    Fasting lipid profile
    Fasting blood glucose and hemoglobin A1c

Coagulation studies
    Fibrinogen, fibrin degradation products, d-Dimer
    Antithrombin
    Proteins C and S
    Antiphospholipid antibodies and lupus anticoagulant
    Factor V Leiden
    Prothrombin gene mutation
    Hemoglobin electrophoresis and sickle-cell preparation

Immunological studies
    Erythrocyte sedimentation rate
    C-reactive protein
    Antinuclear antibodies
    Anticytoplasmic nuclear antibodies

Example Case, cont'd.
Upon return from CT, her blood pressure was 180/105 mm Hg. It was checked on two more occasions, and both measurements showed slightly lower readings. Otherwise, her examination had not changed. She did not receive any antihypertensive medications.

General emergency management

Although many individual components of general emergency management have not been tested in clinical trials, current guidelines provide detailed recommendations [3]. Patients are observed closely

Table 4.10 General emergency treatment acute ischemic stroke

Protect airway (impaired consciousness/bulbar dysfunction)
    Elective intubation
Supplemental oxygen (hypoxic patient)
Treat fever
    Antipyretic agents
    Mechanical hypothermia
Monitor cardiac rhythm and treat arrhythmias
Treat hypotension
    Volume expansion (crystalloids or colloids)
    Hypertensive agents
Treat hypoglycemia
    Glucose (possibly with thiamine)
Treat hyperglycemia
    Administer insulin, glucose, and potassium
    Continuous infusion

with frequent measurements of vital signs, pulse oximetry, and neurological status [47]. The goals are to control acute complications and to stabilize the patient so that stroke-specific interventions can be prescribed [48].

Protecting the airway with elective intubation is often indicated for patients with decreased level of consciousness, severe bulbar dysfunction, or hypoxia necessitating oxygen supplementation [49–52] (Table 4.10). Fever following stroke is associated with an increased risk of morbidity or mortality presumably as the result of increased metabolic demands and other cellular consequences of an elevated temperature [53,54]. While clinical trials have been inconclusive, lowering the body temperature by antipyretics or cooling devices can be prescribed [55,56]. Induced hypothermia may be neuroprotective, and the utility of this intervention is being tested in the setting of acute stroke. Currently, it is considered to be experimental [57–62]. Serious cardiac arrhythmias are a potential complication; these should be treated with medications selected on a case-by-case basis [63,64]. Arterial hypotension, secondary to volume depletion, blood loss, or decreased cardiac output may occur. Aortic dissection is rare, but its presence is associated with an increased likelihood of unfavorable outcomes [65]. Treatment includes volume replacement and vasopressor agents.

An elevated blood pressure is commonly found and is associated with increased risk of neurological worsening and poor outcomes [66,67]. It may represent preexisting disease, but hypertension may also be secondary to the stress of the stroke, nausea, or pain [68]. It may also be a physiological response to increased intracranial pressure or ischemia. Patients with a systolic blood pressure >185 mm Hg or diastolic blood pressure >110 mm Hg cannot be treated with IV tPA, and treating hypertension in order to permit the use of the intervention is recommended by guidelines [3] (Table 4.11). Lowering the blood pressure may lessen the course of brain edema, reduce hemorrhagic transformation, prevent further vascular damage, and forestall recurrent stroke.

Table 4.11 Treatment of arterial hypertension acute ischemic stroke

Management before, during, and after treatment with reperfusion
  therapy

Before treatment:

If systolic pressure is >185 mm Hg or diastolic is >110 mm Hg
  Labetalol 10–20 mg IV over 1–2 minutes, may repeat ×1, or
  Nitropaste – apply 1–2 inches, or
  Nicardipine infusion, 5 mg/h, titrate dose by 0.25 mg/h at 5- to
    10-minute intervals, maximum dose 15 mg/h achieve desired
    blood pressure, reduce to 3 mg/h

During and after treatment:

If systolic pressure is 180–230 mm Hg or diastolic is
  105–120 mm Hg
  Labetalol 10 mg IV over 1–2 minutes, may repeat every 10–20
    minutes, maximum dose of 300 mg, or
  Labetalol 10 mg IV followed by an infusion of 2–8 mg/min

If systolic pressure is >230 mm Hg or diastolic is 121–140 mm Hg
  Labetalol 10 mg IV over 1–2 minutes, repeat every 10–20
    minutes, maximum dose of 300 mg, or
  Labetalol 10 mg IV followed by an infusion of 2–8 mg/min, or
  Nicardipine infusion, 5 mg/h, titrate dose of 0.25 mg/h at 5- to
    10-minute intervals, maximum dose, 15 mg/h achieve desired
    blood pressure, reduce to 3 mg/h

If blood pressure remains elevated, consider infusion of sodium
  nitroprusside

Administration among patients not given reperfusion therapies

If systolic pressure is >220 mm Hg or diastolic pressure is
  >120 mm Hg
  Treat with medications similar to those patients given reperfusion
    therapies

Conversely, the aggressive use of antihypertensive agents may reduce perfusion to the ischemic penumbra and lead to neurological worsening [69]. The level of blood pressure that mandates aggressive treatment and the selection of medications to use in this setting are not established [70]. Cautious lowering of blood pressure in the first hours after stroke is recommended. Medications, which are given parenterally, should have a short duration of action so that the antihypertensive effects can be reduced if the patient deteriorates neurologically [3] (Table 4.11). The time for starting maintenance antihypertensive medications is not established, but most patients probably can be treated at 24–48 hours after stroke.

Hypoglycemia is an important alternative diagnosis and should be aggressively treated. If there is a concern about precipitating Wernicke–Korsakoff syndrome, thiamine can be administered as an adjunct. More than one-third of patients have hyperglycemia, which is associated with poor outcomes [71]. Although elevations of blood glucose complicate more severe strokes, hyperglycemia (blood glucose >200 mg/dL) is an independent predictor of unfavorable outcome [72,73]. The aggressive management of hyperglycemia in other critically ill patients improves outcome. Still, there is uncertainty about the level of blood glucose to treat in the setting of acute stroke. Current guidelines recommend that patients with a blood glucose >140–200 mg/dL should be treated with an insulin infusion [3] (Table 4.10). Most patients are also given potassium and glucose in order to avoid hypoglycemia or hypokalemia [74]. Subsequent treatment should include longer-term measures to treat diabetes mellitus with oral agents or insulin as decided on a case-by-case basis.

Example Case, cont'd.
The patient was screened for treatment with IV tPA. The potential risks and benefits from treatment were discussed. The patient and her husband agreed to treatment. She received 72 mg of tPA with the 10% bolus dose started at 9:05 PM. The subsequent infusion was given over 1 hour. During that time, arrangements were made for her to be admitted to the hospital.

Emergency treatment of the acute ischemic stroke itself

Emergency therapies to treat the acute ischemic stroke include medications that have putative neuroprotective effects and interventions that are used to maintain or restore perfusion to the brain (Table 4.12). A large number of neuroprotective agents given alone or in conjunction with reperfusion therapies have been tested, but they have either an unacceptably high rate of complications or a lack of efficacy in improving outcomes [75,76]. Additional clinical trials testing promising neuroprotective agents are under way. Emergency measures to restore perfusion to the brain have been successful in improving outcomes, most notably IV tPA. Several other therapies aimed at augmenting perfusion to the brain have not been demonstrated as useful (Table 4.13). At present, IV tPA is the only medication that has been approved by the FDA to treat patients with acute ischemic stroke.

IV administration of tPA is the focus of emergency treatment of patients with acute ischemic stroke. A clinical trial found that the administration of tPA within 3 hours of onset of stroke was associated with favorable outcomes in 31–50% of treated patients in comparison to 20–30% of patients treated with placebo [39]. The risk of symptomatic hemorrhage was approximately 6% with a higher risk of bleeding among patients with multilobar infarctions [77]. A meta-analysis of clinical trials testing tPA found that a "cure" could be achieved in 50% of patients treated within 90 minutes of onset of stroke and in 25% of persons treated within 90–180 minutes

[78]. Thus, the goal is to evaluate and treat patients as quickly as possible. A European study looked at the outcomes following the administration of IV tPA among patients treated after regulatory approval and found that safety and efficacy were better than that achieved in the clinical trials [79]. Current guidelines provide recommendations about the selection and treatment of patients with tPA [3] (Tables 4.14 and 4.15). In addition to bleeding (including symptomatic hemorrhagic transformation of the infarction), angioedema of the throat, lips, and tongue may complicate the administration of tPA. The IV administration of other thrombolytic agents, including streptokinase, urokinase, anistreplase, staphylokinase, reteplase, tenecteplase, and desmoteplase, outside the setting of a clinical trial, is currently not recommended.

Intra-arterial administration of thrombolytic agents is a potential alternative to IV treatment (Figure 4.5). The medication would be given following the angiographic demonstration of an arterial occlusion. An advantage is concentrating the medication at the site of thrombus. The intervention could potentially be given to patients who could not be treated with IV therapy (i.e., recent surgery, arrival after 3 hours). Intra-arterial treatment with recombinant prourokinase was beneficial in improving arterial recanalization and clinical outcomes, especially among persons with moderately severe strokes [80]. Other studies have evaluated urokinase

Table 4.12 Neuroprotective therapies

Metabolic protection
  Hypothermia
  Sedatives
Inhibit glutamate release
NMDA/AMPA antagonists
Calcium channel blockers
Membrane active agents
Neurotrophic factors
Nitric oxide modulation
Free radical scavenger

Table 4.13 Therapies to restore or improve perfusion acute ischemic stroke

Pharmacological thrombolysis
  IV
  Intra-arterial
Antiplatelet agents
Anticoagulants
Vasodilation
Induced hypertension
Endovascular treatment
  Angioplasty/stenting
  Clot extraction
  Clot disruption
Surgical reconstruction
Volume expansion

Table 4.14 Treatment of patients with acute ischemic stroke with IV tissue-type plasminogen activator – questions to ask

Did the stroke begin within the last 3 hours?
  This should be the time that the patient was last known to be normal
  Stroke present upon awakening (uncertain time) – not treated
  If previous transient ischemic attack (complete resolution), clock restarts
  Some symptoms before 3 hours and then worsening – not treated
What is the severity of the patient's stroke?
  No measurable neurological impairment – not treated
  Minor and isolated impairments – usually not treated
  A disabling localized impairment (visual loss, aphasia) – treated
  Suggestive of subarachnoid hemorrhage – not treated
  Major improvement or spontaneous recovery – not treated
  Minimal improvement – treated
  Severe impairments (National Institutes of Health Stroke Scale >20) – treat with caution
  Seizure with stroke – treated if impairments are not post-ictal
Recent medical problems associated with bleeding?
  Not treated if the following are present:
    Recent (<3 months) myocardial infarction, stroke, or head trauma
    Recent (<3 weeks) gastrointestinal and urinary tract bleeding
    Recent (<2 weeks) major surgery
    Recent (<1 week) arterial puncture at a noncompressible site
    History of previous intracranial hemorrhage
Any findings on examination associated with increased risk?
  Systolic blood pressure is >185 mm Hg, or diastolic blood pressure is >110 mm Hg – can reduce pressure in order to treat
  Evidence of active bleeding on examination – not treated
Any medications associated with an increased bleeding risk?
  Oral anticoagulants or heparin – need to have coagulation tests
  If international normalization ratio (INR) is ≤1.7, or aPTT (activated partial thromboplastin time) is normal – may be treated
Any abnormalities found on laboratory testing?
  INR is >1.7 or prolonged aPTT – not treated
  Platelet count is <100,000 – not treated
  Blood glucose <50 mg/dL (2.7 mmol/L) – not treated
Any abnormalities found on brain imaging?
  Evidence of hemorrhage – not treated
  Early evidence of multilobar infarction – treat with caution
Does the patient and/or family understand the risks and benefits?

Table 4.15 Treatment of acute ischemic stroke IV administration of tissue-type plasminogen activator (tPA)

Administration of tPA
  Dosage – 0.9 mg/kg up to a maximum of 90 mg
  10% of dosage given as a bolus over 1–2 minutes
  Remainder infused over 1 hour
Monitoring
  Admit to an intensive care or stroke unit for close monitoring
  Neurological assessments every 15 minutes during infusion and first 30 minutes after the completion of infusion, then every 30 minutes for the next 6 hours, then hourly for the next 18 hours
  Measure blood pressure every 15 minutes for 2 hours, then every 30 minutes for the next 6 hours, then hourly for the next 18 hours
Administer antihypertensive medications if:
  Systolic blood pressure is ≥180 mm Hg, or
  Diastolic blood pressure ≥105 mm Hg
Delay placement of nasogastric tubes, bladder catheters, or intra-arterial pressure catheters
Obtain a CT study at 24 hours – before starting anticoagulants or antiplatelet agents

and other thrombolytic agents [81–83]. Current guidelines indicate that intra-arterial thrombolysis is an option for the treatment of patients within 6 hours of a major stroke secondary to an occlusion of the middle cerebral artery who cannot be treated with IV tPA [3]. This therapy should be performed at centers that have the necessary resources and clinical expertise. Unfortunately, the number of centers that can do these interventions is relatively small. Current guidelines also indicate that IV thrombolysis should not be withheld in order to treat with intra-arterial therapy, as this remains unapproved and there is no direct evidence showing that the approach improves patient outcomes as compared with IV tPA. The combination of a lower dose of IV tPA followed by intra-arterial treatment is being tested in a clinical trial [84].

Ancrod, a defibrinogenating enzyme derived from pit viper venom, is being tested, but at present, it is not FDA approved or recommended. Emergency anticoagulation has been tested in several clinical trials. Overall, there is no evidence that these medications halt neurological worsening or improve neurological outcomes following stroke [85–87]. These agents are not effective in preventing early recurrent stroke, including among patients with cardiac sources of embolization [88]. In addition, anticoagulants are associated with an increased risk of bleeding, including symptomatic hemorrhagic transformation of the infarction, especially among patients with severe strokes. As a result, current guidelines do not recommend urgent anticoagulation for the treatment of patients with acute ischemic stroke [3].

Aspirin, administered within 48 hours of onset of stroke, is associated with modest improvement in favorable outcomes and a small increase in the risk of bleeding complications [89,90]. Current guidelines recommend that aspirin be started within 48 hours of stroke in most patients [3]. The initial oral dose is 325 mg, and then subsequent treatment is with a daily dosage of 81 mg. Aspirin is not a substitute for other acute interventions for stroke, and it should not be started within 24 hours of treatment with tPA. There is no information about the utility of clopidogrel, ticlopidine, or dipyridamole in the emergency management of patients with recent stroke. On occasion, intravenously administered antiplatelet agents may be used as an adjunct to endovascular interventions. The glycoprotein IIb/IIIa receptor blocker, abciximab, was not found to be effective in improving outcomes after stroke [91]. Clinical trials have not established the utility of volume expansion, vasodilators, or induced hypertension in the treatment of acute ischemic stroke.

The safety and effectiveness of emergency carotid endarterectomy or other vascular operations are not established. Endovascular mechanical interventions are used increasingly for the treatment of patients with acute ischemic stroke; these may be used in conjunction with thrombolytic medications. Limited data are available about the use of emergency angioplasty and stenting [92–94]. Clot disruption using ultrasound or other devices has also been attempted; in some circumstances, these interventions are being used to complement IV or intra-arterial thrombolysis [95,96]. Devices have also been developed to extract a thrombus from a major intracranial artery [97,98]. While the data for efficacy of some of these interventions are limited, some devices have been approved for the extraction of a thrombus in the setting of acute ischemic stroke. Current guidelines advise that the approved clot-extraction devices may be a reasonable intervention for the treatment of some patients with acute stroke [3].

Example Case, cont'd.
The next day, she was alert but still had left-sided visuospatial neglect. She did not recognize her left arm and leg when she moved them. The sensory loss persisted. The NIHSS score was calculated as 8. Her follow-up CT scan showed a left partial lobe and insular infarction. Upon testing with a swallowing study, the speech pathologist reported that she could take food, fluids, and medications by mouth. Other rehabilitation services were also started. Warfarin was restarted after 24 hours to reduce the likelihood of recurrent embolization related to atrial fibrillation. She was also receiving subcutaneous heparin to prevent deep vein thrombosis (DVT) while she was immobile. The medications to treat her hypertension, diabetes mellitus, and lipids were also restarted.

General treatment after admission to the hospital

The aims of management after admission to the hospital are (a) to continue interventions started in the emergency department; (b) to monitor for and prevent potential complications of acute treatment including IV tPA; (c) to detect changes in the neurological status and initiate therapies to prevent or treat medical and neurological complications of the stroke; (d) to facilitate therapies aimed at improving outcomes after stroke; (e) to evaluate for the cause of stroke and prescribe medical or surgical interventions to prevent recurrent stroke; (f) to start rehabilitation efforts; and (g) to plan for care after discharge from the hospital. Most components of general treatment have not been tested in clinical trials, and current recommendations are based on customary care (Table 4.16). The use of preprinted orders, care maps, or stroke treatment protocols facilitate patient care [99]. These should be developed by physicians, nurses, and other healthcare

Table 4.16 Components of management hospitalization for acute ischemic stroke

Monitor vital signs, cardiac rhythm, and neurological status
Activity
    Initially at bed rest with head of bed flat
        Adjusted to the severity of stroke and medical status
        Mobilization within 24 hours for minor strokes
    Avoid falls
    Measures to prevent skin pressure sores
Hydration and nutrition
    Initially IV fluids to maintain hydration
        Also provides access for giving medications
    Perform swallowing assessment
        If unable to swallow, nasogastric or percutaneous endoscopic gastrostomy feeding
        If able to swallow, may have dysphagic diet
    Avoid constipation, fecal impaction, and diarrhea
    Treat nausea and vomiting
    Prescribe medications to prevent gastritis and peptic ulcers
Prevent and treat medical complications
    Prevent and treat pneumonia
        Avoid aspiration and atelectasis
        Screen if fever develops and treat with antibiotics
    Prevent and treat urinary tract infections
        If possible, avoid indwelling bladder catheters
        Screen if fever develops and treat with antibiotics
    Prevent and treat deep vein thrombosis/pulmonary embolism
        Mobilize as soon as patient is stable
        Administer heparin or low molecular weight heparin, or
        Use external compressive device
Treat concomitant diseases and risk factors
    Heart disease
    Diabetes mellitus, hypertension, smoking, hyperlipidemia
    Medications, diet, and lifestyle changes
Evaluate for cause of stroke and treat to prevent recurrent stroke
    Antiplatelet agents (for most cases of arterial cause of stroke)
    Oral anticoagulants (for most cases of cardioembolic stroke)
    Surgical or endovascular procedures (selected on location and severity of the arterial pathology)
Treat for complication of seizures
    Anticonvulsants for those patients who have seizures
    Prophylactic anticonvulsants not recommended
Observe for complication of hemorrhagic transformation of infarction
Start rehabilitation and plan for discharge
    Integrated multidisciplinary assessment and treatment
Education to the family and patient
    Stroke prevention, warning symptoms, recovery

professionals. Many of the components of general management are included in the quality indicators for stroke care (Table 4.4).

The patient's activity is modified in response to the severity of the stroke and overall medical status. Early mobilization is advised in an attempt to reduce the risk of pneumonia, DVT, pulmonary embolism, pressure sores, and orthopedic complications [100]. Falls are a potential risk during the initiation of standing and walking [101]. Initially, IV fluids are given to maintain hydration and to provide a route for the administration of medications. Because of the risk of aspiration, patients should have their swallowing assessed prior to taking liquids, solid food, or medications by mouth [102,103]. Patients with brainstem or major hemispheric strokes are at the greatest risk for dysphagia; both bedside and more sophisticated tests are available to evaluate swallowing [104]. The placement of a nasogastric tube, or in patients who need prolonged feeding percutaneous endoscopic gastrostomy (PEG), is used to maintain hydration and nutrition. In general, a PEG tube is considered superior to a nasogastric tube [105]. Bowel management is aimed at avoiding constipation, fecal impaction, and fecal incontinence [106,107]. Patients who have nausea and vomiting should also receive symptomatic treatment. Rarely, gastrointestinal bleeding from gastritis or peptic ulcer disease may complicate stroke.

Seriously ill, immobile patients and those who are unable to cough are at high risk for pneumonia, which is a leading cause of morbidity and mortality after stroke [108]. The development of fever following stroke should prompt screening for pneumonia and urinary tract infection. Protecting the airway, avoiding aspiration, and encouraging deep breathing and mobilization may help lower the risk of pneumonia. The prophylactic administration of antibiotics is not recommended, but patients with suspected pneumonia should be treated promptly. Urinary tract infections are also relatively common [108]. Many patients have urinary incontinence or retention, and indwelling catheters are placed to help avoid skin complications and to ease care. However, catheters do increase the risk of infections, and they should be avoided if possible. Intermittent catheterization may be an alternative. The urine should be screened in any patient developing a fever;

with prompt initiation of antibiotics if the urinalysis or urine culture is positive.

DVT and secondary pulmonary embolism are important causes of morbidity or mortality following stroke. Older and bedridden patients with a paralyzed leg are at greatest risk. Prompt institution of measures to prevent DVT is a quality of care marker (Table 4.4). Options include early mobilization, antithrombotic agents, and external compressive devices. In general, anticoagulants are preferred because of the robust evidence of their utility for this indication [3,109–112]. Either unfractionated heparin or low molecular weight heparins may be administered. External compression of the legs is an option when a patient cannot be treated with anticoagulants [113]. A patient who has a pulmonary embolus secondary to DVT in the lower extremity and who cannot receive anticoagulants may require placement of a device to occlude the inferior vena cava.

Cerebral edema with secondary increased intracranial pressure is a leading cause of death among patients with multilobar cerebral infarctions [114–116] (Table 4.17). Increased intracranial pressure causes hypoperfusion that leads to worsening of brain ischemia. In addition, the focal mass effect of the infarction can cause herniation that leads to secondary brainstem injury. A large cerebellar infarction can compress the brain stem and fourth ventricle, leading to secondary hydrocephalus. Generally, cerebral edema peaks at approximately 4–5 days after the stroke, though a very early and malignant course also may occur. Affected patients have a decline in consciousness and worsening of other neurological signs. The appearance of an ipsilateral third nerve palsy (dilated and nonreactive pupil) is a relatively late finding. Management includes prophylactic measures as outlined in Table 4.17 [117,118]. Corticosteroids are not indicated. While osmotherapy has been recommended, data about usefulness are limited [119]. Among patients with neurological deterioration, surgical decompression may be performed as a life-saving procedure [120–123]. Early surgery (before secondary brainstem injury) is preferred [122,124]. Surgical decompression or ventricular drainage is also recommended for the treatment of patients with mass-producing infarctions of the cerebellum [125–127].

Table 4.17 Cerebral edema and increased intracranial pressure following ischemic stroke

Patients at highest risk for this complication
  Cerebellar infarction >2.5 cm in diameter
  Multilobar cerebral infarction
    Occlusion of internal carotid artery
    Occlusion of proximal portion of middle cerebral artery
Preventive measures
  Prevent hypoxia and hypercarbia
  Treat fever
  Modest elevation of head to augment venous drainage
  Fluid restriction and avoid hypo-osmolar fluids
Image findings
  Cerebellar infarction
    Obliteration of fourth ventricle
    Obliteration of prepontine cistern
    Dilation of lateral ventricles
Cerebral infarction
  Loss of sulci of affected hemisphere
  Obliteration of ipsilateral lateral ventricle
  Shift of midline structures to opposite side
  Dilation of contralateral lateral ventricle
Treatment
  Osmotherapy using mannitol or hypertonic saline
  Intubation and hyperventilation
  Placement of intraventricular catheter – drainage of cerebrospinal fluid
    Cerebellar infarction
  Surgical decompression
    With or without resection of necrotic tissue

Spontaneous bleeding into an infarction ranges from the small petechiae found on the brain imaging to a large hematoma that causes neurological worsening (Figures 4.6 and 4.7). This complication occurs most frequently among patients with multilobar infarctions [128]. The risk of hemorrhagic transformation is increased with the use of antithrombotic or thrombolytic agents, especially among patients with high NIHSS scores and the elderly [77,85,129]. There is no specific intervention to prevent this complication, but it should be sought if a patient has neurological worsening on the first days after stroke.

Epileptic seizures, which are more likely to occur with cortical infarctions and which may occur in

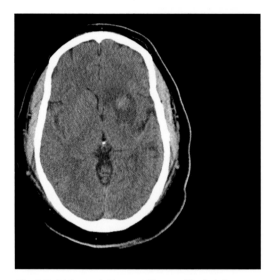

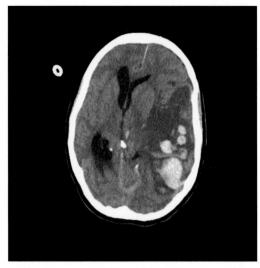

Fig. 4.6 Axial computed tomographic scan of the brain in a patient with a striatocapsular infarction in the left hemisphere. Areas of petechial hemorrhage are seen within the area of infarction.

Fig. 4.7 Axial computed tomographic scan of the brain in a patient previously treated with thrombolytic therapy who subsequently had neurological worsening. A large area of hemorrhage within the infarction is seen. The findings are consistent with symptomatic hemorrhage.

approximately 5% of patients, may occur at the time of the ischemic event or during the first days [130–132]. The seizures may be partial or involve secondary generalization. Status epilepticus is uncommon [133]. While patients who have seizures following stroke should receive anticonvulsants, prophylactic administration of anticonvulsants is not indicated [3].

References available online at www.wiley.com/go/ strokeguidelines.

Intracerebral Hemorrhage

Opeolu Adeoye and Joseph P. Broderick

EXAMPLE CASE

A 68-year-old left-handed male presented by ambulance after onset of a right-sided headache that progressed to left-sided weakness during dinner. Symptoms were witnessed by his wife and began approximately 45 minutes prior to arrival.

MAJOR POINTS

- Emergency evaluation and diagnosis of intracerebral hemorrhage (ICH)
  - Clinical presentation alone is insufficient for distinguishing between stroke subtypes.
  - Both CT and magnetic resonance imaging (MRI) of the head are excellent first choices to detect an ICH.
  - CT is more practical, especially in critically ill and unstable patients.
  - MRI is better at detecting any underlying structural lesions and evidence of prior brain hemorrhage, which is often asymptomatic.
- Treatment of acute ICH/intraventricular hemorrhage (IVH)
  - ICH is a major medical emergency and requires treatment in an intensive care unit with experienced personnel.
  - No randomized trials have shown definitive benefit for any surgical or medical treatment for ICH.
  - Airway, breathing, and circulation should be immediately assessed.
  - Secondary brain injury should be prevented by avoiding hypoxia, controlling blood pressure and

  intracranial pressure (ICP), and preventing/rapidly treating seizures, infection, or thromboembolism.
  - In coagulopathic patients, appropriate agents should be rapidly administered to minimize hemorrhage growth.
  - Ongoing trials should clarify the use of hemostatic agents in patients without coagulopathy.
  - Surgical evacuation may be life-saving in cerebellar ICH, but has a more limited and less clear role in supratentorial ICH. Younger patients with large lobar ICH, or those with an associated structural lesion, may be candidates for surgical evacuation.
- Brain supportive therapy in ICH: ICP and cerebral perfusion pressure/glucose control/prevention and treatment of seizures/body temperature
  - Multimodal monitoring of the ICH patient in the neuroscience intensive care unit aims to rapidly identify and treat abnormalities that may cause secondary brain injury.
  - Treatment of elevated ICP should include appropriate analgesia and sedation, and osmotic therapy and/or cerebrospinal fluid diversion.

A Primer on Stroke Prevention Treatment: An Overview Based on AHA/ASA Guidelines, 1st Edition. Edited by L Goldstein.
© 2009 American Heart Association, ISBN: 9781405186513

- ○ Occult seizures occur commonly in ICH; a high degree of vigilance is required for detecting and appropriately treating seizures after ICH.
- ○ High blood glucose and fever have both been associated with worse ICH outcomes; ongoing trials should clarify appropriate treatment of fever and high blood glucose after ICH.
- Prevention of deep vein thrombosis and pulmonary embolism
  - ○ Pneumatic compression may be used early for venous thrombosis prophylaxis in ICH.
  - ○ Prophylaxis with subcutaneous heparin may be started 3–4 days after onset once hemorrhage stabilization is confirmed.
  - ○ Vena cava filter placement should be considered in ICH patients who develop proximal deep venous thrombosis or subclinical pulmonary emboli *and* who cannot be treated with anticoagulants.
- ICH related to anticoagulation and fibrinolysis: management of acute ICH and restarting antithrombotic therapy

- ○ Warfarin-associated ICH is increasing in incidence.
- ○ Vitamin K and fresh frozen plasma should be administered for the rapid correction of coagulopathy.
- ○ Future trials should clarify the role of prothrombin complex concentrates and/or recombinant activated factor VII for warfarin-associated ICH.
- ○ Reinstitution of antithrombotic therapy must take into account the risk of ICH recurrence versus the risk of thromboembolism.
- Surgical treatment of ICH/IVH
  - ○ Routine evacuation of supratentorial ICH is not associated with improved outcomes.
  - ○ A subgroup of patients with superficial lobar ICH may benefit from surgical evacuation.
  - ○ Emergent evacuation of large cerebellar ICH may be life-saving with good functional outcomes.
  - ○ Ongoing studies should clarify the role of less invasive stereotactic techniques and clot evacuation using thrombolysis.

Emergency evaluation and diagnosis of intracerebral hemorrhage (ICH)

ICH occurs in about 78,000 persons in the United States annually and has a 30-day mortality of 35–50% [1–5]. Only 20% of ICH patients are functionally independent at 6 months [6]. Despite advances in emergency and critical care medicine, ICH outcomes have remained poor over the past 20 years [5]. This chapter will discuss the emergency evaluation and diagnosis of ICH, its medical and surgical treatment, and the impact ongoing trials may have on ICH management.

ICH often presents as a sudden onset of neurological deficits that may be accompanied by headache, vomiting, or depressed level of consciousness. The neurological deficit typically worsens over minutes to hours. Marked hypertension at presentation is more common with ICH than with other stroke subtypes, acute ischemic stroke (AIS), or subarachnoid hemorrhage (SAH) [7].

Emergency medical services (EMS) personnel should triage all suspected stroke patients with the same urgency, and patients should be transported to hospitals capable of rapid evaluation and treatment of any stroke patient. ICH patients may develop elevations in intracranial pressure (ICP) requiring

neurosurgical intervention. Some primary stroke centers are incapable of providing this level of care. All hospitals caring for stroke patients must have adequate staff to provide rapid evaluation, accurate diagnosis, and a plan for quickly transferring patients to tertiary care centers as needed.

Emergency department (ED) staff must communicate with EMS providers and witnesses/family members to confirm the time of onset, history of trauma, history of seizures, other medical history, blood glucose level, warfarin or other antithrombotic use, and initial Glasgow Coma Scale (GCS) score. The physical examination should begin with the assessment of the airway, breathing, and circulation. Retrospective studies suggest that an elevated systolic blood pressure of >160 mm Hg may be associated with hemorrhage growth, neurological decline, and poor outcomes after ICH [8–11], but this has not been confirmed in prospective reports [12,13]. The level of consciousness and the extent of neurological deficit should be determined using the GCS and National Institutes of Health Stroke Scale (NIHSS) scores. Neuroimaging should be rapidly obtained for the identification of ICH.

Both CT and magnetic resonance imaging (MRI) can accurately identify acute ICH. CT may be better at identifying intraventricular hemorrhage (IVH), whereas MRI is better at identifying underlying structural lesions and at evaluating perihematomal edema [14,15]. In a study comparing CT and MRI for detecting acute ICH within 6 hours of symptom onset, gradient-echo MRI was comparable to CT in identifying acute ICH but was more accurate in identifying areas of chronic hemorrhage [14]. CT is more practical than MRI for the rapid evaluation of patients who may have an altered level of consciousness, hemodynamic instability, vomiting, and/or airway compromise. In one study, MRI was not feasible in 20% of 141 acute stroke patients, the majority of whom had an ICH [15]. Thus, CT is often a more practical imaging choice during the first hours after arrival in the ED, but MRI, when available and appropriate, is an excellent imaging modality to evaluate ICH.

Secondary causes of ICH should be ruled out as these may be amenable to interventions, e.g., aneurysm clipping for SAH. Once parenchymal ICH is identified by CT, the hematoma volume may be easily calculated by the ABC/2 formula (A and B are the largest perpendicular diameters of the hematoma in centimeters, and C is the number of vertical CT slices multiplied by the slice thickness in centimeters; Figure 5.1) [16]. ICH volume is a strong predictor of outcome with reported mortality rates of 19% for volumes less than 30 mL and 91% for volumes greater than 60 mL [2].

Complete blood count, glucose, electrolytes, blood urea nitrogen, creatinine, and prothrombin and partial thromboplastin times should be drawn in the ED. A chest X-ray and ECG should also be obtained. A toxicology screen should be performed if cocaine use is suspected, and pregnancy tests should be performed in women of childbearing age.

> **Example Case, cont'd.**
> The example patient should be triaged for rapid evaluation on ED arrival. The following should occur concurrently and as quickly as possible: airway, breathing, and circulation should be assessed; a detailed history should be obtained from EMS providers and the patient's wife; a physical exam should be performed, and the patient's GCS and NIHSS scores should be determined; blood tests should be drawn and sent to the lab; and preparation should be under way to obtain a head CT within 25 minutes of ED arrival, and a report should be obtained from the radiologist within 20 minutes of the test's completion. CT with contrast may also be used at some institutions following the noncontrast study to detect contrast extravasation (a marker of ongoing bleeding) as well as to identify structural abnormalities associated with the ICH. A point-of-care creatinine in the ED is appropriate in these patients to determine any risk to kidney function.
>
> The patient's airway and breathing were intact, and the blood pressure was 210/100 mm Hg. Pulse was irregular with a rate of 66, and the temperature was 99°F. Relevant medical history included atrial fibrillation and hypertension for which the patient had been treated with atenolol and warfarin. The patient had a GCS of 11 (E3, V2, M6) and an NIHSS of 17. Blood tests were sent to the lab, and a head CT was obtained (Figure 5.2).

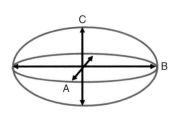

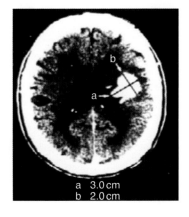

Fig. 5.1 ABC/2 method for determining ICH volume.

Treatment of acute ICH/IVH

Medical treatment of ICH

Medical treatment trials for ICH

Prior to the publication of the 1999 American Heart Association (AHA) guidelines of management of ICH [17], only four small randomized trials of medical therapy for ICH had been published [18–21]. None found the significant benefit of steroids, glycerol, or hemodilution for ICH.

The natural history of ICH is that of ongoing hemorrhage growth in nearly 40% of patients, mostly in the initial 3–4 hours, but up to 24 hours from symptom onset (Figure 5.3) [12,22]. This led to consideration of early administration of hemostatic therapy for acute ICH.

Trials of recombinant activated factor VII (rFVIIa)
rFVIIa has been studied for the management of ICH in hemophilic patients with good results and minimal thromboembolic complications [23,24]. It also promotes hemostasis in patients with normal coagulation [25]. The half-life of rFVIIa is approximately 2.6 hours, and the recommended dose in patients with hemophilia is 90 µg/kg every 3 hours [25].

Two pilot studies of rFVIIa in ICH showed sufficient safety to encourage further testing [22,26]. A large, phase IIB trial randomized ICH patients, diagnosed by CT within 3 hours of symptom onset, to placebo (96 patients) or rFVIIa 40 µg/kg (108 patients), 80 µg/kg (92 patients), or 160 µg/kg (103 patients) [27]. rFVIIa was given within an hour of the baseline CT scan. The primary outcome measure was the change in volume of ICH at 24 hours. Clinical outcomes were determined at 90 days. rFVIIa limited hemorrhage growth, reduced mortality, and improved functional outcomes in a dose-dependent manner [22]. Thromboembolic complications

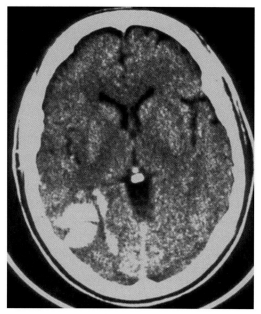

Fig. 5.2 Lobar ICH in a patient on warfarin.

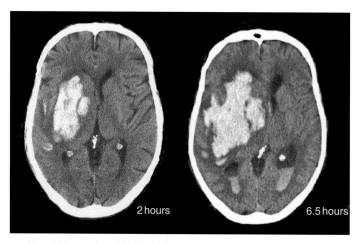

Fig. 5.3 Hemorrhage growth in a patient with basal ganglion ICH.

including myocardial infarction and ischemic stroke occurred in 7% of rFVIIa-treated patients compared with 2% of placebo-treated patients ($P = 0.12$). The administration of rFVIIa within 4 hours of symptom onset limited hemorrhage growth, reduced mortality, and improved functional outcomes. Efficacy and safety of recombinant activated factor VIIa for acute intracerebral hemorrhage trial (FAST) did not confirm that treatment decreased mortality or improved functional outcome for subjects treated with rFVIIa despite replication of the reduction of hemorrhage growth [28].

The use of rFVIIa for the treatment of warfarin-associated ICH has also been reported. In a study of seven patients with warfarin-related ICH, 15–90 μg/kg of rFVIIa was given in addition to standard therapy (fresh frozen plasma [FFP] and vitamin K) [29]. Another study compared 12 patients with warfarin-associated ICH treated with rFVIIa plus vitamin K and FFP with 15 patients treated with vitamin K and FFP alone [30]. Although rapid normalization of the international normalization ratio (INR) occurred with rFVIIa in both studies, rebound increased INR developed, and full doses of FFP and vitamin K were still required. rFVIIa may be a promising therapy for warfarin-associated ICH, but larger prospective studies are required.

Trial of acute blood pressure management

Elevated blood pressure at presentation has been associated with poor outcomes in ICH [31,32]. Hypertension in the setting of hemorrhagic stroke may cause increased bleeding and edema formation [4]. However, rapid blood pressure decline in the first 24 hours from symptom onset has also been associated with poorer outcomes [33]. Elevated blood pressure after ICH is thought to maintain cerebral perfusion pressure (CPP) in the setting of increased ICP. Impaired autoregulation could also compromise cerebral blood flow (CBF) with blood pressure reduction.

CBF was measured by positron emission tomography (PET) in a study of 14 patients with acute supratentorial ICH (1–45 mL in size; 6–22 hours from symptom onset) [34]. Patients then received either nicardipine or labetalol, which reduced mean arterial pressures by 15%, after which CBF was repeated. No change in global or perihematomal CBF was observed, suggesting that autoregulation is preserved in patients with small/medium-sized ICH with modest blood pressure reductions [34].

Trial of hyperosmolar therapy for the treatment of elevated ICP

One trial randomized 128 patients with primary supratentorial ICH to low-dose mannitol or sham therapy within 6 days of onset [35]. Patients were treated with either 100 mL of 20% mannitol ($n = 65$) or sham therapy ($n = 63$) every 4 hours for 5 days, followed by 2 days of tapering. The primary end point was mortality at 1 month with a secondary end point of functional outcome at 3 months as measured by the Barthel Index (BI). There was no mortality difference between groups at 1 month ($P = 0.80$) and no functional outcome difference between groups at 3 months ($P = 0.25$).

Specific medical therapies
Blood pressure management

Elevation of blood pressure after ICH is associated with hemorrhage growth, particularly in hemorrhage secondary to a ruptured aneurysm or arteriovenous malformation. However, the compromise of CBF by blood pressure reduction possibly leading to ischemia of perihematomal tissue could worsen outcome with rapid blood pressure decline [33]. Although both animal and human prospective observational studies question the existence of an "ischemic penumbra" in ICH [34,36], some controversy persists based on human MRI studies that indicate the presence of surrounding tissue at risk for secondary ischemia [37].

Little prospective evidence supports specific blood pressure targets in ICH. The previous AHA recommendation was to maintain a systolic blood pressure of ≤180 mm Hg and/or a mean arterial pressure of ≤130 mm Hg [17]. The reduction in mean arterial pressure by 15% does not significantly impact CBF in humans with ICH as determined by PET [34]. In a small prospective observational study, reduction in blood pressure to <160/90 mm Hg was associated with hemorrhage growth in 9% of patients and neurological decline in 7% but showed a trend toward improved outcomes in patients treated within 6 hours of symptom onset [38]. In the largest prospective study of ICH growth and in the Recombinant Activated Factor VII Intracerebral Hemorrhage trial, baseline blood pressure was not associated with ICH growth [12,13,39]. Hemorrhage growth occurs more frequently in patients with elevated systolic blood pressure, but it remains unclear whether it contributes to hemorrhage growth or whether elevated systolic blood pressure occurs in response to increased ICP from hemorrhage growth [11]. The rapid rate of blood pressure decline in the first 24 hours from symptom onset has been associated with increased death rate in a retrospective study [33]. Experience from traumatic brain injury and ICH supports maintaining CPP >60 mm Hg [40–42].

The Antihypertensive Treatment in Acute Cerebral Hemorrhage pilot study is a three-dose-tiered trial investigating the reduction of systolic blood pressure to 170–200, 140–170, and 110–140 mm Hg. The study was recently completed, and the results are pending. Planning is under way for the large phase III multicenter trial. In addition, the Intensive Blood Pressure Reduction in Acute Cerebral Hemorrhage (INTERACT) pilot study was recently completed [43]. The goal of this study was to determine if lowering blood pressure after ICH would decrease the chance of death or surviving with a severe disability. Patients with spontaneous ICH presenting within 6 hours of onset and with two systolic blood pressure readings ≥150 and ≤220 mm Hg were eligible for enrollment. Two hundred and three patients were randomized to aggressive blood pressure reduction with a goal blood pressure of 140 mm Hg, whereas 201 were randomized to guideline management or goal systolic blood pressure of 180 mm Hg. Early aggressive blood pressure reduction was associated with a nonsignificant decrease in hematoma volume and mortality or severe disability. Mean baseline hematoma volume was 12.7 mL in the guideline blood pressure control group and 14.2 mL in the intensive reduction group. A mean systolic blood pressure reduction of 13.3 mm Hg (95% confidence interval [CI] 8.9–17.6 mm Hg; $P < 0.0001$) was achieved in the intensive reduction compared with the guideline group within an hour of randomization. From 1 to 24 hours, the difference was 10.8 mm Hg (95% CI 7.7–13.9 mm Hg; $P < 0.0001$). Mean hematoma growth was 36.3% in the guideline group and 13.7% in the intensive group (difference 22.6%, 95% CI 0.6–44.5%; $P = 0.04$) at 24 hours [43]. While these findings are promising, the blood pressure parameters for enrollment and a relatively small mean baseline ICH volume (compared with mean volumes of 22–24 mL in the rFVIIa trials [22,28]) render the results of the INTERACT pilot trial difficult to apply to the general ICH population. A phase III trial is in the planning stages.

Example Case, cont'd.
The patient should receive IV antihypertensive treatment with labetalol, nicardipine, esmolol, enalaprilat, or hydralazine. A continuous infusion may be required if target blood pressure is not attained with bolus doses. In this particular patient, a mean arterial pressure goal of 110 mm Hg would be ~15–20% reduction. Lab tests revealed an INR of 2.8 but were otherwise unremarkable. IV vitamin K (10 mg) should be administered and 20 mL/kg FFP infusion begun. The use of rFVIIa is not considered a standard of care and should be considered only as part of a research protocol.

Brain supportive therapy in ICH
Monitoring of neurological and cardiopulmonary function Sudden eruption of hemorrhage into the brain parenchyma causes the destruction of some brain tissue, exerts mass effect on adjacent brain tissue, and can cause increased ICP. In addition to continued bleeding, the physiological and inflammatory response to the hemorrhage results in perihematomal edema and/or ischemia, hydrocephalus, or secondary IVH. All of these can in turn increase ICP, worsen mass effect, and cause neurological deterioration [42].

The ICH patient should be monitored closely, and neurological function should be assessed frequently using the NIHSS [44] and the GCS [45]. Maintaining respiratory and cardiovascular stability is important for preventing secondary brain injury in ICH patients, because these patients have limited autoregulatory capacity. Admission to a neuroscience intensive care unit has been associated with reduced mortality in ICH [46]. This has implications for the organization of critical care services provided by hospitals.

Treatment of elevated ICP
Management of elevated ICP in the neuroscience intensive care unit mostly derives from the trau-

matic brain injury literature. The "Lund protocol" assumes that the blood-brain barrier is disrupted and emphasizes decreasing hydrostatic forces and increasing osmotic forces, thus maintaining fluids within the vascular compartment [47]. CPP-guided therapy, however, focuses on maintaining CPP >70 mm Hg, often necessitating increases in blood pressure [40–42]. No randomized trial has shown either approach to be superior to the other. Thus, a balanced approach to managing elevated ICP in the neuroscience intensive care unit often involves multiple treatments geared toward the particular patient. Initial measures may include simple maneuvers such as head positioning and adequate analgesia. These may progress to aggressive measures including continuous invasive monitoring of ICP and CPP, cerebrospinal fluid (CSF) drainage, osmotic therapy, or induction of barbiturate coma. None of these aggressive treatments have been shown to be effective in a randomized trial of ICH patients.

Head-of-bed elevation Elevating the head of the bed to 30° increases venous outflow and lowers ICP. The head should be maintained in the midline position. Adequate fluid status is necessary since raising the head of the bed may result in a drop in blood pressure, potentially compromising CPP in a hypovolemic patient.

CSF drainage Ventriculostomy placement has not been studied prospectively in ICH, and its use has been associated with increased morbidity and mortality [48,49]. An intraventricular catheter may be used to monitor ICP and for CSF drainage to lower ICP as needed. The main risks of placing a ventriculostomy are hemorrhage and infection. Ventriculostomy-associated bacterial meningitis is reported to have an incidence of 6–22% [50,51].

Analgesia and sedation Adequate sedation and analgesia may blunt increases in ICP. Short-acting agents such as propofol, etomidate, or midazolam may be required for sedation in unstable patients who require intubation or other procedures. Agents such as morphine or fentanyl may be required for pain.

Neuromuscular blockade Prophylactic neuromuscular blockade is associated with increased risk of infections such as pneumonia and can obscure seizure activity. The use of neuromuscular blockade has not been shown to improve outcome after ICH.

Osmotic therapy Mannitol draws fluid into the intravascular space from both edematous and nonedematous brain tissue. Unfortunately, the osmotic effect of mannitol subsequently results in diuresis causing hypovolemia and a hyperosmotic state. A maximum serum osmolality of 320 mOsm/kg has been recommended, but definitive data are lacking to justify this threshold.

Hypertonic saline has been shown to reduce ICP, even in cases refractory to mannitol. However, many issues remain to be clarified, including its exact mechanism of action, the best mode of administration, and the concentration to be used [52,53].

Hyperventilation The broad use of hyperventilation to lower ICP has fallen out of favor due to the concurrent reduction in CBF. Also, its effects on ICP and CBF are transient since the extracellular space of the brain readily adapts to the pH change induced by hyperventilation. After a patient has been hyperventilated for >6 hours, the normalization of arterial pCO_2 can cause rebound intracranial hypertension. The target levels of CO_2 for hyperventilation are 30–35 mm Hg [54].

Barbiturate coma High-dose barbiturates decrease cerebral activity and are effective in lowering refractory intracranial hypertension, but are ineffective and potentially harmful if given prophylactically or as a first-line therapy for elevated ICP. The use of barbiturates for refractory intracranial hypertension requires intensive monitoring and has a high incidence of complications [55]. Continuous electroencephalographic (EEG) monitoring should occur during high-dose barbiturate treatment with the goal of treatment being burst suppression.

Management of glucose

High-admission blood glucose is predictive of 28-day mortality in diabetic and nondiabetic stroke patients [56]. Some studies attribute hyperglycemia in acute stroke to premorbid diabetic glucose metabolism [57,58], whereas others suggest it is a stress reaction to the acute stroke [59]. The AHA guidelines for the management of AIS published in

2007 recommended lowering markedly elevated blood glucose levels to <185 mg/dL (<16.63 mmol/L) [60]. Randomized trials are ongoing to evaluate aggressive glucose reduction in acute stroke.

Antiepileptic drugs

In a series of 761 consecutive ICH patients, early seizures occurred in 4.2% of patients, and 8.1% had seizures within 30 days of onset. Lobar location of ICH was associated with early seizures [61]. In a cohort of 63 ICH patients undergoing continuous EEG monitoring, electrographic seizures occurred in 28% within 72 hours of admission [62]. ICH-related seizures are often nonconvulsive and are associated with higher NIHSS, midline shift, and a trend toward worse outcomes [62]. Clinical seizures in ICH patients should be treated rapidly using IV medications such as lorazepam or diazepam, followed by fos-phenytoin or phenytoin. A brief period of antiepileptic medication after symptom onset may reduce early seizures after ICH, particularly in lobar hemorrhages [61].

Temperature management

Experimental models of brain injury have shown that fever worsens outcome [63,64], and that hypothermia ameliorates brain injury and reduces thrombin-induced brain edema formation [65,66]. Fever duration has been found to be an independent predictor of poor outcome in ICH [67]. These data provide a rationale for aggressive fever reduction in ICH, but while cooling to 32–34°C can be effective in lowering refractory intracranial hypertension, it is associated with a high rate of complications and may result in rebound intracranial hypertension if reversed too quickly [68,69].

Example Case, cont'd.

The patient should be admitted to the neuroscience intensive care unit and closely monitored for neurological deterioration that may warrant endotracheal intubation and/or placement of an ICP monitor. Pneumatic compression boots should be used. This patient's coagulopathy limits the ability to perform invasive cranial procedures and increases the risk of prolonged bleeding. Thus, prompt administration of vitamin K and

---

FFP is necessary. With the lobar location of the ICH, prophylactic administration of an antiepileptic may be considered. Decline in neurological status may also be secondary to edema and mass effect for which osmotic agents may be administered.

Prevention of deep vein thrombosis and pulmonary embolism

Occult venous thrombosis occurs in 10–50% of acute stroke patients with hemiplegia [70], and 1–2% of ICH patients develop pulmonary emboli [22,71]. Little evidence is available to guide the prevention of thromboembolism in the setting of ICH. A recent trial randomized patients with ICH to compression stockings versus compression stockings plus intermittent pneumatic compression. Asymptomatic deep venous thrombosis was detected by ultrasonography at day 10 in 15.9% of patients wearing compression stockings alone compared with 4.7% in the combined group (relative risk 0.29 [95% CI 0.08–1.00]) [71]. Another trial randomized 68 ICH patients to low-dose heparin starting on the 10th day (group 1), the 4th day (group 2), or the 2nd day (group 3) after ICH onset. Group 3 patients had significantly fewer pulmonary emboli than the other two groups without increased bleeding in any of the groups [72].

Recurrent ICH

Recurrent ICH occurs in ~1% of patients during the initial 3 months after an acute ICH [73,74]. A theoretical analysis estimated that anticoagulation increases the risk of ICH recurrence 2-fold [74]. Selecting therapy for an individual patient with a deep vein thrombus or pulmonary embolus must balance the risk of ICH recurrence with the associated mortality rate of >50% against the risk of subsequent thromboembolism. No randomized clinical trial has compared anticoagulation with vena cava filter placement in ICH. Vena cava filters do reduce the risk of pulmonary embolism in patients with proximal deep vein thrombosis in the first several weeks, but have an increased longer-term risk of venous thromboembolism [75]. If the patient is anticoagulated, good blood pressure control is important. The Perindopril Protection against Recurrent Stroke Study trial documented a 50% reduction of the risk of ICH recurrence with a reduction of systolic blood pressure by 11 mm Hg [76].

ICH related to anticoagulation and fibrinolysis: management of acute ICH and restarting antithrombotic therapy

Warfarin treatment accounts for approximately one in every five cases of ICH [77,78]. The main risk factors for warfarin-associated ICH are age, history of hypertension, intensity of anticoagulation, and conditions such as cerebral amyloid angiopathy and leukoaraiosis [79–82]. The degree of INR elevation does correlate with hemorrhage growth and prognosis (death and functional outcome) [82].

Available options to counteract the effects of warfarin include vitamin K_1, FFP, prothrombin complex concentrate (PCC), and rFVIIa. Vitamin K_1 is given intravenously at a dose of 10 mg [83]. A small risk of anaphylaxis with IV vitamin K_1 may be reduced by slow infusion [84]. Vitamin K_1 takes at least 6 hours to normalize the INR [84]. FFP may be given to replenish vitamin K-dependent factors inhibited by warfarin. The recommended dose of 15–20 mL/kg of FFP is effective in correcting INR, but the large volume needed may either cause heart failure with rapid infusion or lead to long delays in normalizing INR due to slow infusion [85]. Varying concentrations of clotting factors are found in different FFP preparations [86]. The FFP approach is impractical for treating life-threatening warfarin-associated ICH.

PCC contains high levels of factors II, VII, and X in contrast to factor IX complex concentrate that contains factors II, VII, IX, and X. These preparations require much smaller volume infusions and correct coagulopathy faster than FFP [87,88]. The disadvantage of these preparations is increased risk of serious thromboembolic events.

rFVIIa also rapidly corrects the INR and is effective in reducing hemorrhage growth [22,28–30]. Due to the short half-life of rFVIIa (2.6 hours), full doses of FFP and vitamin K are still required despite the initial rapid correction of INR [29,30]. Also, increased thromboembolic complications in the

treatment versus placebo arms (7% vs. 2%, respectively) of spontaneous ICH patients treated with rFVIIa raise concerns about the use of the agent in patients prone to embolism, such as those with prosthetic heart valves or chronic atrial fibrillation [22].

Reinstituting anticoagulation after warfarin-associated ICH relates primarily to patients anticoagulated for the prevention of cardiogenic embolism due to prosthetic heart valves or chronic atrial fibrillation. The reported rate of cerebral embolism in patients with nonvalvular atrial fibrillation without a history of stroke is 5% per year [89]; patients with prior stroke have a 12% per year risk of ischemic stroke [90]; and the risk in patients with prosthetic mechanical valves is 4% per year [91]. Thus, the decision to anticoagulate after warfarin-associated ICH must balance the risk of ischemic stroke against the risk of ICH recurrence with anticoagulation. In three clinical series with a total of 114 ICH patients, the reversal of anticoagulation with FFP and discontinuation of warfarin for a mean of 7–10 days were associated with embolism in six patients (5%). Rebleeding occurred in one patient (0.8%) upon the reinstitution of anticoagulation between days 7 and 10 [92–94]. PCCs have been used for a total of 78 patients in seven clinical series [86,95–100]. Four thromboembolic events occurred (5%), and continued hemorrhage expansion occurred in five subjects (6%). Thus, the reinstitution of anticoagulation between days 7 and 10 after warfarin reversal appears to be safe. However, elderly patients and those with lobar ICH that are likely due to amyloid angiopathy have a higher risk of ICH recurrence [74] and may be better treated with antiplatelet agents.

ICH related to fibrinolysis

Symptomatic ICH occurs in 3–10% of patients with AIS treated with tissue plasminogen activator (rt-PA) [57,101–103]. ICH onset after fibrinolysis carries a poor prognosis and is associated with a 30-day death rate of 60% or more [102]. No reliable data are available to guide the treatment of ICH in this setting. Recommended therapy includes the infusion of platelets (6–8 units) and cryoprecipitate that contains factor VIII to correct the fibrinolytic state created by rt-PA [60]. Recommendations for surgical management are the same as for spontaneous ICH, but surgery should only occur after intracranial bleeding has been stabilized.

Surgical treatment of ICH/IVH

Craniotomy

Craniotomy has been the most extensively studied surgical treatment for ICH. Of five randomized trials of ICH conducted with access to contemporary medical and surgical technologies, four were single-center studies that randomized fewer than a total of 125 patients. No study provided convincing evidence of surgical benefit after ICH, but one concluded that patients with mild-to-moderate alteration in consciousness (GCS score 7–10) may have lower mortality rates without clear improvement in functional outcome with surgery [104]. Another suggested that ultra-early evacuation might improve 3-month NIHSS score [105].

The International Surgical Trial in Intracerebral Haemorrhage (STICH) randomized 1,033 ICH patients to surgery within 96 hours of onset or medical management [106]. Patients were only randomized if the neurosurgeon was uncertain of the benefit of surgery. The primary outcome was the Glasgow Outcome Scale (GOS) score at 6 months, and secondary outcomes were death, the BI, and the modified Rankin Scale (mRS) at 6 months. No overall benefit from surgery was found when compared with initial conservative, medical management (26% vs. 24% favorable outcome, $P = 0.41$) [106]. Prespecified subgroup analyses identified subjects with a GCS score of 9–12, those with lobar hemorrhages, and those with clots <1 cm from the cortical surface as subjects who were helped by surgery, although this did not reach statistical significance. Further trials are needed to confirm the findings.

The randomized trials mentioned previously did not include patients with cerebellar hemorrhages. Nonrandomized series have reported good outcomes for patients with large (>3 cm) cerebellar hemorrhages or brainstem compression or hydrocephalus [107–109]. Medical management alone in these patients often results in poor outcomes, while patients with small cerebellar hemorrhages without brainstem compression may be managed medically.

Minimally invasive surgery

Endoscopic aspiration

A small, single-center trial randomized 100 patients aged 30–80 years with hemorrhage volume of at least 10 mL to burr hole and continuous lavage of the hematoma cavity or medical therapy within 48 hours of symptom onset [110]. Patients in the endoscopic aspiration arm had artificial CSF infused at a pressure of 10–15 mm Hg, and suction was administered at regular intervals to remove clots and blood-stained CSF.

The mortality rate of the surgical group (42%) was lower than that of the medical group (70%, $P = 0.01$). Also, more in the surgically treated group had a good outcome with minimal to no deficits. Among patients with large (50 mL) hemorrhages, survival was improved by surgery without improvement in the quality of life. For smaller hemorrhages, endoscopic evacuation resulted in similar survival but a better quality of life in the surgically managed group. The benefit was mainly limited to patients with lobar hemorrhage who were age <60 years [110].

Thrombolytic therapy and aspiration of clots

In a small, single-center pilot trial, 11 subjects were randomized to conservative therapy, and nine subjects were randomized to very early surgical removal of ICH within 24 hours of symptom onset. Subjects with deep hemorrhages who underwent surgery were treated with instillation of urokinase into the bed of the clot ($n = 4$) [111]. These subjects had overall good outcomes (3-month BI scores of 100, 100, 90, and 85). A multicenter randomized controlled trial ($n = 71$) examined the utility of stereotactic urokinase infusion within 72 hours for patients with GCS scores ≥5 or clots of ≥10 mL [112]. Treated patients received 5,000 units of urokinase every 6 hours for 48 hours. The primary outcomes were death and functional handicap at 6 months. The median reduction in volume of ICH from baseline was 40% in the surgical group and 18% in the medical group. Rebleeding occurred in 35% of the urokinase group and 17% in the conservative group. A significant reduction in death (40%) was found in the treated group, but no statistically significant difference was noted in the functional outcomes [112]. Urokinase became unavailable in the United States in 1999, whereupon investigators began to examine the instillation of rt-PA for clot evacuation.

A report on 20 patients with IVH found a quicker disappearance of IVH with rt-PA (1–3 days) than urokinase (5–8 days) [113]. Compared with ventriculostomy alone, the infusion of rt-PA reduced mortality from 60% to 90% to 5% [113]. While no large randomized trials are currently available, one small randomized trial and several small series have had similar safety and efficacy of infusion of thrombolytics for the treatment of IVH [114–116]. Following the successful treatment of parenchymal ICH in a pig model [117], pilot human trials of stereotactically administered rt-PA into the hematoma cavity have been conducted [118–120]. These small studies consistently demonstrate the successful reduction of the hemorrhage with minimal systemic or intracranial bleeding complications [118–120]. A multicenter, randomized, controlled, and stratified study comparing the administration of rt-PA into the clot cavity versus standard medical therapy is ongoing. The Minimally Invasive Stereotactic Surgery + rt-PA for ICH Evacuation study is testing the hypotheses that (a) early use of minimally invasive surgery plus rt-PA for 3 days is safe for the treatment of ICH, and (b) early use of minimally invasive surgery plus rt-PA for 3 days produces clot size reduction compared with medically treated patients. This phase II trial is almost completed.

Early clot evacuation

"Ultra-early" stage

In a retrospective review with historical controls, 100 patients with putaminal hemorrhages had surgery within 7 hours of symptom onset [121]. Sixty of the hemorrhages were treated within 3 hours. These patients had a baseline GCS score of 6–13, and most patients had a hematoma volume of >20–30 mL. Patients with mild symptoms or GCS scores of ≤5 were treated conservatively. At 6 months, 7 (7%) had died, whereas 15 (15%) had fully recovered, and 35 (35%) were living independently at home. Based on these findings, a small, single-center randomized trial of craniotomy within 4 hours was performed [122]. The mean time to the operating room was 191 minutes (range 95–240 minutes), but the 6-month mortality was higher for patients who underwent surgery (36% vs. 29%, P = NS), and

functional outcomes in survivors were no different (P = 0.88). In addition, 4 out of 11 patients who underwent ultra-early operation had acute rebleeding, of whom 75% died. The authors suggested that the early rebleeding seen in the absence of operation might actually be facilitated by craniotomy, and that surgery with the concomitant use of rFVIIa might solve this problem [123].

Within 12 hours

As part of the ultra-early surgical trial, a third group of patients underwent craniotomy within 12 hours of ictus (n = 17) [122]. The mortality rate was 18%, as compared with 29% in the medically managed group (P = NS). Early rebleeding was reduced, but the outcome was not noticeably improved [122].

In the small study by Zuccarello *et al.* [105], those randomized to operation had the surgery at a mean of 8 hours and 25 minutes from symptom onset. The likelihood of a good outcome (primary outcome measure: GOS score >3) for the surgical group (56%) did not differ significantly from the medical treatment group (36%), although it trended in favor of surgery. No significant difference in mortality rate was seen at 3 months. The analysis of the secondary 3-month outcome measures showed a nonsignificant trend toward a better outcome in the surgical treatment group for the median GOS, BI, and mRS scores and a significant difference in the NIHSS score (4 vs. 14; P = 0.04) [105].

Within 24 hours

A prospective trial within 24 hours matched 34 patients with hypertensive basal ganglia hemorrhage and comparable hematoma volume and GCS scores. Seventeen patients were treated surgically. Eight patients died (47%), and no statistical difference was seen in patient survival. At 3, 6, and 12 months, there was no statistical difference in the functional outcomes (using the BI score) between the two groups [124].

Within 48 hours

In a prospective randomized trial of 52 patients with supratentorial ICH, 26 patients were assigned to the surgical group and underwent craniotomy, with the median time from bleeding to operation being 14.5 hours (range 6–48 hours). At 6 months, 12 patients (46%) had died, and only 1 patient (4%) was living independently at home. No statistically significant difference in mortality and morbidity rates was found between the treatment groups [104].

Within 96 hours

In the STICH trial, "early" surgery was compared with initial conservative treatment for 1,033 patients with ICH [106]. The average time from symptom onset to surgery was 30 hours (range 16–49 hours), and the average time for only 16% (74 of 465 patients) was fewer than 12 hours. At 6 months, good functional outcome was 26% ($n = 122$) for the surgical group, which was not significant when compared with the medical group (24%; OR 0.89, 95% CI 0.66–1.19). The absolute 2.3% (−3.2% to 7.7%) and relative 10% (−13% to 7.7%) benefits for early surgery over initial conservative medical treatment were not significant [106].

Decompressive craniotomy

In the single published case series of decompressive craniotomy for ICH, 12 consecutive patients (mean age 50 years [range 19–76 years]) were treated with decompressive hemicraniectomy. Eleven patients (92%) survived to discharge, and six (54.5%) had a good functional outcome, defined as mRS of 0–3 (mean follow-up 17.13 months, range 2–39 months). Of note, three of the seven patients with pupillary abnormalities had good recoveries, as did four of the eight with clots >60 mL. Although these data are uncontrolled and preliminary, they support rigorous controlled trials, which may identify a subgroup of patients in whom this technique might prove to be worthwhile [125].

Example Case, cont'd.

With the superficial location of the patient's ICH (Figure 5.2), early surgical evacuation may be considered. This is again limited by the patient's coagulopathy, emphasizing the need to reverse the coagulopathy as quickly as possible.

Withdrawal of technological support

Withdrawal of life-sustaining support is the most common immediate cause of death in patients with ICH [126]; thus, the use of do-not-resuscitate (DNR) orders biases predictive models of ICH outcomes [127]. Aggressive care during the first 24 hours after ICH onset should be considered, and new DNR orders should be postponed during that time. Patients with previous DNR orders are not included in this recommendation. DNR status relates only to the circumstance of cardiopulmonary arrest and patients should receive all other appropriate medical and surgical interventions.

Prevention of recurrent ICH

Hypertension is the most important target for ICH prevention, and the OR for ICH was 3.5 with untreated hypertension but only 1.4 for treated hypertension in one study [128]. Smoking, heavy alcohol use, and cocaine use are also risk factors for ICH [129,130], and discontinuation should be recommended for the prevention of ICH recurrence.

References available online at www.wiley.com/go/ strokeguidelines.

Subarachnoid Hemorrhage

Jonathan L. Brisman and Marc R. Mayberg

EXAMPLE CASE

A 48-year-old otherwise healthy woman presented to the emergency room because of severe headache associated with nausea that came on suddenly while watching television. There was no prior history of headaches, and the current episode was described as the worst of her life. She felt as if she were going to pass out, but she did not lose consciousness. The patient previously smoked cigarettes and had no other family members with cerebral aneurysms. A noncontrast head CT scan revealed a diffuse subarachnoid hemorrhage (SAH). Physical examination showed a woman with mild nuchal rigidity and photophobia but no focal neurological deficits. She was admitted to the intensive care unit for further diagnostic evaluation and definitive care.

MAJOR POINTS

- Non-traumatic subarachnoid hemorrhage (SAH) is an important cause of morbidity and mortality, caused by the rupture of a cerebral aneurysm in most (80%) cases.
- MRA, CTA, and digital subtraction angiography (DSA) are excellent modalities with which to diagnose ruptured and unruptured cerebral aneurysms, DSA remaining the gold standard.
- SAH is a medical emergency requiring ICU management to detect and treat the numerous potential medical and neurological complications.
- Ruptured cerebral aneurysms should be treated promptly (within 72 hours) to prevent disastrous rehemorrhage.
- Treatment of ruptured aneurysms should be performed by teams experienced in the two major treatment modalities: microsurgical "clipping" and endovascular "coiling."

- Unruptured cerebral aneurysms are managed very differently from ruptured lesions as the natural history is comparatively benign; decision to treat must carefully weigh risks and benefits, taking into account patient and aneurysm-specific factors.
- Cerebral arteriovenous malformations (AVMs) are congenital vascular lesions that can present with SAH and should be treated if they bleed; treatment of unruptured AVMs is controversial as there is debate about the natural history risk of a lesion that has not bled.
- Treatment of brain AVMs includes endovascular embolization, stereotactic radiosurgery, surgical excision, or most often some combination of these modalities, with complete angiographic obliteration as the goal to prevent future hemorrhage.

A Primer on Stroke Prevention Treatment: An Overview Based on AHA/ASA Guidelines, 1st Edition. Edited by L Goldstein.
© 2009 American Heart Association, ISBN: 9781405186513

Introduction and definitions

Spontaneous (i.e., atraumatic) intracranial hemorrhage into the subarachnoid space is a neurological emergency and an important form of hemorrhagic stroke that results in significant morbidity and mortality. Although the most common cause (80%) of nontraumatic SAH is rupture of a cerebral aneurysm, other etiologies such as ruptured arteriovenous malformation (AVM), vasculitis, dural arteriovenous fistula, hemorrhagic brain tumors, and hemorrhagic transformation of ischemic stroke exist and need to be considered.

It should be kept in mind that SAH is frequently associated with head trauma, and because of the frequency of traumatic head injury, this is still the leading cause of SAH. This chapter focuses on spontaneous SAH and, in particular, SAH caused by a ruptured intracranial aneurysm (IA), a focal abnormal outpouching of a cerebral artery. Brief attention will also be given to AVMs, another potentially life-threatening cause of spontaneous SAH. The elective management of unruptured IAs, in which therapies to avert a disastrous SAH must be weighed against the risk of intervention, will also be discussed.

In 1994, the American Heart Association (AHA) published guidelines for the management of aneurysmal SAH [1]. A recent retrospective study of 100 centers demonstrated that there has been significant compliance with these guidelines [2]; whether this has translated into improved outcomes has not been studied. Because of recent advances in the field, such as the development and mainstream incorporation of endovascular treatment of aneurysms, better imaging capabilities, and publication of several important randomized trials, the AHA formed another writing group to reassess the recommendations for the management of aneurysmal SAH. This chapter summarizes some of these new guidelines (AHA guidelines, in press, 2008). The new guidelines, including the level and class of evidence supporting those recommendations, are replicated in Table 6.1.

Epidemiology, risk factors, and genetics

Although IAs are surprisingly common, estimated at 1–5% of the population, most are small and often not discovered, and do not cause harm during the lifetime of the individual. A small percent of aneurysms do rupture, leading to SAH, which is estimated to occur in 27,000 persons in the United States yearly and represents 5% of all strokes [3–6]. Why aneurysms form and what causes them to bleed are not certain, but hypertension, heavy alcohol use, cocaine use, tobacco use, and genetic factors are believed to play a role (Table 6.1, Section 1). SAH has a mean age of presentation of 55–60 years of age and is more common in women than men (1.6–2:1) and more common in blacks (2.1–1) than whites [7]. Most IAs are located at branch points along the circle of Willis within the subarachnoid space at the base of the brain (Figure 6.1). Hemodynamic factors associated with branching of the arteries may contribute to the formation and rupture of these lesions that have a reduction in the tunica media, the middle muscular layer of cerebral arteries.

Although aneurysms are felt to be sporadically acquired lesions, they occur in association with fibromuscular dysplasia, Ehlers–Danlos type IV, Marfan's syndrome, AVMs of the brain, and most commonly autosomal dominant polycystic kidney disease (ADPKD) [7]. An estimated 5–30% of patients with ADPKD harbor aneurysms, which are multiple in 10–30%. A familial inheritance pattern, independent of the mentioned conditions, is found in 10% and is often associated with multiple aneurysms and increased risk of hemorrhage [7]. Screening with magnetic resonance angiography (MRA) is recommended for all patients with ADPKD and for anyone with two first-degree relatives with IAs [8].

Rupture of an IA leading to SAH is a devastating event, with a 30-day mortality of 45%. An estimated 30% of survivors will have a moderate to severe disability [9]. These figures translate into an estimated 6,700 in-hospital deaths in the United States yearly [9]. Because of the relatively young age of those affected, 27% of all stroke-related years of potential life lost before age 65 are attributable to SAH [9].

Imaging characteristics

Diagnosis of SAH

The initial imaging examination in the evaluation of SAH is the noncontrast CT scan (Table 6.1, Section 3). CT scanning performed within 72 hours of SAH has a high sensitivity and specificity for detecting blood in the subarachnoid space, whereas magnetic

Table 6.1 Guidelines for the management of aneurysmal subarachnoid hemorrhage (in press, 2008)

Section 1

Prevention of subarachnoid hemorrhage: summary and recommendations

1 The relationship between hypertension and aneurysmal SAH is uncertain. However, treatment of high blood pressure with antihypertensive medication is recommended to prevent ischemic stroke and intracerebral hemorrhage, cardiac, renal, and other end-organ injury (Class I, Level of Evidence A).

2 Cessation of smoking is reasonable to reduce the risk of SAH, although evidence for this association is indirect (Class IIa, Level of Evidence B).

3 Screening of certain high-risk populations for unruptured aneurysms is of uncertain value (Class IIb, Level of Evidence B); advances in noninvasive imaging may be used for screening, but catheter angiography remains the "gold standard" when it is clinically imperative to know if an aneurysm exists.

Section 2

Natural history and outcome of aneurysmal SAH: summary and recommendations

1 The severity of the initial bleed should be determined rapidly as it is the most useful indicator of outcome following aneurysmal SAH, and grading scales which heavily rely on this factor are helpful in planning future care with family and other physicians (Class I, Level of Evidence B).

2 Case review and prospective cohorts have shown that for untreated, ruptured aneurysms, there is at least a 3% to 4% risk of rebleeding in the first 24 hours and possibly significantly higher, with a high percentage occurring immediately (within 2 to 12 hours) after the initial ictus, a 1% to 2% per day risk in the first month, and a long-term risk of 3% per year after 3 months. Urgent evaluation and treatment of patients with suspected SAH are therefore recommended (Class I, Level of Evidence B).

3 In triaging patients for aneurysm repair, factors that may be considered in determining the risk of rebleeding include severity of the initial bleed, interval to admission, blood pressure, gender, aneurysm characteristics, hydrocephalus, early angiography, and the presence of a ventricular drain (Class IIb, Level of Evidence B).

Section 3

Manifestations and diagnosis of subarachnoid hemorrhage: summary and recommendations

1 SAH is a medical emergency that is frequently misdiagnosed. A high level of suspicion for SAH should exist in patients with acute onset of severe headache (Class I, Level of Evidence B).

2 CT scanning for suspected SAH should be performed (Class I, Level of B), and lumbar puncture for analysis of cerebrospinal fluid is recommended when the CT scan is negative (Class I, Level of Evidence B).

3 Selective cerebral angiography should be performed in patients with documented SAH to document the presence and anatomic features of aneurysms (Class I, Level of Evidence B).

4 MRA or infusion CT (CTA) may be considered when conventional angiography cannot be performed in a timely fashion (Class IIb, Level of Evidence B).

Section 4

Emergency evaluation and preoperative care: summary and recommendations

1 The degree of neurological impairment using an accepted SAH grading system can be useful for prognosis and triage (Class IIa, Level of Evidence B).

2 A standardized ED management protocol for the evaluation of patients with headaches and other symptoms of potential SAH does not currently exist and should probably be developed (Class IIa, Level of Evidence C).

Section 5

Medical measures to prevent rebleeding after SAH: summary and recommendations

1 Blood pressure should be monitored and controlled to balance the risk of strokes, hypertension-related rebleeding, and maintenance of cerebral perfusion pressure (Class I, Level of Evidence B).

2 Bed rest alone is not enough to prevent rebleeding after SAH. It may be considered as a component of a broader treatment strategy along with more definitive measures (Class IIb, Level of Evidence B).

3 Although older studies demonstrated an overall negative effect of antifibrinolytics, recent evidence suggests that early treatment with a short course of antifibrinolytic agents, when combined with a program of early aneurysm treatment followed by discontinuation of the antifibrinolytic and prophylaxis against hypovolemia and vasospasm may be reasonable (Class IIb, Level of Evidence B), but further research is needed. Furthermore, antifibrinolytic therapy to prevent rebleeding may be considered in certain clinical situations, e.g., patients with a low risk of vasospasm and/or a beneficial effect of delaying surgery (Class IIb, Level of Evidence B).

Table 6.1 *Continued*

Section 6

Surgical/endovascular treatment of ruptured aneurysms: summary and recommendations

1 Surgical clipping or endovascular coiling should be performed to reduce the rate of rebleeding after aneurysmal SAH (Class I, Level of Evidence B).

2 Wrapped or coated aneurysms as well as incompletely clipped or coiled aneurysms have an increased risk of rehemorrhage compared to those completely occluded, and therefore require long-term follow-up angiography. Complete obliteration of the aneurysm is recommended whenever possible (Class I, Level of Evidence B).

3 For patients with ruptured aneurysms judged by an experienced team of cerebrovascular surgeons and endovascular practitioners to be technically amenable to both endovascular coiling and neurosurgical clipping, endovascular coiling can be beneficial (Class IIa, Level of Evidence B). Nevertheless, it is reasonable to consider individual characteristics of the patient and the aneurysm in deciding the best means of repair, and management of patients in centers offering both techniques is probably indicated (Class IIa, Level of Evidence B).

4 Although previous studies showed that overall outcome was not different for early versus delayed surgery after SAH, early treatment reduces the risk of rebleeding after SAH, and newer methods may increase the effectiveness of early aneurysm treatment. Early aneurysm treatment is reasonable and is probably indicated in the majority of cases (Class IIa, Level of Evidence B).

Section 7

Hospital characteristics and systems of care: summary and recommendations

1 Early referral to high-volume centers that have both experienced cerebrovascular surgeons and endovascular specialists is reasonable (Class IIa, Level of Evidence B).

Section 8

Anesthetic management: summary and recommendations

1 Minimizing the degree and duration of intraoperative hypotension during aneurysm surgery is probably indicated (Class IIa, Level of Evidence B).

2 There are insufficient data on pharmacological strategies and induced hypertension during temporary vessel occlusion to make specific recommendations, but there are instances where their use may be considered reasonable (Class IIb, Level of Evidence C).

3 Induced hypothermia during aneurysm surgery may be a reasonable option in some cases but is not routinely recommended (Class III, Level of Evidence B).

Section 9

Management of cerebral vasospasm: summary and recommendations

1 Oral nimodipine is indicated to reduce poor outcome related to aneurysmal subarachnoid hemorrhage (Class I, Level of Evidence A). The value of other calcium antagonists, whether administered orally or intravenously, remains uncertain.

2 Treatment of cerebral vasospasm begins with early management of the ruptured aneurysm, and in most cases maintaining normal circulating blood volume and avoiding hypovolemia is probably indicated (Class IIa, Level of Evidence B).

3 One reasonable approach to symptomatic cerebral vasospasm is volume expansion, induction of hypertension, and hemodilution [Triple-H therapy] (Class IIa, Level of Evidence B).

4 Alternatively, cerebral angioplasty and/or selective intra-arterial vasodilator therapy may also be reasonable, either following, together with, or in the place of, Triple-H therapy depending on the clinical scenario (Class IIb, Level of Evidence B).

Section 10

Management of hydrocephalus: summary and recommendations

1 Temporary or permanent CSF diversion is recommended in symptomatic patients with chronic hydrocephalus following SAH (Class I, Level of Evidence B).

2 Ventriculostomy can be beneficial in patients with ventriculomegaly and diminished level of consciousness following acute SAH (Class IIa, Level of Evidence B).

Section 11

Management of seizures: summary and recommendations

1 The administration of prophylactic anticonvulsants may be considered in the immediate posthemorrhagic period (Class IIb, Level of Evidence B).

2 The routine long-term use of anticonvulsants is not recommended (Class III, Level of Evidence B) but may be considered for patients with risk factors such as prior seizure, parenchymal hematoma, infarct, or MCA aneurysms (Class IIb, Level of Evidence B).

Section 12

Management of hyponatremia: summary and recommendations

1 Administration of large volumes of hypotonic fluids and intravascular volume contraction should generally be avoided following SAH (Class I, Level of Evidence B).

2 Monitoring volume status in certain patients with recent SAH using some combination of central venous pressure, pulmonary artery wedge pressure, fluid balance, and body weight is reasonable, as is treatment of volume contraction with isotonic fluids (Class IIa, Level of Evidence B).

Table 6.1 *Continued*

3 The use of fludrocortisone acetate and hypertonic saline is reasonable for correcting hyponatremia (Class IIa, Level of Evidence B).

4 In some instances, it may be reasonable to reduce fluid administration to maintain a euvolemic state (Class IIb, Level of Evidence B).

Rating levels of evidence and recommendations

Quality of evidence

Class I: conditions for which there is evidence for and/or general agreement that the procedure or treatment is useful and effective.

Class II: conditions for which there is conflicting evidence and/or a divergence of opinion about the usefulness/ efficacy of a procedure or treatment.

Class IIa: the weight of evidence or opinion is in favor of the procedure or treatment.

Class IIb: usefulness/efficacy is less well established by evidence or opinion.

Class III: conditions for which there is evidence and/or general agreement that the procedure or treatment is not useful/effective and in some cases may be harmful.

Therapeutic recommendations

Level of Evidence A: data derived from multiple randomized clinical trials.

Level of Evidence B: data derived from a single randomized trial or nonrandomized studies.

Level of Evidence C: consensus opinion of experts.

Diagnostic/prognostic recommendations

Level of Evidence A: data derived from multiple prospective cohort studies employing a reference standard applied by a masked evaluator.

Level of Evidence B: data derived from a single Grade A study or one or more case-control studies or studies employing a reference standard applied by an unmasked evaluator.

Level of Evidence C: consensus opinion of experts.

CSF, cerebrospinal fluid; CTA, CT angiography; ED, emergency department; MCA, middle cerebral artery; MRA, magnetic resonance angiography; SAH, subarachnoid hemorrhage.

resonance imaging (MRI) is less accurate. The sensitivity of detecting SAH from a ruptured aneurysm using CT scans is dependent on the slice thickness, the scanner resolution, and the technician's and interpreting radiologist's expertise, as well as the interval between the hemorrhage and when the CT scan was obtained. For example, the expected sensitivity of 100% when a CT scan is obtained within 12 hours of rupture drops to 93% when the scan interval is extended to 24 hours [10]. In addition, CT scan can also show the presence of conditions that may require emergent treatment, such as intraventricular blood and hydrocephalus, or parenchymal hemorrhage with mass effect. The absence of subarachnoid blood on the CT scan does not rule out SAH, and a lumbar puncture may be indicated when the clinical suspicion is high (see further discussion) (Table 6.1, Section 3).

Diagnosis of IAs

Technological advances have been made in recent years that have improved the detection and characterization of IAs. The three radiological examinations used for this purpose are CT angiography (CTA), MRA, and catheter-based digital subtraction angiog-

raphy (DSA). Although standard head CT scans and brain MRI may detect aneurysms that are large, particularly if they are calcified or thrombosed, these are not optimal. The head CT of the example patient revealed a diffuse hemorrhage with blood in the suprasellar cistern and interhemispheric fissure but did not show an aneurysm (Figure 6.2a). CTA, MRA, and DSA are each excellent modalities with which to study aneurysms (Figure 6.3a–6.3e). Each has advantages and disadvantages, and the decision regarding which test to employ depends upon the specific clinical situation. Often, obtaining more than one of these tests is helpful and complementary.

MRA, which is an MRI with special sequences used to study the vasculature, is the least invasive modality to study aneurysms (Table 6.1, Section 3). It is also the least sensitive, particularly for smaller aneurysms. Reports have documented a sensitivity of 0.69–0.99 and a specificity of 1.00. The sensitivity dropped to as low as 0.38 in one series for aneurysms smaller than 3 mm in diameter [7,11–13]. A disadvantage of MRA is that it takes longer to acquire images (30–90 minutes) as compared with CTA, making it cumbersome and often impractical in critically ill patients. Individuals with pacemakers or

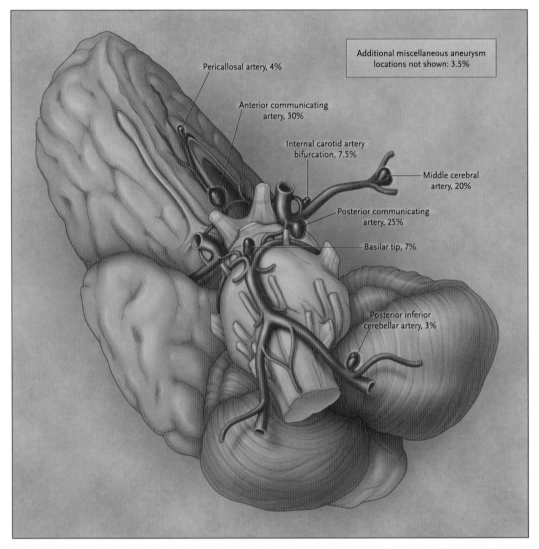

Fig. 6.1 The intracranial vasculature showing the most frequent locations of intracranial aneurysms. Percentages indicate the incidence of intracranial aneurysms. Reprinted with permission, Massachusetts Medical Society. From Brisman JL, *et al*. N Engl J Med. 2006;355:928–939.

other metallic implants or with severe claustrophobia often cannot undergo MRA examination.

CTA is a CT scan obtained after an IV injection of contrast in which thin-section images are reconstructed using a computer software to optimize the imaging of blood vessels (Table 6.1, Section 3). Images are acquired within a few minutes, and in less than a minute, a routine noncontrast head CT scan can be simultaneously obtained. CTA has the advantage of demonstrating the vasculature relative to the bones of the skull base, which is important for surgical planning (Figure 6.3a and 6.3b). Additionally, special commercially available software permits manipulations of the reconstructed images in three dimensions.

Sensitivity and specificity of CTA for the detection of IAs have been reported as 0.77–0.97 and 0.87–1.00, respectively. As with MRA, the sensitivity drops precipitously for smaller lesions with estimated sensitivity rates of 0.40–0.91 for aneurysms smaller than 3 mm [12,14]. In recent years, newer generation CT scanners (16-slice and 64-slice multidetectors) have claimed increased ability to visualize IAs, and recent data demonstrate even higher sensitivity and specificity [15]. The major disadvantages of CTA are the need for IV contrast, which may be harmful in

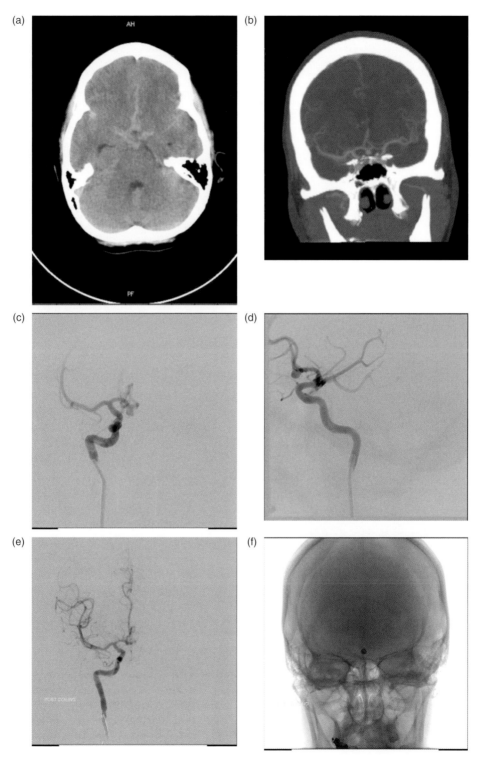

Fig. 6.2 (a) Noncontrast head CT scan shows a diffuse subarachnoid hemorrhage with blood in the interhemispheric fissure and suprasellar cistern. (b) CT angiography, coronal cut, clearly shows a small anterior communicating artery aneurysm. Angiography in the anteroposterior (c) and lateral projection (d) confirms this finding. No residual aneurysm is apparent postcoiling (e). The coil mass is best seen on an unsubtracted anteroposterior skull radiograph (f).

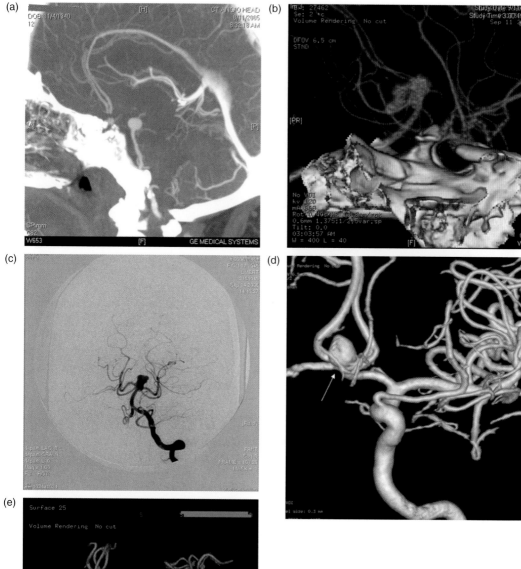

Fig. 6.3 The three major imaging modalities for intracranial aneurysms. Saggital 2D (a) and reformatted oblique view 3D (b) CT angiography shows two different patients with basilar tip aneurysms. The associated bony anatomy is appreciated. The anteroposterior 2D digital subtraction angiography (DSA) (vertebral artery injection) (c) and 3D DSA (carotid injection) (d) show a basilar tip and anterior communicating artery aneurysms, respectively. The 3D magnetic resonance angiography shows a distal middle cerebral artery aneurysm (e).

patients with impaired renal function, an allergic reaction to the dye, and radiation exposure.

The gold-standard test for cerebral aneurysm detection and characterization is catheter-based DSA (Table 6.1, Section 3). The test has the highest sensitivity and specificity provided that the angiographic equipment is capable of performing three-dimensional rotational angiography, a form of catheter-based angiography in which images are sequentially acquired as the fluoroscopic gantry rotates 360 degrees around the patient's head, enabling reformatted images to be manipulated in three dimensions (Figure 6.3d). This is the most expensive of the radiographic tests for aneurysms and also requires physicians trained in techniques of angiography. The procedure requires skilled operators to introduce catheters into the arterial system (generally from the transfemoral route) using radiographic guidance. Catheters are selectively advanced into the carotid and vertebral arteries, contrast is injected, and images are obtained (Figure 6.3c and 6.3d). Increased experience has led to lower complication rates; yet this remains an invasive technique. Minor risks include groin hematoma (6.9–10.7%), arterial puncture site injury (0.05–0.55), allergic dye reaction, contrast-induced renal toxicity (1–2%), and radiation exposure. Major risks include thromboembolic stroke or vascular dissection (less than 1% with experienced operators) [16–18].

Management of ruptured aneurysms

Initial evaluation
Rupture of an IA generally presents with acute onset of severe headache that patients often describe as the "worst headache of their life." This is often accompanied by nausea, emesis, photophobia, and neck stiffness. Syncope and seizures are not infrequently the initial manifestation, and approximately 10% of patients present with coma or die before reaching medical attention. The Hunt and Hess Grading Scale (Table 6.2) is a commonly used scoring system for aneurysmal SAH to describe the neurological condition on admission. In addition to providing a common parlance for healthcare providers, it is a good predictor of outcome (Table 6.1, Section 4). Approximately 40% of patients with SAH will experience a headache of less magnitude 7–21 days prior to the presenting hemorrhage, referred to as a "warning leak" or "sentinel bleed," which represents a small rupture [19]. The example patient was given the admitting diagnosis of a grade I aneurysmal SAH because of her good neurological condition.

People presenting with symptoms suggestive of SAH should first undergo a noncontrast head CT scan, which is the recommended initial procedure of choice (Table 6.1, Section 3). An estimated 50% of patients with SAH are misdiagnosed during the first physician encounter, perhaps reflecting the commonness of headaches as a complaint, a lack of awareness of the presenting signs and symptoms of the disease, and the fact that other diagnoses such as tension and migraine headaches can mimic that of a ruptured aneurysm. If the rupture is significant enough, leading to intracerebral hematoma in addition to subarachnoid blood, the presentation can mimic that of the common nonhemorrhagic stroke (Figure 6.4d). A grading score, the Fisher Score, is commonly used to describe the extent of the blood on an initial noncontrast CT scan. The Fisher Score correlates with the chances of developing delayed vasospasm, one of the most serious consequences of SAH (described in more detail later).

When there is a suspicion for SAH and the CT scan is negative for blood, a lumbar puncture should be obtained (Table 6.1, Section 3). As with the CT scan, timing is critical as a lumbar puncture obtained within the first 6 hours or beyond 3 weeks after rupture may have less sensitivity. Four tubes of cerebrospinal fluid (CSF) should be collected and properly numbered based on the order in which the fluid was collected, as a progressive decrease in the number of red blood cells can help suggest a traumatic tap as opposed to a true SAH, in which there

Table 6.2 Hunt and Hess Grading Scale for Subarachnoid Hemorrhage

Grade	Clinical description
1	Asymptomatic or minimal headache and slight nuchal rigidity
2	Moderate-to-severe headache, nuchal rigidity, and no neurological deficit other than cranial-nerve palsy
3	Drowsiness, confusion, or mild focal deficit
4	Stupor, moderate-to-severe hemiparesis, and possibly, early decerebrate rigidity and vegetative disturbances
5	Deep coma, decerebrate rigidity, and moribund appearance

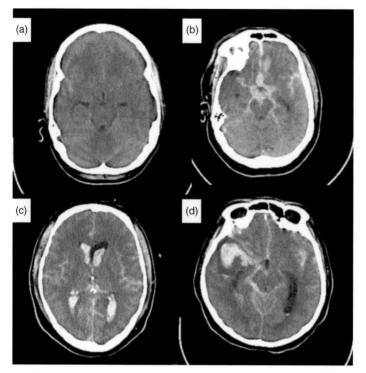

Fig. 6.4 CT scan after aneurysmal rupture almost always shows varying amounts of subarachnoid hemorrhage (a–d), although additional intraventricular (c) or intraparenchymal (d) blood is not infrequently seen and often suggests the location of the aneurysm.

is generally no significant difference in the number of red blood cells between the first and fourth tubes. Xanthochromia of the CSF supernatant is the most reliable way to differentiate an aneurysmal SAH from a traumatic lumbar puncture. This yellowish discoloration of the CSF represents bilirubin from hemoglobin breakdown and would not be expected to be present if the blood were fresh (less than 6 hours) as is the case in a traumatic spinal tap. Guidelines for interpreting CSF results in this setting have been published [20]. If the CT scan shows no blood and the CSF is normal, the likelihood of SAH is very low.

Acute management

The initial assessment of the patient with SAH should focus on maintaining airway, breathing, and circulation. Rapid sequence intubation is recommended for those requiring ventilator support. Aneurysmal SAH is an emergency, and any patient with this diagnosis, once cardiovascular and respira-

tory stability is achieved, should be referred to a facility with familiarity in treating this disease, as patients cared for in high-volume centers have better outcomes (Table 6.1, Section 7) [21]. Dedicated neurological intensive care units and neurointensivists have also been associated with improved outcome in SAH patients. The accepting institution should have surgeons capable of performing aneurysm clipping and coiling (described later). Upon admission to an intensive care unit, blood pressure should be kept in the normal range, and this is often achieved with the assistance of an arterial line and an IV agent such as labetalol or nicardipine (Table 6.1, Section 5). Anticonvulsants are given, particularly if there is an intracerebral hematoma in addition to SAH or if craniotomy is planned (Table 6.1, Section 11). The duration of anticonvulsant usage, the choice of anticonvulsant agent, and whether to administer such medication at all for patients with SAH without intracerebral hematoma are currently being re-evaluated [22].

The most important issue on admission is the identification of the ruptured aneurysm and treatment of the lesion to prevent a potentially disastrous rehemorrhage. Based on the prospective Cooperative Aneurysm Study, rebleeding from an unrepaired aneurysm is estimated at 4% within 24 hours of the initial bleed followed by approximately 1–2% per day for the first 4 weeks (Table 6.1, Section 2) [23]. Bed rest and antifibrinolytic therapy are no longer considered adequate therapy to prevent rebleeding (Table 6.1, Section 5). Securing the aneurysm is achieved by either endovascular coiling or microsurgical clipping (described later), which should be attempted within 72 hours of the hemorrhage in almost all patients (Table 6.1, Section 6). Hunt and Hess Grade 5 patients or those at the extremes of age (>85) are a complex subset of patients for whom no specific guidelines are available, and treatment must therefore be individualized.

Many physicians obtain an emergent CTA on admission, which has a very high degree of sensitivity in disclosing the site and morphology of the aneurysm. The example patient had a CTA performed the evening of admission that clearly showed an anterior communicating artery aneurysm (Figure 6.2b). Regardless of the results of this test, catheter-based cerebral angiography is usually indicated to determine the source of the SAH, which will be a ruptured cerebral aneurysm in most (80–85%) cases. Angiography in this patient confirmed the findings of CTA and showed a small anterior communicating artery aneurysm that was presumed to have ruptured (Figure 6.2c and 6.2d). Four-vessel angiography (both vertebral arteries and both carotid arteries) is recommended as multiple aneurysms are present in up to 15% of patients [24], and this provides a baseline of the intracranial blood vessels that can aid in diagnosing vasospasm (discussed later) should it develop. Some centers use CTA alone if clipping is the chosen treatment modality, but there is insufficient data to support this strategy [16]. If four-vessel angiography does not reveal a lesion, angiography of the external carotid arteries bilaterally should be performed to rule out a dural arteriovenous fistula, a rare but important cause of SAH (Figure 6.5a–6.5d). If properly performed angiography is negative (10–20% of SAH), the study is repeated in 1 week, and MRI with and without gadolinium of the brain and cervical spine is obtained

to rule out small tumor, thrombosed aneurysm, which may not appear with angiography, or other more rare entities.

"Benign perimesencephalic nonaneurysmal SAH" is a recognized condition in which the same clinical signs and symptoms of aneurysmal SAH are present and the CT scan shows a very small amount of blood strictly localized anterior to the brain stem, usually in the region of the midbrain [25]. Angiography is negative, and this is almost always a benign condition. Because of the increasing resolution of CTA, some have recommended this as the sole test when the CT appearance is classic for perimesencephalic SAH [26]. Adequate data are not available to support CTA as the sole imaging modality, and DSA is indicated. A second DSA, however, is not necessary.

Repair of cerebral aneurysms: microsurgical clipping and endovascular coiling

There are two main treatment options to secure a ruptured aneurysm: endovascular coiling and microsurgical clipping. In the former, a neurosurgeon, neurologist, or neuroradiologist with special training performs a cerebral angiogram followed by the placement of very small microcatheters into the aneurysm through which metallic coils of varying sizes and shapes are deployed (Figure 6.6). The coils are thrombogenic and cause an acute occlusion of the aneurysm while preserving flow in the surrounding normal vessels. The procedure is generally performed under general anesthesia, although some physicians prefer to keep the patients awake to monitor their neurological status. The use of IV heparinization during the procedure is variably used and continued for 12–36 hours. Microsurgical clipping is performed by neurosurgeons under general anesthesia. After a craniotomy is performed, permanent clips made from MRI-compatible alloys with a spring-loaded mechanism are ideally placed across the neck of the aneurysm, excluding it from the circulation (Figure 6.7). Although some aneurysm morphologies and locations are better suited to one technique or the other, many aneurysms can be successfully secured with either method, and the decision to use one or the other is made based on other patient-, institutional-, and operator-specific factors. In general, the decision should be made by a team with expertise in both treatment modalities (Table 6.1, Section 6).

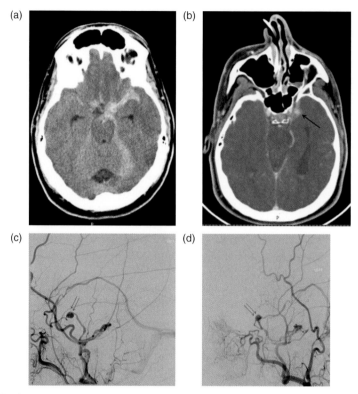

Fig. 6.5 Four-vessel angiography was negative in this 50-year-old man who presented with a diffuse subarachnoid hemorrhage (a) and a CT angiography suggestive of a ruptured aneurysm (b, arrow). Angiography of the external carotid arteries in the anteroposterior (c) and lateral projection (d) clearly shows a dural-based arteriovenous fistula with an associated venous aneurysm (double arrows).

Comparing outcomes for clipping and coiling

Although clipping techniques have been used and improved upon for over 50 years, the first description of coil placement within aneurysms was in 1991, followed by the Food and Drug Administration approval in 1995. Whereas coiling was initially used as a last resort for aneurysms that could not be clipped in the mid-1990s, the techniques and coils have improved dramatically such that it is now considered a safe and less invasive alternative to clipping. Coiling is now first-line therapy in many centers.

The exact risks of coiling are somewhat difficult to quantify due to technical advances in recent years leading to increased safety, and the inability to divorce the consequences of a coiling procedure from the consequences of the SAH. Minor risks associated with coiling are similar to that of diagnostic angiography. More serious risks include arterial dissection, a thromboembolic event with stroke, and aneurysm rupture (1.0–2.7%) [27]. With increased experience, operators are now learning how to manage these complications to keep adverse outcomes acceptably low [28,29]. Approximately 5–14.5% of aneurysms at one large volume center could not be coiled because of unusual vascular tortuosity or failure of coils to properly sit within the aneurysm, usually due to a broad base of the aneurysm in relation to the dome [30]. Advanced techniques in which balloons are inflated or stents are deployed across the neck of the aneurysm, as well as newer complex-shaped coils, permit the treatment of many wide-neck lesions previously felt not to be candidates for this technique (Figure 6.8a–6.8c). Risks of surgery include those associated with any craniotomy, such as bleeding and infection, as well as the risks associated with the direct attack of an aneurysm requiring brain retraction, vessel manipulation, aneurysm dissection, and clipping.

One disadvantage of coiling is that complete occlusion is not always guaranteed. Complete or

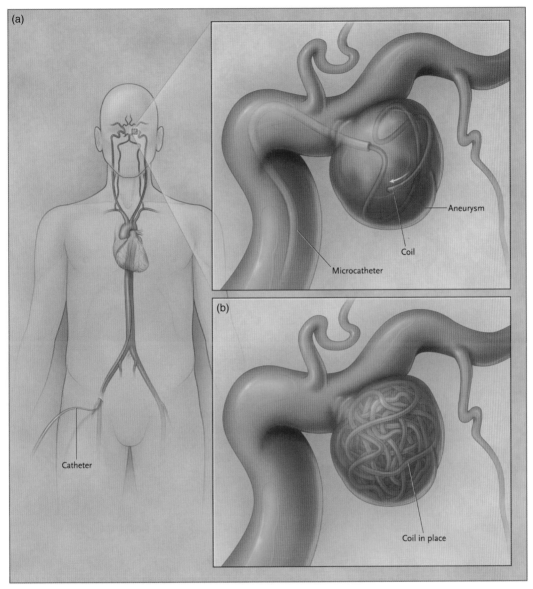

Fig. 6.6 Endovascular occlusion of an aneurysm of the posterior communicating artery with Guglielmi detachable coils. (a) The microcatheter is inserted into the femoral artery and navigated through the aorta, the left carotid artery, and then into the aneurysm where coils are deployed. (b) At the end of the coiling, the aneurysm no longer fills with blood. Reprinted with permission, Massachusetts Medical Society. From Brisman JL, *et al.* N Engl J Med. 2006;355:928–939.

near complete occlusions in 85–90% can be expected, with lower rates of success with larger aneurysms [27]. Another disadvantage to coiling is that over time, the coil mass can compact in response to blood flow and result in aneurysm recanalization, which places such patients at risk for recurrent hemorrhage. Recurrence secondary to aneurysm recanali-

zation, estimated at 20.9–33.6%, is more common in larger aneurysms [31]. Rehemorrhage after coiling was noted in 0.8% with a mean follow-up of 31.32 $\pm$ 24.96 months [31]. Vigilant angiographic follow-up is required after coiling as repeat coiling can be safely performed. Newer coils embedded with biological agents to promote neointima formation and

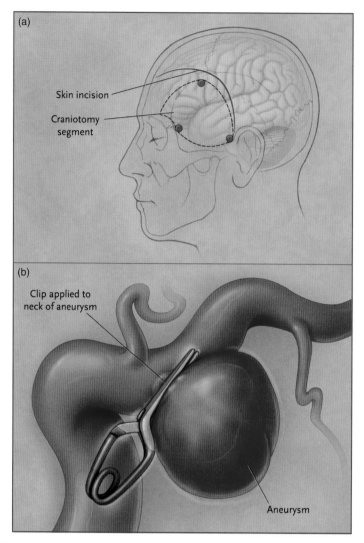

Fig. 6.7 Microsurgical clipping of an aneurysm of the posterior communicating artery. (a) The skin incision (unbroken curved line) and craniotomy (dashed lines) needed to approach the aneurysm are depicted. (b) The application of the clip blades to the neck of the aneurysm to achieve occlusion. Reprinted with permission, Massachusetts Medical Society. From Brisman JL, *et al.* N Engl J Med. 2006;355:928–939.

prevent recurrence are under clinical investigation. Residual aneurysm and aneurysm recurrence is also possible with clipping but significantly less so, making this a more definitive and durable treatment [32].

The International Subarachnoid Aneurysm Trial (ISAT) was a prospective multicenter study conducted primarily in Europe, which compared outcomes at 1 year for 2143 SAH patients randomized to microsurgical clipping versus endovascular coiling. The trial was stopped after a planned interim analysis at 1 year found a 23.7% risk of dependency or death in the endovascular cohort compared with a 30.6% risk (relative risk of 22.6% and absolute risk of 6.9% difference) in the surgical arm [33]. It should be noted that to be randomized in the study, an aneurysm had to be deemed equally treatable by either technique, a condition met by only 2143 out of 9559 patients screened, or 22.4% of all SAH evaluated at participating centers. Second, the great

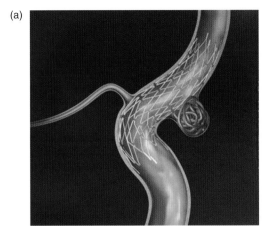

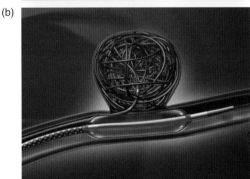

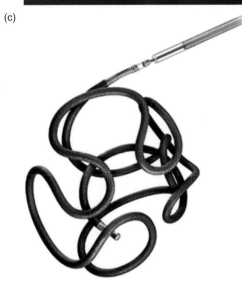

Fig. 6.8 Advanced techniques for endovascular occlusion of aneurysms using stent-assistance (a), balloon-assistance (b), and three-dimensional coils (c).

majority of the lesions treated were in patients in good clinical grade (>90%), who harbored anterior circulation aneurysms (97.3%) and whose aneurysms were less than 10 mm (almost 95%). The generalization of this study to all aneurysms, or even to all ruptured aneurysms, would not be valid.

A separate publication confirmed these findings at the 1 year follow-up for all randomized patients [34]. A third publication from the ISAT study investigators reanalyzed the data substratified for age and found that the findings were not as robust for patients less than 50 years and may not be valid for patients less than 40 years old, again due to poorer durability and slightly increased rehemorrhage risk of coiling [35]. A proposed algorithm for the treatment of ruptured aneurysms is presented (Figure 6.9).

The example patient's aneurysm was evaluated by an endovascular neurosurgeon who performs both clipping and coiling. It was deemed to be equally treatable using either modality. Based on the ISAT data, the patient was offered coiling as the recommended treatment. If the aneurysm could not be safely coiled, clipping would be recommended. The patient agreed to undergo coiling, which was performed uneventfully with complete occlusion (Figure 6.2e and 6.2f). She was discharged home 10 days later, neurologically intact. Her first follow-up angiogram was performed 6 months later and showed no aneurysm recanalization.

In-hospital care and complications

Although securing the aneurysm by clipping or coiling is performed to prevent rebleeding and its devastating consequences, it does little to offset the immediate and delayed effects of the SAH on the injured brain. Complications from SAH can be divided into *neurological* and *medical* with significant overlap.

Neurological complications
Hydrocephalus
Hydrocephalus occurs in about 15–20% of patients who have an aneurysmal SAH [7], and may occur in an acute or delayed fashion. Symptomatic acute hydrocephalus (generally obstructive hyrocephalus) is usually treated with a ventriculostomy to relieve

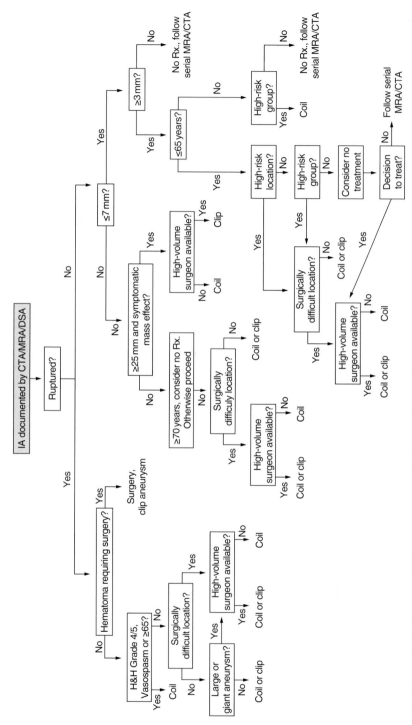

Fig. 6.9 Algorithm for the treatment of intracranial aneurysms (IAs). For simplicity, the following categories are defined based on the International Study of Unruptured Intracranial Aneurysms and the International Subarachnoid Aneurysm Trial studies and the available literature: high-risk group = patients who have suffered subarachnoid hemorrhage (SAH) from another IA, patients who are very anxious about having an untreated IA, and patients who have a family history of SAH from an IA, or patients with adult polycystic kidney disease; high-risk location = posterior communicating artery aneurysm or aneurysms located on the vertebrobasilar system (i.e., posterior inferior cerebellar artery, basilar tip); surgically difficult location = aneurysms located on the vertebrobasilar system, paraclinoid aneurysms (i.e., ophthalmic, superior hypophyseal), or large (>12 mm)/giant (>25 mm) aneurysms. CTA, CT angiography; DSA, digital subtraction angiography; MRA, magnetic resonance angiography.

the increased intracranial pressure and to permit intracranial pressure measurements during the acute period (Table 6.1, Section 10). Asymptomatic acute hydrocephalus is usually followed conservatively as it will ultimately resolve spontaneously in many patients. Patients who are initially asymptomatic from hydrocephalus may also begin to show signs of increased intracranial pressure [3]; a CT scan should be obtained for all SAH patients who experience a neurological decline. The example patient had neither radiographic nor symptomatic hydrocephalus and did not require ventriculostomy placement. Delayed hydrocephalus (generally communicating hydrocephalus) can occur at any time in the first 1–4 weeks after SAH; it may spontaneously resolve or require ventriculoperitoneal shunt placement (Table 6.1, Section 10).

Vasospasm

Cerebral vasospasm, a diffuse or focal narrowing of the cerebral arteries occurring between day 3 and day 14 following SAH, is responsible for the majority of morbidity and mortality in patients surviving the initial bleed [36]. As many as 70% of patients will have angiographic vasospasm on day 7 after a hemorrhage (the peak incidence for vasospasm), but only 20–30% of patients develop symptomatic cerebral ischemia (temporary or permanent) from the arterial narrowing that decreases blood flow to the brain [36]. The etiology of vasospasm is unknown.

Patients with symptomatic vasospasm often have signs including decreased level of arousal, confusion, or focal neurological deficit, such as aphasia and/or hemiparesis. There is no good preventive therapy for vasospasm, although many agents have been tried. Avoiding hypovolemia is recommended as it may permit vasospasm treatment if it develops (see further discussion). The detection of vasospasm is crucial, as treatment is available. The use of the calcium-channel blocking agent nimodipine improved the outcome related to vasospasm in several prospective randomized trials [37]. Oral nimodipine (60 mg every 4 hours for 21 days) is administered beginning immediately after SAH and is continued for 21 days. Transcranial Doppler (TCD) ultrasonography is a very sensitive test to detect vasospasm and is generally performed on a daily basis or every other day after SAH during the acute period. Increasing velocities by TCD suggest

onset of vasospasm and will direct the management based on the clinical scenario [24]. DSA is generally employed to confirm the diagnosis and may enable endovascular therapy (see further discussion). Once vasospasm has been diagnosed, medical treatment consists of the "triple H" therapy: *h*ypertension, *h*ypervolemia, and *h*emodilution (Table 6.1, Section 9). Those failing medical treatment with persistent neurological deficit (given a trial of 1–2 hours of aggressive hypertensive therapy) are urgently taken for angiography and angioplasty of the stenotic vessels (Table 6.1, Section 9) [36]. On post-bleed day 5, the example patient developed increasing TCD velocities in the left middle cerebral artery consistent with mild-moderate vasospasm. There was no clinical deterioration, however, and the patient's blood pressure was permitted to rise up to 200 mm Hg systolic. She was hydrated, and a central venous line was placed with a central venous pressure goal of 8–12 mm Hg. Her TCD velocities were unchanged until day 9 after the SAH, at which point the velocities normalized within the left middle cerebral artery and the triple "H" therapy was weaned.

Medical complications

Numerous medical complications afflict patients in the first 2 weeks following aneurysmal SAH [24]. Some, such as hyponatremia, seizures, neurogenic pulmonary edema, or cardiogenic dysfunction, are caused by the intracranial insult, whereas others (deep vein thrombosis, pulmonary embolism, pneumonia, malnutrition) are often the result of a generalized debilitated state and prolonged intensive care unit stay. Hyponatremia is almost always a result of cerebral salt wasting and not SIADH (syndrome of inappropriate antidiuretic hormone secretion), although a mixed picture is possible. Fluid restriction should not be attempted, particularly in the face of vasospasm where it might lead to decreased circulating volume and stroke (Table 6.1, Section 12).

Once the aneurysm is secured, blood pressure can be moderately elevated to improve cerebral perfusion. The utility of decadron is unsupported, although it seems to alleviate headaches in some patients and is commonly used for a short period if the patient undergoes craniotomy. Hyperglycemia and hyperthermia should be corrected as they have a negative impact on outcome [38]. Deep vein thrombosis prophylaxis can be achieved with sequential compression devices and subcutaneous heparin can be safely administered in most cases as soon as the aneurysm is secured.

Cardiac abnormalities after SAH are common and include eclectrocardiographic changes, cardiac enzyme elevations, and left ventricular dysfunction with or without pulmonary edema [39–41]. These cardiac markers do not necessarily portend myocardial damage and should not delay early operative intervention to treat the aneurysm [42]. Findings of markedly decreased ejection fraction with wall motion abnormalities that do not match the electro-cardiographic vascular distribution of ischemia help make the diagnosis [39,40].

Management of unruptured aneurysms

Aneurysms that are unruptured, particularly those that are asymptomatic, are managed differently than those that present with SAH. A very small subgroup of patients with unruptured aneurysms present with syndromes related to brain or cranial nerve compression by local mass effect, such as acute third nerve palsy associated with a posterior communicating artery aneurysm. Such aneurysms are often treated promptly because of the increased risk of rupture in this group [7]. For the remainder of patients with unruptured aneurysms, recent data suggest that previous estimates of yearly risk of rupture of 1–2% per year were incorrect. The International Study of Unruptured Intracranial Aneurysms (ISUIA) was a retrospective analysis of 2,621 patients with unruptured aneurysms from 53 centers who were followed without intervention. For small (<10 mm) aneurysms of the anterior cerebral circulation (intracranial carotid artery, anterior communicating artery, and middle cerebral artery), the rate of rupture was 0.05% per year [43]. Aneurysms at other locations such as the posterior communicating artery and basilar tip as well as aneurysms in patients that had additional aneurysms that had previously ruptured had considerably higher rupture rates, ranging from 0.26% to 0.69% annually. A prospective cohort of patients from this same study group showed that aneurysms less than 7 mm had a 5-year cumulative risk of 0% [44]. Recent prospective single-center studies have demonstrated signifi-

cantly higher risks of rupture for unruptured aneurysms [45].

Risk of rupture must be balanced against risks of treatment, which have not been well characterized, are multifactorial, and seem to be operator- and institution-specific. Although the risks associated with unruptured aneurysm clipping had been recorded as 4.0–10.9% morbidity and 1.0–3.0% mortality in experienced centers [46,47], ISUIA found a 15.7% surgical risk for clipping an unruptured aneurysm among a broader cohort of surgeons with variable experience [43].

Johnston *et al.* recently reviewed the morbidity and outcomes associated with clipping versus coiling of unruptured aneurysms using hospital discharge data from a variety of sources [48–50]. Coiling resulted in better outcomes, lower mortality, and shorter length of stay, and was less expensive. This advantage of coiling for unruptured aneurysms may be offset by the higher recurrence rate compared with clipping, with an associated increased risk of bleeding. The risk of partial treatment or recurrence is lower with clipping (incomplete occlusion, 5.2%, recurrence, 1.5%) [32], rendering this treatment option somewhat more definitive and durable. Additionally, coiled aneurysms generally require repeat angiography at time intervals to evaluate for recurrence, which may contribute to overall morbidity, hospitalization time, and cost. In 2000, the Stroke Council of the AHA published guidelines for the management of unruptured IAs [51]. Two factors, namely the continued evolution of endovascular technology and a re-evaluation of the ISUIA by the study authors resulting in a restratification of natural history risk, suggested that some modification of these guidelines was necessary. One algorithm for managing unruptured aneurysms based on generally accepted practice is offered here (Figure 6.9).

Management of brain AVMs

AVMs are congenital abnormalities of the brain in which the capillary bed is developmentally lacking, with resultant arteriovenous shunting. In addition to abnormally dilated and tortuous arteries that feed the malformation, and hypertrophied draining veins carrying arteriolar blood under high pressure, there is often a tangle of vessels within the brain itself that is referred to as the AVM nidus. Over time, AVM veins receiving arterial pressure blood develop fibromuscular thickening with deficiency of the elastic lamina, making them susceptible to rupture. Although brain AVMs are estimated to have a population prevalence of 0.1%, only a small fraction (1–2%) of those people will develop symptoms during their lifetime [52]. Most cases are sporadic, although some familial conditions such as Osler–Weber–Rendu are associated with brain AVMs.

Brain AVMs most often present with headaches, seizures, or hemorrhage, with hemorrhage being the most frequent (30–82%) [53]. As mentioned, the great majority of AVMs are asymptomatic and detected incidentally when a CT scan or MRI of the brain is performed for unrelated reasons (Figure 6.10a and 6.10b). Although CTA and MRA are good noninvasive tests to demonstrate the vascular nature of the lesion [52], DSA is the gold-standard test for defining the lesion and plan treatment (Figure 6.10c).

Both sexes are affected equally, and presentation is usually before age 40 [51]. The hemorrhage is typically intraparenchymal, although SAH is often seen, particularly if the bleeding site is from part of the AVM adjacent to a sulcus or an associated aneurysm, which is present in about 10% of AVMs. Hemorrhage from a brain AVM is associated with a 10–15% mortality and 30–50% permanent neurological morbidity [52]. AVMs that have bled are generally treated, as the estimated rehemorrhage risk is approximately 6% per year for the first year, with risk returning to 2–4% thereafter [54]. AVMs that have not bled pose a more difficult management dilemma, as the true natural history risk of hemorrhage is not well defined. Hemorrhage risks of 2–4% per year have been historically accepted, but more recent data suggest that it may be possible to risk-stratify AVMs based on numerous factors including drainage into deep venous sinuses, deep location, and associated aneurysms, with certain AVMs demonstrating bleeding risk at approximately 1% per year [55]. Because of the uncertainty regarding which patients with unruptured AVMs should undergo treatment, a current ongoing multicenter randomized prospective trial is studying this question. A Randomized Trial of Unruptured Brain Arteriovenous Malformations (ARUBA) is prospectively randomizing patients with brain AVMs that

(a)
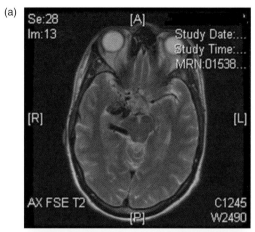

(b)
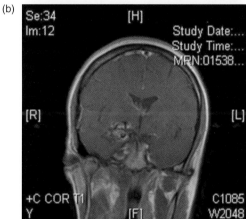

(c)
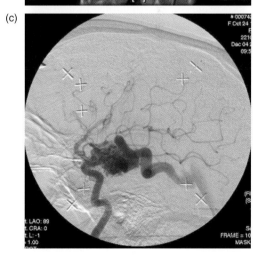

Fig. 6.10 A right medial temporal arteriovenous malformation is seen on this T2-weighted axial (a) and coronal (b). Radiosurgery was performed using this lateral projection right internal carotid angiogram (c). The "X" marks represent the radiosurgical head holder placed on the patient's head prior to the angiogram and needed for radiosurgical planning.

have not hemorrhaged either to treatment or to conservative management [56].

The treatment of brain AVMs requires complete angiographic obliteration of the nidus, as partial therapy has not been shown to decrease future bleeding risk and may increase it. Treatment options for AVMs are surgical excision, radiosurgery, and endovascular embolization; often, a combination of treatment modalities incorporating more than one procedure is needed. Surgical excision is the most curative approach and is recommended if it can be accomplished with acceptable risk. A grading system based on AVM size, location, and venous drainage pattern is generally predictive of surgical outcome [57]. This grading scale, suggests that small (<3 cm) AVMs that drain superficially in noneloquent cortex are associated with the lowest surgical risks, whereas large lesions with central drainage in eloquent cortex have higher risk and may be considered inoperable. Complications, including minor and major, and transient and permanent, have been recorded as 3.9–14% [52,58], depending upon the nature of the lesion and the experience of the treatment team. Endovascular embolization is a rapidly evolving technology that, although not curative, may reduce the arterial flow and the size of the AVM, thereby enabling surgery or radiosurgery. Stereotactic radiosurgery utilizes computer-generated algorithms to precisely apply highly conformal focused radiation to the AVM in a single fraction, minimizing radiation exposure to adjacent brain structures. Obliteration after radiosurgery takes an average of 18 months to 3 years, and protection against hemorrhage is not afforded during this period. For lesions less than 3 cm (a commonly used cutoff for radiosurgery of AVMs), cures of approximately 80% can be expected [59,60]. Guidelines for the management of intracranial AVMs were published in 2001 [61]. It is anticipated that increased experience with radiosurgery and newer embolic agents as well as the results of the ARUBA trial may necessitate the modification of these guidelines.

Gaps in current knowledge

Several areas of uncertainty exist regarding the management of SAH. In particular, to what extent and how quickly endovascular approaches such as coiling will replace clipping as the primary and perhaps favored therapy for IAs are questions that may take some time to answer. It is hoped that longer-term follow-up on coiled aneurysms will disclose whether or not the slightly increased risk of aneurysm compaction, recanalization, and hemorrhage associated with coiling will be outweighed by the increased risks of clipping, which offers a more definitive and durable therapy. What is the true natural history risk of an unruptured asymptomatic aneurysm and at what point should intervention be offered? Despite continued research both clinically and in the laboratory, the cause and optimal treatment of vasospasm are still not known.

Future directions

Continued growth of the endovascular industry is likely to bring new technologies, such as newer stents and coils that reduce the incidence of recurrence after coiling. The safety and durability of both endovascular techniques and microsurgery will continue to be evaluated by further analysis of ongoing trials such as the ISAT and ISUIA as well as new trials. Continued and rapid improvements in CTA and MRA may make catheter-based DSA less critical in the evaluation and treatment of SAH and IAs. Lastly, as more aneurysms are treated conservatively based on the ISUIA data, there will be an opportunity to prospectively follow these untreated aneurysms to gain a better understanding of the true rupture risk and factors that may affect rupture.

References available online at www.wiley.com/go/ strokeguidelines.

Prevention of Recurrent Ischemic Stroke

Jose G. Romano and Ralph L. Sacco

EXAMPLE CASE

A 72-year-old woman woke up with speech difficulties and right-sided weakness. She had a history of hypertension. Her medications included aspirin and an angiotensin-converting enzyme inhibitor (ACE-I). She had given up tobacco 3 years previously and did not exercise. On examination, her body mass index (BMI) was 31 kg/m^2, her blood pressure (BP) was 170/100 mm Hg, and her pulse was regular, and no neck bruits or precordial murmurs were noted. There was dysarthria and a right hemiparesis with 4/5 arm and leg strength. Imaging revealed a small 9-mm left pontine infarct.

Echocardiogram showed left ventricular hypertrophy, no segmental wall motion abnormality or valvular disease, and normal ejection fraction. Neck and brain magnetic resonance angiography (MRA) showed normal vertebral and basilar arteries and irregular plaques at both carotid bifurcations causing 30% stenoses. Cholesterol was 253 mg/dL, triglycerides was 294 mg/dL, high-density lipoprotein cholesterol (HDL-C) was 30 mg/dL, and low-density lipoprotein cholesterol (LDL-C) was 160 mg/dL. Fasting glucose was 240 mg/dL, and hemoglobin A1C (HbA1C) was 9%.

MAJOR POINTS

- One in four strokes is a recurrent event; recurrent stroke is preventable.
- Hypertension is a major, treatable risk factor for recurrent stroke.
- Treatment of dyslipidemia with statins is effective in preventing recurrent stroke.
- Although there is no definite evidence that tight glycemic control prevents recurrent stroke, antidiabetic medication reduces the risk of other adverse outcomes.
- Lifestyle modification such as tobacco cessation, weight loss, exercise, and alcohol in moderation should be encouraged.
- Carotid endarterectomy should be recommended in significant symptomatic carotid stenosis.
- Antiplatelet therapy is indicated in non-cardioembolic stroke.
- Anticoagulants reduce the risk of recurrent cardioembolic stroke.

Introduction

Of the estimated 780,000 strokes occurring in the United States each year, about 180,000 are recurrent events [1]. In addition, about 15–26% of all strokes are preceded by a transient ischemic attack (TIA) [2]. The risk of stroke after TIA or minor ischemic stroke is 8.4% [3] to 10% at 3 months [4]. Although,

A Primer on Stroke Prevention Treatment: An Overview Based on AHA/ASA Guidelines, 1st Edition. Edited by L Goldstein.
© 2009 American Heart Association, ISBN: 9781405186513

traditionally, a distinction has been made between TIA and stroke, magnetic resonance imaging (MRI) data have revealed that many individuals with clinically diagnosed TIA, particularly after prolonged events, have imaging evidence of cerebral infarction [5]. Thus, the approach to secondary prevention after ischemic stroke or TIA is similar. More importantly, with the advent of MRI, silent cerebral infarcts are increasingly detected in asymptomatic individuals; a recent population study described silent cerebral infarcts in 17.7% of asymptomatic adults [6]. Therefore, secondary stroke prevention is critical to prevent clinical and subclinical stroke recurrence and the high mortality and morbidity associated with cerebrovascular diseases.

This chapter will summarize the American Heart Association/American Stroke Association (AHA/ASA) secondary stroke prevention guidelines [7,8] and review the evidence that supports them. The classification of the recommendations and the level of supportive evidence are defined in Table 7.1, and the specific AHA/ASA recommendations are given after each section. Hemorrhagic stroke will not be addressed, as it is reviewed in other chapters. Similarly, certain topics in secondary stroke prevention such as stroke related to patent foramen ovale, sickle-cell disease, cerebral vein and sinus thrombosis, and hypercoagulable states, and stroke in pregnancy and associated with hormonal therapy are also addressed elsewhere in this book.

Table 7.1 American Stroke Association (ASA) classification of recommendations and levels of evidence

---

AHA/ASA Classification of Recommendations

I   Evidence for or general agreement that treatment or procedure is useful and effective.

II Conflicting evidence or divergence of opinion about usefulness or effectiveness of treatment or procedure.

IIa Weight of evidence or opinion for treatment or procedure.

IIb Usefulness and effectiveness less well established.

III Evidence or general agreement that treatment or procedure is not useful or effective and may be harmful.

AHA/ASA Level of Evidence

A   Based on multiple randomized clinical trials.

B   Based on single randomized trial or nonrandomized studies.

C   Based on expert opinion or case studies.

AHA, American Heart Association.

We will first discuss the modifiable risk factors for the prevention of stroke recurrence. Subsequently, the management of large-vessel disease and the use of antithrombotic agents will be addressed.

Hypertension

Hypertension is the most important modifiable risk factor for stroke. Although a linear relationship has been described between systolic and diastolic BP and the risk of stroke [9,10], most of these data come from individuals without stroke. Only few randomized studies have evaluated BP control in secondary stroke prevention. A meta-analysis of seven randomized controlled studies studying individuals with prior stroke or TIA suggested that BP reduction resulted in a reduction in stroke (odds ratio [OR] 0.76, 95% confidence interval [CI] 0.63, 0.92) and myocardial infarction (MI) (OR 0.79, 95% CI 0.63, 0.98) [11].

The target BP to optimally decrease stroke recurrence is uncertain. A progressive reduction in BP was correlated with better outcomes in the Perindopril Protection against Recurrent Stroke Study (PROGRESS); in this study of patients with stroke or TIA in which the main outcome was stroke recurrence, a 9/4 mm Hg reduction in BP resulted in a 24% relative risk reduction in ischemic stroke (95% CI 9%, 37%) and a 50% hemorrhagic risk reduction (95% CI 26%, 67%), whereas a greater decrease of 12/5 mm Hg improved outcomes to a relative risk reduction of 36% (95% CI 19%, 49%) for ischemic stroke and 76% (95% CI 55%, 87%) for hemorrhagic stroke [12]. Most secondary prevention studies, however, have achieved only modest BP reductions (10/5 mm Hg on average), with few reaching prespecified BP targets [11]. Therefore, a significant reduction in BP to the normal range of <120/80, as defined by the Joint National Committee on Prevention, Detection, Evaluation and Treatment of High Blood Pressure (JNC 7) [13], has not been adequately studied. Ongoing trials such as the Secondary Prevention of Small Subcortical Strokes (SPS3) Study will address this issue [14]. Nonetheless, reduction of BP in normotensive subjects in the Heart Outcomes Prevention Evaluation (HOPE) and PROGRESS trials [12,15] has suggested that the concept of hypertension needs to be redefined and that individuals who have had a stroke or TIA without a clear diagnosis of hypertension should be placed on antihypertensive medication.

Because of a general lack of direct comparative data, there is no preferred antihypertensive medication for secondary stroke prevention, but there are data supporting ACE-Is. In the HOPE study, individuals with vascular disease treated with ramipril had a relative risk reduction of 32% ($P < 0.001$) in stroke (although this was not the primary outcome) with a very small reduction of BP of 3/1 mm Hg [15], although this may be an underestimation of the true BP reduction because of the manner in which BP was measured [16]. In PROGRESS, perindopril plus indapamide resulted in significant reduction in stroke [12]. This led some to invoke non-BP reduction effects of ACE-I such as vascular protection as the mechanism of stroke prevention [17]. Other agents have also been evaluated in stroke prevention, such as the angiotensin receptor blocker (ARB) agents; these showed benefit over a calcium channel blocker in secondary stroke prevention [18]. Recent studies have not been encouraging in secondary stroke prevention. The Ongoing Telmisartan Alone and in Combination with Ramipril Global Endpoint Trial showed noninferiority of the ARB telmisartan compared with the ACE-I ramipril, but the combination of telmisartan and ramipril over ramipril alone showed no advantage in preventing cardiovascular events or stroke in patients with vascular disease or diabetes [19]. The Prevention Regimen for Effectively avoiding Secondary Strokes (PRoFESS) study did not find benefit of the ARB telmisartan versus placebo in secondary stroke prevention [20]. Diuretics have also been studied in stroke prevention: they are superior to placebo in secondary stroke prevention [21], similar to ACE-I in primary prevention [22], and the combination of an ACE-I and a diuretic is superior to an ACE-I alone [12]. Beta-blocker receptor agents have not shown efficacy in secondary stroke prevention [23,24]. At this point, the available evidence suggests that effective BP reduction rather than a particular agent are required for secondary stroke prevention; ACE-I plus a diuretic is one appropriate first option.

It is unclear whether similar benefits of BP reduction occur for all stroke subtypes. A greater benefit for hemorrhagic stroke compared with ischemic stroke was found at similar BP reductions in the PROGRESS trial [12]. Some might be concerned that lowering BP excessively could result in impaired cerebral perfusion in certain ischemic stroke subtypes such as large artery intracranial atherosclerosis. However, the Warfarin–Aspirin Symptomatic Intracranial Disease (WASID) study did not find any increase in recurrent stroke in the territory of the stenotic intracranial artery in individuals with BPs <140/90 mm Hg, including individuals with >70% stenosis [25]. A similar concern exists for individuals with cerebral small-vessel disease, particularly as it pertains to periventricular ischemia and cognitive outcomes; this premise is being studied in the SPS3 study, in which intensive versus usual BP control is being compared [14].

Summary of recommendations

1 Antihypertensive treatment is recommended for the prevention of recurrent stroke and other vascular events in persons who have had an ischemic stroke or TIA and are beyond the hyperacute period (Class I, Level of Evidence A).

2 Absolute BP target level and reduction is uncertain and should be individualized, but benefit has been associated with an average reduction of ≈10/5 mm Hg, and normal BP levels have been defined as <120/80 mm Hg by the JNC 7 (Class IIa, Level of Evidence B).

3 As benefit extends to persons with and without a history of hypertension, this recommendation should be considered for all ischemic stroke and TIA patients (Class IIa, Level of Evidence B).

4 Optimal drug regimen remains uncertain; the available data support the use of diuretics and the combination of diuretics and an ACE-I (Class I, Level of Evidence A).

5 Lifestyle modifications have been associated with BP reductions and should be included as part of comprehensive antihypertensive therapy (Class IIb, Level of Evidence C).

6 The choice of specific drugs and targets should be individualized with consideration of specific patient characteristics (e.g., extracranial cerebrovascular occlusive disease, renal impairment, cardiac disease, and diabetes) (Class IIb, Level of Evidence C).

Example Case, cont'd.

Our patient's BP remained elevated during her 5-day hospital stay with systolic BPs in the 150–180 mm Hg range; that she had chronic hypertension was evident by the presence of left ventricular hypertrophy. She was treated with a higher dose of ACE-I and the addition of diuretic. The use of this combination is supported by the findings of the PROGRESS trial [12].

Dyslipidemia

Current recommendations indicate that patients with ischemic stroke or TIA should follow the National Cholesterol Education Program III guidelines that include diet, exercise, and statin therapy to achieve an LDL level of <100 mg/dL for individuals with previous vascular events, and <70 mg/dL for very high-risk individuals, including those with acute coronary syndromes, multiple vascular risk factors, especially diabetes mellitus (DM), and severe and poorly controlled risk factors such as current tobacco use, and individuals with the metabolic syndrome [26]. A recent Guidelines Update [8] recommends consideration of statin therapy in individuals with an ischemic cerebrovascular event even in the absence of coronary disease.

Until recently, most antilipidemic studies enrolled very few patients with preexistent cerebrovascular disease, with the exception of the Heart Protection Study [27] in which 16% of all patients had cerebral ischemic disease. Although there was an overall reduction in stroke recurrence, this difference was only significant for individuals without preexisting cerebrovascular disease. The recently published Stroke Prevention by Aggressive Reduction in Cholesterol Levels (SPARCL) study [28] provides guidance on the role of statins in secondary stroke prevention. In this study, 4,731 patients with no known coronary heart disease (CHD) who had a stroke or TIA in the preceding 1–6 months, and who had LDL-C levels between 100 and 190 mg/dL, were randomized to atorvastatin 80 mg/d or placebo and followed for 5 years. The mean LDL-C for the atorvastatin-treated group was 73 mg/dL and for the placebo-treated group 129 mg/dL during follow-up. The risk of stroke (primary outcome) decreased

from 13.1% to 11.2% (HR 0.84, 95% CI 0.71, 0.99, $P = 0.03$). There was also a reduction in acute coronary events (hazard ratio 0.65, 95% CI 0.50, 0.84, $P = 0.001$). High-dose statins were well tolerated, with only 2.2% experiencing a significant increase in liver enzymes, and there was no significant difference with placebo in the occurrence of myalgias or rhabdomyolysis. The SPARCL study showed that achieving a lower LDL-C level resulted in progressive decrease in stroke and coronary events. Compared with levels >100 mg/dL, achieving a level of <70 mg/dL was associated with a 28% reduction in stroke ($P = 0.0018$) without an increase in hemorrhagic stroke [29]. Similarly, the Treat to New Targets study randomized patients to either atorvastatin 10 mg or atorvastatin 80 mg; individuals on a higher dose (achieving lower LDL-C levels) had a significant reduction in major cardiovascular events (primary outcome) (HR 0.78, $P = 0.0002$) and stroke (HR 0.75, $P = 0.02$) [30].

Statins are helpful for atherosclerotic stroke, based upon the large body of evidence showing their benefit in coronary artery disease (CAD) [31] and by reports of stabilization of carotid plaques [32]. However, not all beneficial effects of statins are explained solely by LDL-C reduction [33], and other mechanisms may be active such as mild BP reduction [34], improvement of vasomotor reactivity [35], and neuroprotection [36,37]. These effects might be mediated by nitric oxide-related vasodilation and anti-inflammatory properties due to cytokine and isoprenoid inhibition [38]. The effect of statins on non-atherosclerotic stroke subtypes has also been explored in the SPARCL trial: in a post hoc analysis, atorvastatin 80 mg/d was found to reduce stroke and cardiovascular events for all ischemic stroke subtypes [39].

One of the concerns raised by the SPARCL study relates to the potential risk of hemorrhagic stroke with statins. A post hoc analysis [40] showed that the risk of ischemic stroke decreased from 11.6% to 9.2%, but there was a small increase in hemorrhagic stroke from 1.4% to 2.3% (HR 1.6, 95% CI 1.1, 2.6) with atorvastatin. The risk of hemorrhage was also more frequent among individuals with a baseline hemorrhagic stroke, in men, and with increasing age, as well as in individuals with less well-controlled hypertension. There was no association between hemorrhage risk and baseline LDL-C level or recent

LDL-C level in treated patients. Moreover, no increase in hemorrhagic stroke was observed in almost 48,000 patients from multiple statin trials in CHD cohorts analyzed in a large meta-analysis [33].

Although the role of other cholesterol particles in stroke is not as well understood as that of LDL-C, there is increasing attention placed on HDL-C. This lipoprotein protects against atherosclerosis not only by extracting cholesterol from the arterial wall, but also through anti-inflammatory, antioxidant, and antithrombotic effects [41]. HDL-C levels are inversely associated with coronary events [42], and large cohort studies [43] and case-control studies [44] have confirmed this association, particularly for large-vessel disease-related strokes [45,46]. HDL-C increases can be achieved with lifestyle modifications [47], niacin [48], statins [49], and fibrates [50]. The Veterans Affairs High-Density Lipoprotein Cholesterol Intervention Trial study [50] evaluated gemfibrozil in patients with CAD with low HDL levels and found a reduction in atherthrombotic strokes after adjustment for baseline variables. The combination of a statin and niacin appears to be effective in reducing cardiovascular events and remodeling the arterial wall [51,52]. Novel interventions to manipulate HDL-C are emerging. With the recognition that HDL-C variants may confer varying degrees of protection [53,54], there has been an effort to supplement a protective Apo A-I peptide, the most important protein in HDL-C. Infusions of apoA-I Milano has led to a regression of aortic atherosclerotic lesions in mice and coronary lesions in humans [55,56].

Summary of recommendations

1 Ischemic stroke or TIA patients with elevated cholesterol, comorbid CAD, or evidence of an atherosclerotic origin should be managed according to the NCEP III guidelines, which include lifestyle modification, dietary guidelines, and medication recommendations (Class I, Level A).
2 Statin agents are recommended, and the target goal for cholesterol lowering for those with CHD or symptomatic atherosclerotic disease is an LDL-C of <100 mg/dL and an LDL-C of <70 mg/dL for very

high-risk persons with multiple risk factors (Class I, Level A).
3 On the basis of the SPARCL trial, the administration of statin therapy with intensive lipid-lowering effects is recommended for patients with atherosclerotic ischemic stroke or TIA and without known CHD to reduce the risk of stroke and cardiovascular event (Class I, Level B).
4 Ischemic stroke or TIA patients with low HDL-C may be considered for treatment with niacin or gemfibrozil (Class IIb, Level B).

Example Case, cont'd.
Our patient had significant dyslipidemia. In the presence of a new stroke and with multiple risk factors, including hypertension, obesity, and poorly controlled DM, the goal LDL-C is <70 mg/dL. In order to achieve this LDL-C level, she was counseled on an appropriate diet and started on high-dose statin therapy.

Diabetes mellitus

DM is diagnosed if a patient has a fasting plasma glucose of ≥126 mg/dL, a casual plasma glucose of ≥200, or a 2-hour oral glucose tolerance test of ≥200 [57]. Over 20 million Americans have diabetes; among individuals older than 60 years, the group most affected by stroke, 21% have diabetes, with African-Americans, Hispanics, and Native Americans having a greater prevalence than whites. Its incidence has exploded in the last two decades, reaching almost epidemic proportions [1].

Population studies show diabetes to be a clear risk factor for first stroke [58–60] as well as for stroke recurrence [61–63], particularly for small- and large-vessel disease-related stroke [64]. Hyperglycemia also increases the risk of poor outcomes in the acute stroke setting [65,66], and poor glycemic control increases the risk of stroke fatality (OR 1.37 per 1% HbA1C, 95% CI 1.09–1.72, $P = 0.0071$) [67].

The proposed mechanisms by which diabetes results in vascular events are varied and include the enhancement of atherogenesis through generation of free radicals, glycosylation of end products, diversion into the aldolase reductase pathway, and vascular smooth muscle cell proliferation, as well as the impairment of nitric oxide-mediated vasodilation and platelet activation [68].

Secondary stroke prevention in patients with diabetes focuses on the treatment of hypertension and dyslipidemia. Randomized trials have shown that BP reduction in diabetics results in a decrease in vascular outcomes including stroke. In the UK Prospective Diabetes Study, a 10-point systolic BP reduction to 144 mm Hg resulted in a 44% RRR for stroke [69]. Although most studies evaluating BP reduction in diabetics have failed to reach very low BP levels, the present recommendation is to tightly control BP to a target of <130/80 mm Hg [13]. The analysis of the Action to Control Cardiovascular Risk in Diabetes (ACCORD) trial [70] will contribute to the knowledge of greater BP reduction in diabetics. ACE-Is and ARBs are preferred as first-line agents in diabetics due to beneficial effects on vascular outcomes and progression of diabetic nephropathy [57,71–73].

Lipid control recommendations are more stringent for diabetics; the target LDL-C in diabetics after stroke is <70 mg/dL [26]. Statin treatment decreases vascular outcomes [74,75] and, in particular, stroke recurrence in diabetics [28,75].

There is no definite evidence that glycemic control reduces the risk of recurrent stroke; in the UK Prospective Diabetes Study, lower baseline plasma glucose levels at the diagnosis of diabetes did not correlate with improved stroke outcome [76], and more intensive glycemic control did not result in a lower stroke risk [77], although metformin may be beneficial in overweight diabetics [78]. Whether more intensive glycemic control than currently recommended is beneficial has been considered; however, in the ACCORD trial, which was stopped for safety reasons, there was increased mortality in individuals randomized to very low HbA1C levels of <6% [79]. Although there was no increased mortality in the Action in Diabetes and Vascular Disease: Preterax and Diamicron Modified Release Controlled Evaluation (ADVANCE) trial, macrovascular diseases, including stroke, were not significantly reduced, whereas microvascular disease was significantly lower in the aggressive glycemic control group [80]. Given the evidence that glycemic control decreases microvascular complications and the pos-

sibility that it may be beneficial to prevent macrovascular complications including stroke, it is reasonable to target an HbA1C level of ≤7%.

Summary of recommendations

1 More rigorous control of BP and lipids should be considered in patients with diabetes (Class IIa, Level B).

2 Although all major classes of antihypertensives are suitable for the control of BP, most patients will require more than 1 agent. ACE-Is and ARBs are more effective in reducing the progression of renal disease and are recommended as first-choice medications for patients with DM (Class I, Level A).

3 Glucose control is recommended to near-normoglycemic levels among diabetics with ischemic stroke or TIA to reduce microvascular complications (Class I, Level A).

4 The goal for HbA1C should be ≤7% (Class IIa, Level B).

Example Case, cont'd.
This patient had newly diagnosed DM. She was referred to a comprehensive diabetes program for dietary and exercise counseling and for screening for kidney and retinal disease. In addition to tight control of hypertension and dyslipidemia, she was treated with oral hypoglycemic agents with a goal HbA1C of ≤7. Given that she was overweight, she was started on metformin.

Lifestyle modification

The following section addresses habits and lifestyle modification including tobacco use, alcohol abuse, obesity, and physical inactivity. The data that support these measures in *secondary* stroke prevention are scarce. Nonetheless, given the strong epidemiological association between these risk factors and stroke, and their adverse impact on other conditions, it is reasonable to extrapolate the data from primary prevention studies. In addition, it appears as if the initiation of these stroke prevention strategies while the patient is still in the hospital increases adherence [81,82].

Tobacco use

About 21% of all US adults are current smokers [1]; 438,000 individuals die of smoking-related diseases each year, a third of these deaths are due to vascular events, and the annual health-related cost of smoking is estimated at $167 billion [84]. The epidemiological association of cigarette smoking and stroke is established and sufficient to infer a causal relationship. A meta-analysis of 32 studies found a relative risk for ischemic stroke of 1.9 and for subarachnoid hemorrhage (SAH) of 2.9 [85]. Subsequent studies have validated these results: the British Doctors Study found a relative risk of 1.31 for ischemic stroke and 2.14 for SAH in men [86], and a Finnish study reported an increased risk in SAH in men (RR 2.4, 95% CI 1.6–3.7) and women (RR 2.5, 95% CI 1.5–4.1) [87]. The combination of oral contraceptives and smoking is associated with greater risk [88]. The association between smoking and intracerebral hemorrhage has not been as well established [85]. Stroke-related mortality is also increased in smokers (RR 2.5, $P < 0.001$) [89]. There is a clear dose relationship between the daily number of cigarettes consumed and both stroke incidence and stroke mortality [86,90,91].

Smoking cessation results in a decreased risk of a first stroke to the level of nonsmokers within 2–5 years [92,93] as well as in a decrease in stroke-related mortality [94], which justifies efforts to enhance tobacco cessation. That more effort is needed in this area is exemplified by the findings of a national survey in which cigarette smoking was continued by 18% of individuals who had experienced a previous stroke or MI [95]. Nicotine replacement, social support, and skills training are the recommended interventions to promote smoking cessation [96].

Alcohol consumption

The effects of alcohol on stroke risk is related to the amount consumed. Alcohol consumption is typically described in number of drinks. One drink is commonly defined as 14 g of alcohol, 12 oz of beer, 5 oz of wine, or 1.5 oz of hard liquor [97].

Although excessive alcohol use and binge drinking results in an increase in all vascular events, it is now becoming clear that light to moderate consumption is protective. A meta-analysis of over 1 million subjects in 34 studies found a "J"-shaped relationship between the amount of alcohol and

mortality. Light to moderate use of 0.5–2 drinks a day was associated with an 18% reduction in total mortality driven by a decline in vascular events [98]. That this is independent of the possible interaction with other vascular risk factors is highlighted by the finding of a decrease in MI with one to two drinks a day in men who already followed a healthy lifestyle (healthy diet, exercise, normal weight, and no smoking) [99]. The "J"-shaped relationship between the amount of alcohol and stroke risk has been reported by multiple studies. A meta-analysis of 35 studies found that compared with nondrinkers, the consumption of <1 drink per day was associated with a reduced ischemic stroke risk (RR 0.8), 1–2 drinks per day with an RR of 0.72, 2–5 drinks per day with an RR of 0.96, and >5 drinks per day increased the risk (RR1.69) [100]. In the Northern Manhattan Stroke Study, the beneficial effects of moderate drinking and the adverse outcome with heavy drinking were confirmed for various ethnic groups [101,102]. Although the consensus is that the specific alcoholic beverage is less important than the amount of alcohol ingested [103], some have suggested that red wine may have added benefits [104].

The beneficial effects of moderate drinking appear to be multifactorial and include elevation of HDL [105], reduction in plasma viscosity [106], decrease in inflammatory markers [107], decreased platelet aggregation [108], and interestingly, enhancement of insulin sensitivity, which may result in decreased postprandial glucose changes [109]. In addition, flavonoids and resveratrol contained in red wine may have beneficial effects [110]. The adverse events of large doses of alcohol are mediated through hypertension, arrhythmias, and cardiomyopathy

Obesity

Obesity, characterized by excess body fat, is defined as a BMI of $\geq 30 \text{ kg/m}^2$, whereas overweight is defined as a BMI between 25 and 29.9 kg/m² [111]. Two-thirds of the adult population in the United States is either overweight or obese, and this proportion appears to be increasing [112]. It is estimated that by 2015, there will be 1.5 billion overweight and obese individuals worldwide [113].

Although obesity is closely related to hypertension, diabetes, and dyslipidemia, it is an independent risk factor for stroke. The association between obesity and stroke in men has been confirmed by various studies [114,115]. The Physician's Health Study found that compared with individuals with a BMI of <23 kg/m^2, obese men had a relative risk of stroke of 2 (95% CI 1.48–2.71), and estimated that each unit increase of BMI resulted in a 6% increase in risk [114]. The association between obesity and stroke in women is less consistent. In the Women's Health Study, obese women had an HR of 1.5 (1.16–1.94) compared with individuals with normal weight [116], and in the Nurses' Health Study, there was a greater than 2-fold increase in stroke risk for BMI ≥32 kg/m^2 compared with <21 kg/m^2 [117], but other reports were unable to document this association [118–121]. Abdominal obesity is more closely related to the risk of stroke than general obesity. Waist circumference, a useful measure of abdominal obesity, is defined as >102 cm (40 inches) in men and >88 cm (35 inches) in women. It was closely related to stroke risk in the Northern Manhattan Stroke Study [122]. The mechanisms by which obesity is independently associated with an increased risk of stroke are incompletely understood but may involve prothrombotic [123] and inflammatory [124] states.

Weight reduction interventions include dieting, exercise, behavioral modification therapy, pharmacotherapy, and surgical or laparoscopic approaches. Although no trials have assessed the impact of weight reduction on stroke risk [125], it is also clear that reductions of 5–15% of baseline weight result in better control of hypertension, diabetes, and dyslipidemia [126]. Fruit- and vegetable-rich diets, such as the Mediterranean diet, reduce vascular events [127].

Physical activity

The levels of physical activity have remained stable for adults in the United States in the last decade [128], and only about half of all adults engage in frequent regular vigorous exercise; this proportion is lower for minorities and the elderly, and youth engagement in physical activity is poor [1].

A recent meta-analysis of 18 cohort and 5 case-control studies found a protective effect of physical activity on stroke. Compared with low levels of activity, highly active individuals had a significant decrease in stroke incidence and mortality (RR 0.73, 95% CI 0.67–0.79); the effect was still present but of lesser magnitude for individuals who engage in moderate intensity activity (RR 0.80, 95% CI 0.74–0.86). This effect was seen for both ischemic and hemorrhagic strokes [129]. The protective effect of physical activity has also been documented in older individuals with vascular risk factors [130] and in different ethnic groups [131].

The beneficial effects of physical activity are mediated through various factors, including BP reduction [132], improved glycemic control [133] and lipidic profiles [134], weight reduction, and decreased viscosity [135] and platelet aggregability [136].

Summary of recommendations

1 All ischemic stroke or TIA patients who have smoked in the past year should be strongly encouraged not to smoke (Class I, Level C).

2 Counseling, nicotine products, and oral smoking cessation medications have been found to be effective for smokers (Class IIa, Level B).

3 Avoid environmental smoke (Class IIa, Level C).

4 Patients with prior ischemic stroke or TIA who are heavy drinkers should eliminate or reduce their consumption of alcohol (Class I, Level A).

5 Light to moderate levels of ≤2 drinks per day for men and 1 drink per day for nonpregnant women may be considered (Class IIb, Level C).

6 Weight reduction may be considered for all overweight ischemic stroke or TIA patients to maintain the goal of a BMI of 18.5–24.9 kg/m^2 and a waist circumference of <35 inches for women and <40 inches for men. Clinicians should encourage weight management through an appropriate balance of caloric intake, physical activity, and behavioral counseling (Class IIb, Level C).

7 For those with ischemic stroke or TIA who are capable of engaging in physical activity, at least 30 minutes of moderate-intensity physical exercise on most days may be considered to reduce risk factors and comorbid conditions that increase the likelihood of recurrence of stroke. For those with disability after ischemic stroke, a supervised therapeutic exercise regimen is recommended (Class IIb, Level C).

Example Case, cont'd.

The patient does not currently smoke, but her husband is an active smoker. She does not drink. She is overweight and does not exercise regularly. Both she and her husband were counseled on the risks of smoking, and her husband accepted a referral to a smoking cessation clinic. She was seen by the dietitian who placed her on a low-sodium, low-fat, low-cholesterol, and reduced-calorie diet. She was instructed on the importance of daily exercise. After discharge from rehabilitation 2 weeks later, she started stationary bicycle training 30 minutes a day.

Carotid atherosclerotic disease

Atherosclerotic extracranial carotid disease may account for as many as one in five ischemic strokes although some population-based studies have found a lower frequency; in a multiethnic population, the proportion of extracranial carotid stenosis-related strokes ranged from 8% to 11% [137]. The natural history of previously symptomatic carotid disease has been detailed by large clinical trials. The North American Symptomatic Carotid Endarterectomy Trial (NASCET) defined a 26% risk of ipsilateral stroke at 2 years in the presence of stenosis of 70% or more for individuals treated medically, with increasing risk at a greater degree of stenosis [138]. The risk of stroke after purely ocular symptoms (amaurosis fugax) was less than in individuals with cerebral symptoms [139]. For stenosis of 50–69%

in symptomatic patients, the risk of ipsilateral stroke on antiplatelet therapy was 22.2% over 5 years [140]. Stenosis under 50% is unlikely to result in stroke.

The benefits of endarterectomy in individuals who present with a stroke, hemispheric TIA, or amaurosis fugax are well known. The results of NASCET are summarized in Table 7.2; these results have been reinforced by similar findings from the European Carotid Surgery Trial and the Veterans Affairs Cooperative Study [141,142]. Based on these studies, despite an overall perioperative risk of stroke and death of 7.1% across studies [143], carotid endarterectomy (CEA) is recommended for recently symptomatic patients with 70–99% stenosis; endarterectomy is also recommended for individuals with a recently symptomatic 50–69% stenosis, but other factors such as age, gender, and comorbidities should be considered [7,143].

The benefits of endarterectomy diminish with increasing time from the ischemic event in patients with TIA or nondisabling stroke. For patients with a symptomatic carotid stenosis between 50% and 99%, the number needed to treat to prevent one ipsilateral stroke at 5 years is five for patients treated with endarterectomy within 2 weeks (vs. medical therapy) but 125 for patients treated after 2 weeks. The decrease in efficacy of endarterectomy is more pronounced for individuals with a moderate carotid stenosis of 50–69% compared with individuals with a more severe 70–99% stenosis [144]. This is probably due to the fact that plaque destabilization that leads to artery-to-artery embolism constitutes a dynamic factor, with plaque

Table 7.2 Benefit of carotid endarterectomy in symptomatic patients in the North American Symptomatic Carotid Endarterectomy Trial (NASCET) study (136,138)

Population	% Stenosis*	Nonsurgical†	Surgical†	Absolute risk reduction	NNT‡
Symptomatic	50–69%	22.2%	15.7%	6.5% at 5 years	20
Symptomatic	70–99%	26%	9%	17% at 2 years	8

*Angiographic measurement according to the NASCET method.

†Risk of ipsilateral stroke.

‡Numbers needed to treat (NNT) to prevent one stroke at 2 years.

inflammation and destabilization followed by remodeling and subsequent decrease in embolic risk [145]. Also, greater age, male gender, higher degree of stenosis, and ulceration of the plaque increase the likelihood that endarterectomy will be efficacious in decreasing the risk of subsequent events [146].

Stenting of the carotid artery is increasingly performed in the United States. The Stenting and Angioplasty with Protection in Patients at High Risk for Endarterectomy Study evaluated patients with coexisting conditions, mainly cardiovascular, that placed them at high risk; this study enrolled mostly asymptomatic patients and found better outcomes for patients treated with stenting [147]. Two subsequent class 1 evidence studies have compared stenting and endarterectomy in symptomatic carotid stenosis [148,149]. Both were designed as noninferiority studies with 30-day stroke and death as the primary outcome. The Stent-Supported Percutaneous Angioplasty of the Carotid Artery versus Endarterectomy trial enrolled 1,200 cases with carotid stenosis ≥50% within 6 months from symptoms and found similar rates of death or ipsilateral stroke 30 days with stenting (6.8%) and endarterectomy (6.4%) ($P = 0.09$) [149]. The Endarterectomy versus Angioplasty in Patients with Symptomatic Severe Stenosis was stopped after the enrollment of 527 patients with ≥60% stenosis within 4 months of the index event because of futility and increased risk associated with stenting. The incidence of any stroke or death at 30 days was 9.6% after stenting and 3.9% after endarterectomy [148]; this difference persisted at 6 months (6.1% for endarterectomy and 11.7% with stenting). Further caution comes from the lead-in data from the Carotid Revascularization Endarterectomy versus Stent Trial study in which the 30-day complications rate in individuals treated with stenting with distal protection increased significantly with age; octagenerians had a 12.1% complication rate compared with 3.2% in younger individuals [150]. Therefore, at this time, there is insufficient evidence to recommend endovascular therapy for symptomatic carotid stenosis except for select patients at very high surgical risk or other technical reasons. Ongoing studies will contribute to the clarification of the role of endovascular treatment of symptomatic carotid stenosis.

Summary of recommendations

1 For patients with recent TIA or ischemic stroke within the last 6 months and ipsilateral severe (70–99%) carotid artery stenosis, CEA is recommended by a surgeon with a perioperative morbidity and mortality of <6% (Class I, Level A).

2 For patients with recent TIA or ischemic stroke and ipsilateral moderate (50–69%) carotid stenosis, CEA is recommended, depending on patient-specific factors such as age, gender, comorbidities, and severity of initial symptoms (Class I, Level A).

3 When degree of stenosis is <50%, there is no indication for CEA (Class III, Level A).

4 When CEA is indicated, surgery within 2 weeks rather than delayed surgery is suggested (Class IIa, Level B).

5 Among patients with symptomatic severe stenosis (>70%) in whom the stenosis is difficult to access surgically, medical conditions are present that greatly increase the risk for surgery, or when other specific circumstances exist such as radiation-induced stenosis or restenosis after CEA; carotid artery stenting (CAS) is not inferior to endarterectomy and may be considered (Class IIb, Level B).

6 CAS is reasonable when performed by operators with established peri-procedural morbidity and mortality rates of 4–6%, similar to those observed in trials of CEA and CAS (Class IIa, Level B).

7 Among patients with symptomatic carotid occlusion, extracranial circulation/intracranial circulation bypass surgery is not routinely recommended (Class III, Level A).

8 Endovascular treatment of patients with symptomatic extracranial vertebral stenosis may be considered when patients are having symptoms despite medical therapies (antithrombotics, statins, and other treatments for risk factors) (Class IIb, Level C).

Example Case, cont'd.
Our patient had mild asymptomatic internal carotid artery plaques for which no revascularization procedure was indicated. Tight vascular risk factor control and antiplatelet therapy were recommended.

Intracranial stenosis

In the United States, it is estimated that between 8% and 10% of all strokes are due to intracranial atherosclerotic disease [151], but this condition has clear ethnic differences, affecting Asians, African-Americans, and Hispanics more frequently than Caucasians. Some reports have cited that as many as one quarter of all strokes in Asians are due to intracranial stenoses [152]. At present, it is recommended that patients be treated with antiplatelet agents and appropriate control of existing vascular risk factors; endovascular therapy remains of uncertain benefit for this condition [7,153].

The gold standard to detect intracranial arterial disease remains conventional catheter angiography. The recent Stroke Outcomes and Neuroimaging of Intracranial Atherosclerosis study evaluated the role of transcranial Doppler (TCD) ultrasound and MRA in detecting 50–99% stenosis of the large intracranial arteries [154]. When using commonly employed criteria for intracranial stenosis, both TCD and MRA had strong negative predictive values of 83% and 87%, respectively, but the positive predictive values were lower at 55% and 66%. The accuracy of CT angiography appears to be excellent in evaluating intracranial disease [155,156]. Therefore, a normal TCD or MRA is a relatively trustworthy indication that there is no significant intracranial large-vessel stenosis, but an abnormal result has a suboptimal predictive value. If a risky or invasive procedure is planned, then confirmatory conventional angiography is required. On the other hand, if medical treatment will not be significantly altered by the test results, it is reasonable to rely on noninvasive diagnostics.

The WASID study [153] randomized patients with a recent stroke or TIA due to intracranial arterial disease of 50–99% to aspirin 1300 mg/d versus warfarin international normalization ratio (INR) of 2–3. There was no difference in the primary outcome of ischemic stroke, intracerebral hemorrhage, or vascular death between the treatment arms, which occurred at a staggering 22% over the 1.8-year average follow-up period. Most of the events occurred over the first few weeks. There was, however, a more than 2-fold incidence of major hemorrhage or death in the anticoagulated group. There was no subgroup of patients for whom warfarin was superior to aspirin [157]. Therefore, warfarin appears to be no more effective and riskier than aspirin for this disease. This study also allowed the identification of a group at high risk of recurrent stroke in the territory of the stenotic vessel, including individuals with a severe stenosis (70–99%), women, and individuals who enrolled soon after the onset of symptoms [158]. Therefore, an individual presenting with a stroke due to a 70–99% intracranial stenosis would have a 2-year risk of recurrent stroke of 25%, whereas a lower degree of stenosis of 50–69% would only carry an 11% risk.

Given the elevated risk of recurrence, there has been considerable interest in endovascular approaches for the treatment of intracranial stenosis. Initial experience with balloon-expandable stents was associated with a high risk of peri-procedural complications [159], but the development of self-deployed stents appears to provide a safer alternative [160]. The efficacy of endovascular therapy as compared with the best medical therapy will be studied in the Stent Placement versus Aggressive Medical Management for the Prevention of Recurrent Stroke in Intracranial Stenosis trial. At this time, intracranial stenting outside of a clinical trial should be reserved for patients at high risk who have had recurrent events despite medical therapy.

> The usefulness of endovascular therapy (angioplasty and/or stent placement) is uncertain for patients with hemodynamically significant intracranial stenoses who have symptoms despite medical therapies (antithrombotics, statins, and other treatments for risk factors) and is considered investigational (Class IIb, Level C).

Antithrombotic therapy

Antithrombotic drugs used for stroke prevention include anticoagulants and antiplatelet agents. Anticoagulants are prescribed for cardioembolic strokes, venous strokes, and arterial dissections; they have not shown benefit for most non-cardioembolic strokes [153,161,162]. Antiplatelet agents are reserved for individuals with large- or small-vessel-related strokes. Recent studies have contributed to the extensive literature on the role of antithrombotic therapy in cerebrovascular diseases.

Cardioembolic strokes

Atrial fibrillation (AF), the most important cardioembolic cause of stroke, affects about 2.2 million individuals in the United States and is more common with increasing age [163]. Given the aging population, it is estimated that by the year 2050, there may be as many as 10 million individuals with AF in the United States [164]. Many studies have confirmed the superiority of anticoagulants over placebo and antiplatelet agents in AF. A recent meta-analysis of over 28,000 individuals with nonvalvular AF [165] concluded that warfarin reduced the risk of stroke by 64% compared with placebo, whereas antiplatelet agents reduced the risk by 22%. Direct comparison of anticoagulants versus antiplatelet agents showed a 39% relative risk reduction in favor of warfarin.

A prior stroke or TIA is the most important predictor of recurrent stroke in AF. Across various studies, the risk of stroke in individuals with a prior cerebrovascular event is 2.5 (95% CI 1.8–3.5); in this population, the stroke rate with aspirin is estimated at 10% per year [166]. The absolute risk reduction for recurrent stroke for warfarin is 6%, certainly greater than the 1.5% risk of major hemorrhage [167]. This benefit appears to extend to the very old

[168]. As a prior cerebrovascular event increases the prospect of cerebral hemorrhage, tight BP control and avoidance of elevated INR are important as these measures have a substantial benefit in preventing warfarin-related hemorrhages [169].

Nonetheless, the use of warfarin is burdensome, as its bioeffects are variable and there is a need for frequent blood testing. This has led to a growing interest in direct thrombin inhibitors, which offer stable dosing, few interactions with other medications, no dietary restrictions, and no need for INR testing. Ximelagatran was evaluated in randomized trials [170] and found to be as effective as warfarin in preventing recurrent strokes (2.83% per year with ximelagatran and 3.27% per year with warfarin, $P = 0.625$), with similar rates for hemorrhagic complications. However, 6% of individuals treated with ximelagatran had a significant increase in liver enzymes; therefore, this agent is not currently recommended for secondary stroke prevention. Another direct thrombin inhibitor, dabigatran, has shown efficacy and safety in small trials [171], and larger studies with this agent are being conducted.

There is a variety of other cardioembolic stroke sources. However, their review is beyond the scope of this chapter. The following recommendations summarize the prevalent thought on the management of various conditions that result in cardioembolic strokes.

Summary of recommendations

Atrial fibrillation

1 For patients with ischemic stroke or TIA with persistent or paroxysmal (intermittent) AF, anticoagulation with adjusted-dose warfarin (target INR, 2.5; range, 2.0–3.0) is recommended (Class I, Level A).
2 In patients unable to take oral anticoagulants, aspirin 325 mg/d is recommended (Class I, Level A).

Acute MI and left ventricular thrombus

1 For patients with an ischemic stroke caused by an acute MI in whom LV mural thrombus is identified by echocardiography or another form of cardiac imaging, oral anticoagulation is reasonable, aiming for an INR of 2.0–3.0 for at least 3 months and up to 1 year (Class IIa, Level B).

2 Aspirin should be used concurrently for the ischemic CAD patient during oral anticoagulant therapy in doses up to 162 mg/d, preferably in the enteric-coated form (Class IIa, Level A).

Cardiomyopathy

1 For patients with ischemic stroke or TIA who have dilated cardiomyopathy, either warfarin (INR, 2.0–3.0) or antiplatelet therapy may be considered for the prevention of recurrent events (Class IIb, Level C).

Valvular heart disease

Rheumatic mitral valve disease

1 For patients with ischemic stroke or TIA who have rheumatic mitral valve disease, whether or not AF is

present, long-term warfarin therapy is reasonable, with a target INR of 2.5 (range, 2.0–3.0) (Class IIa, Level C).

2 Antiplatelet agents should not be routinely added to warfarin in the interest of avoiding additional bleeding risk (Class III, Level C).

3 For ischemic stroke or TIA patients with rheumatic mitral valve disease, whether or not AF is present, who have a recurrent embolism while receiving warfarin, adding aspirin (81 mg/d) is suggested (Class IIa, Level C).

Mitral valve prolapse

1 For patients with MVP who have ischemic stroke or TIAs, long-term antiplatelet therapy is reasonable (Class IIa, Level C).

Mitral annular calcification

1 For patients with ischemic stroke or TIA and MAC not documented to be calcific, antiplatelet therapy may be considered (Class IIb, Level C).

2 Among patients with mitral regurgitation resulting from MAC without AF, antiplatelet or warfarin therapy may be considered (Class IIb, Level C).

Aortic valve disease

1 For patients with ischemic stroke or TIA and aortic valve disease who do not have AF, antiplatelet therapy may be considered (Class IIa, Level C).

Prosthetic heart valves

1 For patients with ischemic stroke or TIA who have modern mechanical prosthetic heart valves, oral anticoagulants are recommended, with an INR target of 3.0 (range, 2.5–3.5) (Class I, Level B).

2 For patients with mechanical prosthetic heart valves who have an ischemic stroke or systemic embolism despite adequate therapy with oral anticoagulants, aspirin 75–100 mg/d, in addition to oral anticoagulants, and maintenance of the INR at a target of 3.0 (range, 2.5–3.5) are reasonable (Class IIa, Level B).

3 For patients with ischemic stroke or TIA who have bioprosthetic heart valves with no other source of thromboembolism, anticoagulation with warfarin (INR, 2.0–3.0) may be considered (Class IIb, Level C).

Non-cardioembolic strokes

Antiplatelet therapy is indicated for most patients with non-cardioembolic stroke or TIA. Aspirin, aspirin plus extended-release dipyridamol, and clopidogrel are all appropriate options for secondary stroke prevention, and act by inhibiting platelet function. Meta-analysis of patients on antiplatelet therapy with prior stroke or TIA found a 22% reduction in the combined risk of recurrent stroke, MI, and vascular death [172], whereas others found a 13% reduction (RR 0.87, 95% CI 0.81–0.94) in the combined end point with aspirin alone compared with placebo [173]. Many other individual antiplatelet agents have been compared with aspirin in stroke prevention. Triflusal, a compound structurally related to aspirin, was found to have similar effects on the combined end point of stroke, MI, and vascular death, but with fewer hemorrhagic complications; however, it is not available in the United States [174,175]. Ticlopidine, a thienopyridine, was found to be more effective than aspirin in one study [176], but another report found no difference between ticlopidine and aspirin in African-Americans [177]. Given the side effects of diarrhea, rash, and neutropenia, this drug is now rarely used in the United States. Another thienopyridine commonly used is clopidogrel. Treatment with clopidogrel was associated with an 8.7% relative risk reduction for the combined end point of stroke, MI, and vascular death in patients with a history of either stroke, MI, or symptomatic peripheral arterial disease. The benefit did not reach statistical significance in the subgroup that had stroke as a qualifying event [178]. A novel thienopyridine, prasugrel, has not been studied in stroke patients, but in patients with acute coronary syndromes, when compared with clopidogrel, it resulted in a reduction in MI, stroke, and cardiovascular death, with a slight increase in hemorrhagic events [179].

Given the limited effects of single antiplatelet agents, there has been an interest in combination therapy. The combination of aspirin and clopidogrel has been utilized successfully in patients with acute coronary syndromes. The Management of Atherothrombosis with Clopidogrel in High-Risk Patients study [180] evaluated the combination of aspirin and clopidogrel versus clopidogrel in patients with a recent stroke or TIA and an additional risk factor such as previous stroke, MI, peripheral vascular disease, or DM. There was a nonsignificant relative risk reduction of 6.4% for the combination but a significant excess of bleeding complications (life-threatening bleeding 2.6% combination, 1.3% clopidogrel, $P<0.0001$; major bleeding 1.9% combination, 0.6% clopidogrel, $P < 0.0001$). The Clopidogrel for High Atherothrombotic Risk and Ischemic Stabilization, Management, and Avoidance (CHARISMA) study [181] evaluated patients with cerebrovascular disease, coronary disease, peripheral vascular disease, or with multiple vascular risk factors, who were randomized to receive aspirin or aspirin plus clopidogrel. There was a statistically non-significant 7% relative risk reduction in the combined end point of stroke, MI, and vascular death. Combination therapy resulted in a greater incidence of bleeding than with aspirin alone (severe bleeding 1.7% combination, 1.3% aspirin, $P = 0.09$; moderate bleeding 2.1% combination, 1.3% aspirin, $P < 0.001$). At this point, data suggest that the combination of aspirin and clopidogrel is not superior to either agent alone in secondary stroke prevention, and results in a greater frequency of hemorrhages. Ongoing studies will further contribute to the understanding of the role of the combination of aspirin and clopidogrel in stroke reduction [14].

Studies have shown that the combination of aspirin and extended-release dipyridamole is more effective than aspirin in decreasing stroke recurrence. In the European Stroke Prevention Study 2 (ESPS-2) [182], a 23% relative risk reduction in stroke recurrence was obtained when compared with aspirin alone ($P = 0.006$). The European/Australasian Stroke Prevention in Reversible Ischaemia Trial study [183] compared aspirin plus extended-release dipyridamol and aspirin alone and found an HR of 0.8 (0.66–0.98) for the combined end point of stroke, MI, vascular death, and major hemorrhage for the combination; the HR for stroke alone was 0.84 (0.67–1.17). This study was limited by the open treatment assignment (although outcome evaluation was blinded), the nonstandard aspirin dose, and the discrepancy between the intention to treat and on-treatment analysis. Nonetheless, these results are consistent with the findings of the ESPS-2 study. Direct comparison of clopidogrel versus aspirin plus extended-release dipyridamol was evaluated in the PRoFESS trial. In this large study, recurrent stroke occurred at similar rates for each treatment arm (9% aspirin + extended-release dipyridamol vs. 8.8% clopidogrel, $P = $ not statistically significant) [2].

Summary of recommendations

1 For patients with non-cardioembolic ischemic stroke or TIA, antiplatelet agents rather than oral anticoagulation are recommended to reduce the risk of recurrent stroke and other cardiovascular events (Class I, Level A).
2 Aspirin (50–325 mg/d) monotherapy, the combination of aspirin and extended-release dipyridamole, and clopidogrel monotherapy are all acceptable options for initial therapy (Class I, Level A).
3 The combination of aspirin and extended-release dipyridamole is recommended over aspirin alone (Class I, Level B).
4 Clopidogrel may be considered over aspirin alone on the basis of direct-comparison trials (Class IIb, Level B).
5 For patients allergic to aspirin, clopidogrel is reasonable (Class IIa, Level B).
6 Addition of aspirin to clopidogrel increases the risk of hemorrhage and is not routinely recommended for ischemic stroke or TIA patients unless they have a specific indication for this therapy (i.e., coronary stent or acute coronary syndrome) (Class III).

Example Case, cont'd.
Our patient had a small pontine infarct while on aspirin with no evidence of cardioembolism or significant large-vessel extracranial or intracranial disease. Her stroke was thought to be related to small-vessel disease, and therefore, antiplatelet therapy was indicated. We recommended the combination of aspirin and extended-release dipyridamole. This combination was selected given its superiority versus aspirin alone in preventing recurrent stroke [182,183]. Another option would have been monotherapy with clopidogrel [20,178].

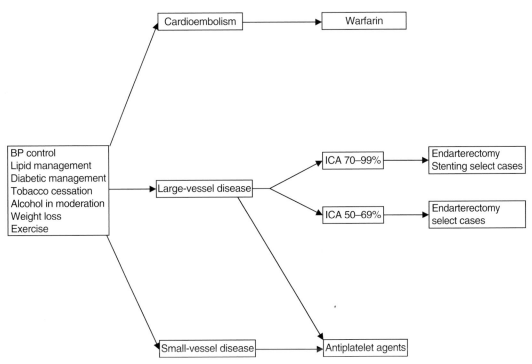

Fig. 7.1 Algorithm for secondary stroke prevention.
BP, blood pressure; ICA, internal carotid artery.

Conclusion

Advances in the understanding of stroke risk factors and mechanisms of cerebral injury afford the possibility of modifying the course of cerebrovascular diseases, thus preventing its devastating personal and societal consequences. Figure 7.1 provides an algorithm for secondary stroke prevention in the non-acute phase. These recommendations ought to be used as general guidelines, but management should consider individual characteristics. Numerous clinical trials continue to add new evidence to our approach in preventing stroke among survivors of cerebral ischemic events, and existing recommendations quickly get outdated when new evidence becomes available. The data reviewed in this chapter, with major points summarized at the beginning of the chapter, offer the clinician therapeutic options to reduce the incidence of stroke recurrence and to improve outcomes.

References available online at www.wiley.com/go/ strokeguidelines.

Post-Stroke Rehabilitation and Recovery

Pamela Woods Duncan, Danielle Blankenship, and Nicol Korner-Bitensky

EXAMPLE CASE

J is a 72-year-old right-handed, English-speaking, retired salesperson with no medical history other than hypertension. J was transferred to a rehabilitation inpatient facility, 14 days after experiencing a right middle cerebral artery distribution ischemic stroke.

Prior to the stroke, J was living with a spouse in a two-story home that they own. The couple shared domestic activities, and J enjoyed swimming, golfing, socializing, and driving to various activities. They have two adult children. Their daughter lives close by and visits frequently. Their other child has very little contact with the couple.

The report from the acute care hospital indicated that J presented with a dense left hemiplegia, disorientation, and somnolence. The emergency room nurse reported adequate spoken and listening skills. By discharge, J was participating in 45 minutes of daily rehabilitative therapy and had progressed to using a wheelchair for short distances, but tended to bump into obstacles on the left. J was walking with maximum assistance of one person while using a quad cane, with a tendency for the left knee to buckle and for the left foot to drag.

During an initial interview with J on the day after admission, he was sitting slumped in a wheelchair

MAJOR POINTS

- The primary goals of rehabilitation is to prevent complications, to minimize impairments, and to maximize function.
- Secondary prevention is fundamental to preventing stroke recurrence.
- Early assessment and intervention are critical to optimize rehabilitation.
- Standardized evaluations and valid assessment tools are essential to the development of a comprehensive treatment plan.
- Evidence-based interventions should be based on functional goals.

- Every candidate for rehabilitation should have access to an experienced and coordinated rehabilitation team to ensure optimal outcome.
- The patient and family and or caregiver are essential members of the rehabilitation team.
- Patient and family education improves the likelihood of informed decision making, social adjustment, and maintenance of rehabilitation gains.
- The rehabilitation team should utilize community resources for community reintegration.
- Ongoing medical management of risk factors and comorbidites is essential to ensure survival.

A Primer on Stroke Prevention Treatment: An Overview Based on AHA/ASA Guidelines, 1st Edition. Edited by L Goldstein.
© 2009 American Heart Association, ISBN: 9781405186513

with his left arm dangling over the sidearm. During the conversation, J provided some accurate and basic information but was easily distracted and repeatedly mentioned pain while pointing to his left shoulder. J periodically provided irrelevant answers to questions and spoke with little emotional expression. J expressed a desire to get back to walking and was anxious to return home, becoming tearful during this part of the discussion.

J fell from his wheelchair on the day of the admission while trying to get up alone. Since admission, he required personal assistance with morning care and the help of one person for transfers to and from the wheelchair, bed, and toilet. He coughed during and after meals. The nursing staff noted that J was often in a great hurry to get to the bathroom and did not always make it on time.

Introduction and background

Stroke is a leading cause of long-term disability, with over 4 million individuals in the United States living with the effects of stroke [2]. Stroke can cause a variety of neurological impairments (Table 8.1), can lead to several potential complications, and may result in limitations in activities of daily living (ADLs) and quality of life. Stroke is a *chronic* disease that requires interdisciplinary coordination to provide seamless treatment across the spectrum of acute care, post-acute rehabilitation, and community-based programs.

Ten percent of stroke survivors recover almost completely, 25% recover with minor impairments, 40% experience moderate-to-severe impairments that require special care, and 10% require care in a long-term facility [2,3]. Over 60% of stroke survivors are limited in community ambulation and are at a substantial increased risk for falls and fractures [4]. Fourteen percent experience a second stroke in the first year, and rehospitalization rates are greater than 30% [2,3]. The trajectory of recovery following stroke depends on severity and is often modified by comorbid conditions (i.e., cardiac disease, preexisting cognitive impairments, and diabetes) [5].

Table 8.1 The effects of stroke

Impairments	Limitations in activities of daily living
1 Hemiparesis or hemiplegia	1 Self-care limitations (bathing, dressing, and feeding)
2 Impaired balance and coordination	2 Impaired mobility (transfers, walking)
3 Spasticity	3 Instrumental activities of daily living (cooking/cleaning, managing finances, medication management, and self-care management)
4 Sensory impairments (e.g., proprioception and touch)	
5 Visual deficits (e.g., hemianopsia)	4 Driving
6 Pain (e.g., shoulder/hand syndrome)	
7 Hemi-neglect or inattention	Quality of life (participation)
8 Apraxias	1 Social and physical role functions
9 Dysphagia (trouble swallowing)	2 Work
10 Language impairments (aphasia)	3 Leisure activities
11 Impairments of articulation (dysarthria)	
12 Problems in learning, attending, or remembering; impaired executive function	Most common post-stroke complications
13 Emotional lability	1 Aspiration pneumonia
14 Depression	2 Deep vein thrombosis
15 Bladder and bowel dysfunction	3 Falls
16 Fatigue and limited cardiovascular endurance	4 Skin breakdown
	5 Malnutrition
	6 Painful shoulder
	7 Contractures

Recovery usually plateaus around 3–6 months [6]. Whereas many stroke survivors experience recovery immediately following stroke, functional decline often occurs due to intervening comorbidities, physical inactivity, deconditioning, and social isolation [7]. Recent studies demonstrate that with specific therapies to improve the use of the upper extremity, balance, strength, and mobility, stroke survivors may experience motor recovery beyond the traditional plateau and have improved use of the upper extremity, walking, improved endurance, less depression, and better quality of life [8–10].

Stroke carries a large societal and economic burden [2]. In addition to the direct effects of stroke on individuals, millions of spouses, children, family, and friends of stroke survivors are also affected. The quality of life of these caregivers often declines, and caregiver depression is common. The direct and indirect cost of stroke care in the United States is estimated to be over $65 billion. The mean lifetime cost of ischemic stroke is over $140,000 [2]. These costs include inpatient care, rehabilitation, and follow-up care for lasting deficits. The cost of stroke is expected to escalate exponentially over the next decade with the aging of society and the inherent increased risk of stroke in the elderly.

It is extremely important that stroke survivors have access to high-quality post-acute rehabilitation programs. The goals of rehabilitation and recovery programs are to prevent complications, minimize impairments, improve function, and optimize quality of life. Care should be individualized for each person and guided by evidence-based recommendations for assessments and interventions. Substantial evidence exists that individuals do better with a well-organized multidisciplinary approach to post-acute stroke care [11]. Based on this evidence, every major stroke rehabilitation guideline recommends that individuals who are admitted to a hospital with stroke and need rehabilitation should be treated in a comprehensive or rehabilitation stroke unit by an interdisciplinary team. If no interdisciplinary team is available, consideration should be given to transferring the person with a stroke to a facility that offers interdisciplinary stroke care. After discharge from post-acute rehabilitation, stroke survivors should engage in community support and wellness programs that include physical and leisure activities.

There are several evidence-based clinical guidelines established for stroke rehabilitation and recovery [12–19]. All of the guidelines recommend similar evidence-based strategies for early access to rehabilitation care, organization of in-hospital care, and integrated community programs and services to enhance health and quality of life. The guidelines emphasize the importance of engaging the family in the patient's care as well as educating patients and their families for improved self-management. Each guideline makes similar recommendations for the management of the secondary stroke risk factors, risks of post-stroke complications, as well as strategies for the management of impairments and functional consequences of stroke. Better adherence to post-acute rehabilitation guidelines is associated with improved patient outcomes [20].

The recommendations in this primer are integrated from the following evidence-based guidelines and updated by several new sources of evidence-based interventions [10,21] and a recommended blueprint for stroke rehabilitation [22].

1 American Heart Association (AHA)/American Stroke Association Endorsed Practice Guidelines: Veteran Affairs/Department of Defense Clinical Practice Guideline for Management of Adult Stroke Rehabilitation Care http://stroke.aha.journals.org/cgi/content/full/36/9/e/100 or www.oqp.med.va.gov/cpg/STR/G/StrokeSum508.pdf
2 Canadian Stroke Strategy Best Practice for Stroke Care http://www.canadianstrokenetwork.ca/eng/tools/downloads/CSSManualENG_short.pdf
3 Australian Clinical Guidelines for Stroke Rehabilitation and Recovery www.nhmrc.gov.au/publications/synopses/cp105syn.htm
4 Stroke Canada Optimization of Rehabilitation through Evidence http://www.canadianstrokenetwork.ca/eng/tools/downloads/SCORE_EBR_Aug2307.pdf

Numerous resources are available on the Internet to guide evidence-based post-acute rehabilitation practices. The Canadian Stroke Network has made invaluable contributions to evidence-based rehabilitation practice by supporting Internet resources:

1 Evidence-Based Review of Stroke Rehabilitation www.ebrsr.com
2 StrokeEngine http://www.strokengine.org

3 Bedside Test Screens for Swallow Disorders http://swallowinglab.uhnres.utoronto.ca/order.html

Other useful resources include:

1 Montreal Cognitive Assessment http://www.mocatest.org/
2 National Institute of Health Stroke Scale http://www.nihstrokescale.org/
3 Stroke Impact Scale US English version: www2.kumc.edu/coa/SIS/Stroke-Impact-Scale.htm; international versions: www.mapi-research.fr/t_03_serv_dist_Cduse_sis.htm

The *key indicators* of the outcomes of post-acute rehabilitation and recovery should be measured at 3 months post-stroke and include [1,14]:

1 functional status (including ADLs and instrumental ADLs);
2 post-stroke complications;
3 rehospitalizations (related to the stroke or stroke-related complications);
4 community-dwelling status;
5 quality of life (Stroke Impact Scale – participation domain);
6 mortality.

Recommendations for post-acute stroke rehabilitation and recovery

Organization of post-acute rehabilitation care

Stroke rehabilitation and recovery programs should begin as soon as the patient has achieved medical stability. Care is best offered in interdisciplinary organized stroke units. Rehabilitative care can also be offered in skilled nursing facilities, in outpatient settings, and in the home. It is important that wherever care is provided that the services be comprehensive, coordinated, and delivered by clinical providers experienced in stroke management. Where interdisciplinary community rehabilitation services and caregiver support are available, early supported discharge services may be provided for those with mild-to-moderate disability.

Standardized assessments

Comprehensive standardized assessments of individuals with stroke are required for appropriate clinical management, referrals for services, discharge planning and caregiver support, and for monitoring

progress. Standardized assessments document neurological disability, levels of function, family support, and quality of life (also see Chapter 18). These assessments should be performed by members of the interdisciplinary team and each discipline should accept responsibility for using standardized assessments for its respective stroke evaluations. *Clinicians should differentiate between screening and assessment tools and use each where appropriate. When using an evaluative measure to detect change over time, clinicians should insure that the assessment is responsive to patient change. It is important to use evaluative measures at indicated times during rehabilitation to detect patient progress.*

Recommended standardized assessments are:

1 neurological impairments: National Institute of Health Stroke Scale [23];
2 dysphagia: Toronto Swallowing (TOrr-BEST) [24];
3 cognition: Cognitive Harmonization Measures [25] or Montreal Cognitive Assessment [26];
4 visual perception: the Motor Free-Visual Perception Test [27];
5 depression screen: patient health questionnaire (PHQ)-9 [28] or Geriatric Depression Scale [29];
6 motor function: Fugl-Meyer Motor [30] Assessment or Chedoke-McMaster Stroke Assessment [31];
7 balance and mobility scales: Berg Balance Scale [32], Gait Velocity [33], or Timed Up and Go [34];
8 functional status: Functional Independence Measure [35,36] or Barthel Index [37], instrumental ADLs [38,39];
9 endurance: Six-Minute Walk [40];
10 quality of life: Stroke Impact Scale [41,42].

In addition to using standardized assessments, the medical history should include assessment of comorbidities, stroke risk factors, medications, hemispatial neglect, and prior functional status. Within 24–48 hours, each patient should have screening for swallowing and risk assessments for skin breakdown, deep vein thrombosis, and falls. Social history needs to document prior living arrangement, potential discharge (home) environment, and availability of social support.

These evaluations should be used to assess the probability of outcomes, determine the most appropriate level of care, develop interventions, and establish discharge plans. The assessment findings and probability of outcomes should be shared with the patient and family. It is also critical that the results of standardized assessments be consistently integrated and available throughout the continuum of care.

Intensity and duration of therapies

There is controversy about the timing of initiation of therapy and the intensity of therapy required for stroke recovery. It is recommended that rehabilitation therapy start as early as possible, once medical stability is reached. The frequency and intensity of therapies (occupational therapy, physical therapy, speech-language pathology) in usual care are generally less than those used to establish evidence-based recovery in randomized controlled trials. The active therapy time during the usual rehabilitation session is very limited, and the intensity of activities is not consistently progressed. Currently, the intensity and duration of therapy are often driven by payment policies or challenges in the mechanisms or delivery of care. It is recommended that several strategies be considered to increase the intensity and duration of therapy care including (a) teaching family members to assist in delivery of care; (b) using therapy aids, robotics, and assistive technologies to increase therapy times; and (c) expanding the hours and availability of rehabilitation care [22]. Extending the duration (weeks or months) of care will require the development of expanded models of care that integrate medically supervised care therapists with more systematic community-based exercises and activities [22]. Adequate, well-resourced, community-based programs integrated with chronic care management and consultation by rehabilitation therapists should graduate stroke patients to self-management of their health.

Patient and family/caregiver education

Family and caregivers of individuals with stroke should be involved in all decision making and treatment planning. They should attend team meetings with rehabilitation providers with one team member identified as the primary coordinator of care and point of contact for the family. Family and caregivers should be provided with written and interactive materials that describe stroke risk, stroke impair-

ments, the nature of rehabilitation, and expected recovery. They should also receive materials about available community resources that can provide assistance, needed services, physical activity, and leisure programs for the stroke survivor *and* the caregivers. Patient and family education should be documented in the medical record to avoid conflicting recommendations from different disciplines.

Discharge planning

During post-acute rehabilitation care, the patient's primary care provider should be contacted and given the results of all assessments, expected outcomes, recommended discharge and self-management plans, provision of equipment, follow-up appointments, and availability of and recommendations for community-based services. Each patient and the primary caregiver should be given a contact person from the post-acute rehabilitation team for any follow-up.

Management of the consequences of stroke

Motor impairments

1 Progressive resistive exercise

2 Electrical stimulation in conjunction with therapeutic exercises and activities (e.g., walking)

3 Task-specific training – engage in repetitive, progressive exercises and tasks that challenge the patient to acquire motor skills by using the involved limbs during functional tasks and activities

4 Constraint-induced movement should be considered for a selected group of patients with 20 degrees of wrist extension and 10 degrees of finger extension, who do not have sensory or cognitive deficits

5 Body weight-supported treadmill training may be used in selected patients

6 Functional gait task varying surfaces, environments, inclines, steps, speeds, cadence, and dual tasks

7 Lower extremity orthotic devices should be considered if ankle or knee stabilization is needed to help the patient walk

8 Walking assistive devices should be considered to help with mobility, efficiency, and safety when needed

9 Programs should be structured to be progressive and include challenging exercises and activities

10 Group therapies, self-practice, or robot-assisted devices may provide more opportunity for practice

Spasticity

1 Prevent by positioning, range of motion, stretching, and splinting
2 Consider use of tizanidine or baclofen for spasticity that results in pain, poor skin hygiene, or decreased function
3 Use of botulinum toxin, phenol/alcohol neurolysis, or intrathecal baclofen should be considered for selected patients with most disabling or painful spasticity

Range of motion and shoulder pain/subluxation

1 Do not use overhead pulleys
2 Bed positioning to prevent shoulder impingement
3 Modalities: ice and soft tissue massage
4 Gentle stretching and mobilization, self-range of motion
5 For shoulder range of motion and pain, focus on external rotation and abduction for 90 degrees
6 Educate patient, caregiver, and staff to provide support for a subluxated shoulder during activities
7 External support for hemiplegic upper extremity during mobility and transfers
8 Reduction of hand edema; active range of motion in conjunction with elevation, or pressure garments
9 Functional electrical stimulation

Sensory training

1 Sensory-specific training and cutaneous electrical stimulation may be considered. For hemianopsia, patients should be taught compensatory scanning techniques. Prism glasses may be used to improve visual function in people with homonymous hemianopsia, but there is no evidence of a benefit in ADL function.

ADLs (self-care and mobility)

1 Occupational and physical therapy programs to train and practice self-care activities (i.e., dressing, bathing, feeding)
2 Practice specific mobility tasks (rolling, come to sit, transfer, sit to stand, walk)

Cardiovascular fitness (endurance)

1 Include interventions to increase cardiovascular fitness once individuals have sufficient strength in the lower limb muscle groups and have been evaluated for exercise tolerance. The exercise evaluation and interventions should follow the recommendations established by the AHA Guidelines on Physical Activity Post-Stroke [43].

Dysphagia

1 Each stroke patient's swallowing should be assessed
2 Keep all patients NPO (nothing per oral intake) until a healthcare professional trained to administer and interpret a simple, valid, bedside protocol screens patient for swallowing difficulty
3 Consider enteral feeding for the stroke patient who is unable to maintain adequate oral nutrition
4 Consider feeding tube
5 Swallowing treatment and management by speech and language pathologist when a treatable disorder in swallow anatomy of physiology is identified

Bowel and bladder function

1 Incontinence is a major burden and should be managed using an organized functional approach. Routine use of indwelling catheter is not recommended. However, if urinary retention is severe, then intermittent catherization should be used. For individuals with urge incontinence, a prompted voiding regime program and bladder training should be considered.
2 Constipation and fecal impaction are more common after stroke than bowel incontinence. Goals of management are to ensure adequate intake of fluid, bulk, and fiber, and to help the patient establish a regular toileting routine. Stool softeners and judicious use of laxatives may be useful.

Communication

1 Patients with communication disorders should receive early treatment and monitoring of change in communication abilities in order to optimize the recovery of communication skills, to develop useful compensatory strategies when needed, and to facilitate improvements in functional communication.

2 Speech and language pathologists should educate the rehabilitation staff and family/caregivers in techniques to enhance communication with patients who have communication disorders.

3 Interventions may include treatment of phonological and semantic deficits following models derived from cognitive neuropsychology, constraint-induced therapy, and the use of gesture.

4 Patients may be considered for group therapy.

5 Volunteers (including family or staff) trained in supported conversation techniques may be useful.

6 Patients with severe aphasia may benefit from augmentative and alternative communication devices used in functional activities.

Depression

1 All patients with stroke should be considered to be at high risk for depression. There should be an assessment of patients' prior history of depression, and they should be screened for depression using a validated tool.

2 Once diagnosed, the treatment of depression and other emotional disorders can improve rehabilitation outcomes. If not contraindicated, treatment with psychotherapy and or pharmacotherapy can stabilize mood and improve ability to participate in therapies. Patients should be given the opportunity to participate in support groups and the opportunity to talk about their illness and impact of stroke on their lives.

Cognitive deficits

1 Cognitive deficits after stroke are common and heterogeneous. All patients should be screened for cognitive impairments using validated screening tools. Screening should establish a patient's cognitive status in domains including arousal, alertness, attention, orientation, memory, language, agnosia, visual–spatial/perceptual function, praxis, and executive function.

2 Patients who demonstrate cognitive impairments should be referred to professionals with specific expertise in the areas of cognitive function and intervention strategies. Rehabilitation should be tailored to the cognitive impairments identified. Attention training may have a positive effect on targeted outcomes; compensatory strategies may be used to improve memory and apraxia.

Community reintegration

The post-discharge period is consistently reported by patients and their families to be difficult. The patients and their families lose social and emotional support. Patients are at high risk for a recurrent stroke, falls, fractures, and functional decline. Patients and their families should be made aware of community-based outpatient rehabilitation programs, day programs, support groups, and centers for physical and social activity programs. Several studies establish that patients can continue to improve their balance, strength, and endurance with progressive and well-developed exercise programs. In some patients, motor and functional recovery may also continue with highly repetitive training programs, such as constraint-induced movement.

The AHA has developed guidelines for Physical Activity and Exercise for Post-Stroke Survivors [43]. These guidelines provide specific recommendations for evaluation of patients for post-stroke aerobic exercise and have made the recommendations for exercise programs. The reader is referred to the following site to download the recommendations for preexercise evaluation and the summary of exercise recommendations for stroke survivors (http://circ. ahajournals.org/cgi/content/full/109/16/2031).

Because stroke patients who return to the community are at an increased risk of falls, they should be assessed for a history of falls and risk for falls on visits to their primary care physician. The falls risk assessment may be guided by the American Geriatrics Society for Guidelines for Falls Prevention in the Elderly [44]. The Canadian Stroke Best Practice Guidelines recommend for follow-up and community reintegration after stroke that:

1 Stroke survivors and their caregivers should have their individual psychosocial and support needs reviewed on a regular basis.

2 Any stroke survivor with reduced activity at 6 months or later after stroke should be assessed for appropriate targeted rehabilitation.

3 People living in the community who have difficulty with ADLs should have access as appropriate to therapy services to improve or prevent deterioration in ADL.

4 Stroke survivors should continue to be screened and managed for depression.

Patient example, continued: best practice assessments, interventions, and plans

J was in good health, active, and socially engaged prior to his stroke. He has good social support from his wife and child. He presented with the most common risk factor for stroke – hypertension. Otherwise, his prior medical history was unremarkable. He had a severe stroke with dense hemiplegia and a risk of subluxation and a painful left shoulder. He presents with symptoms of dysphagia and has cognitive impairments, left visual–spatial neglect, an attention deficit, impulsiveness, memory problems, and a hemianopsia. His psychological symptoms include flat affect, anxiety, and most likely depression.

Because J has severe motor deficits (including lack of wrist extension and individual finger movements), sensory impairments, as well as visual–spatial neglect, the prognosis is that J will not experience full recovery of function. His recovery will occur over months and will need to be sustained by continued physical and social activities. Depression could also modify recovery and decrease the trajectory of functional recovery. Good family support will contribute to the likelihood that J can be discharged home from inpatient rehabilitation. J is also at risk for several post-stroke complications. Dysphagia can lead to malnutrition and aspiration. Limited mobility can lead to pressure ulcers in sitting and in deep vein thrombosis. J is at high risk of falling, which could cause further injury, fear of falling, and fractures. J is also at risk for recurrent stroke. Currently, J is dependent in ADLs, including the need for assistance with toilet transfers, bed transfers, and morning care. He is walking with maximal assistance and has significant difficulty using a self-propelling wheelchair. J's spouse is concerned about managing at home after discharge, and the family is unsure of what to expect.

J's care should be managed by a multidisciplinary team. Better clinical outcomes will be achieved if his post-acute rehabilitation and recovery care are coordinated and organized. J will need a multidisciplinary team including a physician, nurse, physical therapist, occupational therapist, speech language pathologist, neuropsychologist, and social worker. One of the members of the team should assume the primary case management role and be a liaison between the rehabilitation team, the family, and J's primary care physician. The manager should assist the family in coordinating any future care and identify community-based resources.

Appropriate clinical management and selection of interventions should be guided by comprehensive assessments. The assessments should include well-validated, standardized assessments to document J's neurological condition, levels of disability, family support, quality of life, and progress over time. J should be screened for depression and motor, sensory, cognitive, communication, and swallowing deficits by appropriately trained clinicians from the multidisciplinary team. Standardized assessments that should be performed during the rehabilitation admission are listed in Table 8.2. The results of the standardized assessments should be used to assess the probability of J's outcome, to determine the appropriate level of care and to develop interventions (also see Chapter 18). The assessment findings and expected outcomes should be discussed with J, his family, and his primary care provider. In addition to these primary assessments, J should receive a comprehensive language evaluation by speech and language pathologists and neuropsychological assessments to more explicitly assess his communication and executive functions. The most challenging symptoms for J and his family on his returning home will be his impaired cognitive function. Comprehensive assessment of cognition will assist the family in understanding these deficits and adapting to J's new functional status.

J's spouse is concerned about managing at home after his discharge. The case manager should interview the spouse and children to assess available social support, insurance and finances available to support continued therapies, transportation, and assistants to aid in the home. The interview should include an assessment of the home to identify any modifications or equipment required prior to discharge. The family needs to be included in all decision-making processes for J's care and needs to understand all of the options for discharge care. The family also needs to be informed about available support services when J returns home. All members of the rehabilitation team need to be aware and supportive of the family as they go through this difficult transition. Caregiver stress may be decreased by a social worker or case manager regularly evaluating

Table 8.2 Standardized assessments

Standardized assessment	Measures
National Institutes of Health Stroke Scale [23]	**1** Assesses stroke severity and predicts likelihood of recovery **2** Should be administered at the time of hospital admission or within 24 hours of start of stroke **3** Scale should be repeated at the time of acute care discharge and results available or repeated at admission to rehabilitation facility
Montreal Cognitive Assessment (MoCA) [26]	The MoCA is a cognitive screening test designed to assist health professionals for the detection of mild cognitive impairment. It is more sensitive in detecting mild cognitive impairment than the Mini Mental State Examination.
Fugl-Meyer [45]	Measures upper and lower extremity motor and sensory impairment. It "assesses the ability to move the arm and its segments selectively as well as sensation and passive joint mobility with an array of qualitatively rated items."
Grip strength [46]	Hand strength
Berg Balance Scale [32]	Assesses static and dynamic posture as well as helps determine risk for falling
Wolf Motor Function Test [9]	Assesses upper-extremity function and improvement in stroke patients
Ten-Meter Walk Test [33]	Assesses and measures change in the patient's speed of walking
Six-Minute Walk Test [40]	Assesses and measures endurance
Standardized swallowing assessment [24]	Toronto Bedside Swallow
Geriatric Depression Scale [29]	Screens patient for depression
Pain	Visual Analog Scale: 0–10
Line Bisection Test [47]	A screening tool for the presence of unilateral neglect
Motor Free-Visual Perception Test [27]	Perceptual tasks include spatial relationships, visual discrimination, figure–ground, visual closure, and visual memory. Performance in these areas provides a single score that represents the individual's general visual perceptual ability.
Functional Independence Measure	Assesses and measures changes in patient's functional status

family needs, introducing them to community-based programs prior to discharge and communication with J's primary care provider.

Short-term interdisciplinary goals for J include:

1 improve swallowing;
2 decreased frequency of urinary incontinence;
3 controlled hypertension;
4 improved cognition and communication;
5 decreased depressive symptoms;
6 decrease caregiver stress;

7 implementation of prevention plans to:
   • prevent skin breakdown;
   • prevent deep vein thrombosis;
   • implement secondary prevention of recurrent stroke;
   • prevent shoulder pain and limitations in range of motion;
   • prevent falls;
8 independence in basic ADLs;
9 supervised gait, increased walking velocity, and improved endurance for walking;

Table 8.3 Best practice recommendations for interventions

Problem	Recommended best practice guideline
Left upper-extremity motor weakness	• Initiate range of motion, strengthening program, position arm in view of patients • Assess patient as candidate for constraint-induced movement therapy
Left lower-extremity motor weakness	• Functional strengthening training • Assess patient as candidate for body weight-supported treadmill training (include assessment of cardiovascular function prior to participating)

Shoulder pain	• Task-specific gait training
	  ○ ROM – lateral rotation and assisted ROM in pain-free range. Do not move the shoulder above 90 degrees of flexion and abduction unless the scapula is upwardly rotated.
	  ○ Positioning and protection of the limb during functional tasks
	  ○ Avoid the use of overhead pulleys
	  ○ Educate staff and family to protect the shoulder
	  ○ Modalities: ice, heat, massage
	  ○ Strengthening of shoulder muscle groups
	  ○ Physician may need to prescribe analgesics

Sensory loss (left UE and LE)	• Use sensory stimulation to regain sensation
Visual/spatial neglect	• Need to differentiate between visual field deficits and attention deficits • Evaluate for neglect using standardized assessments • If neglect is present, suggest treatment to teach patient to manage with the neglect. This includes visual scanning, adapting the environment, and educating the patient and family. • Cognitive retraining is indicated (visual–spatial rehabilitation)
Dysphagia	• Recommend swallow assessment using the Toronto Swallow Assessment (TOrr-BEST) • If abnormal, refer to SLP for evaluation for prevention of aspiration (which could lead to aspiration pneumonia) • Video fluoroscopy swallowing study or a modified barium swallow study may be performed. • Consult dietetics if patient will require a special food consistency
Cognitive impairment (attention, neglect, flat affect)	• Assess learning, memory, attention, visual neglect, apraxia, problem solving • Recommend cognitive retraining/compensation
Dependence in ADLs/IADLs	• Functional mobility training, rolling, transfers, wheelchair mobility, dressing, hygiene, etc. • Recommend adaptive technology for safety and function • Assess safety awareness, medicine management, and meal preparation
Decreased walking speed/severe gait impairment	• Task-specific mobility training, which incorporates functional strengthening, balance and aerobic exercises, and practice on a variety of walking tasks on different walking surfaces and in different environments • A combination of task-specific training with a and treadmill training may be optimal. • Assess for use of assistive devices/orthoses
Falls risk	• Assess with Berg Balance Test • History and conditions of falls • Balance training, including walking under conditions of divided attention
Communication impairment	• Refer to SLP for assessment and treatment • Assess listening, speaking, reading, writing, pragmatics • Follow up for long-term communication difficulties
Caregiver stress	• Patient and caregiver education/train caregiver to assist patient • Evaluate needs • Refer to social worker • Provide support and community resources assessment • Share assessment findings and expected outcomes with family/caregivers • Family conference

Table 8.3 *Continued*

Problem	Recommended best practice guideline
Risk for skin breakdown	• The patient is at risk for skin breakdown because of decreased mobility.
	• Skin integrity should be monitored daily.
	• Proper attention must be paid to turning and positioning if patient has poor bed mobility.
Risk for DVT	• Patient should be mobilized as soon as much as possible (out of bed, sitting, standing, and walking).
	• Compression stockings
	• Recommend use of subcutaneous low-dose unfractionated heparin
Risk for malnutrition	• Patient is at risk for malnutrition due to swallowing problems.
	• Consult dietetics to develop a healthy diet based on necessary food consistencies as recommended by SLP and assist with feeding if necessary.
Urinary incontinence	• Frequent, prompted voiding schedule
Recurrent stroke risk	• Patient and family counseling to identify signs and symptoms of stroke
	• Recommend programs to maintain and increase physical activity and healthy diet
Risk for depression	• Routine screening for depression
	• Refer out for a comprehensive psychosocial assessment
	• Include families and caregivers in the process
Hypertension	• Check blood pressure (desired BP 130/90)
	• Re-evaluate medications used to control hypertension
	• Recommend exercise/physical activity
Patient/family education	• StrokEngine at www.strokengine.org is a very valuable educational tool for the patient and family. The family could be provided the link so they can research all of the information for family and caregivers on their own.
	• The patient and family should be educated and be made aware of all safety precautions that need to be taken for J.
	• Hold a family conference with the rehabilitation team
	• Provide patient with educational materials and identify someone who can be a point of contact for questions and concerns. Education is more effective when it can be an interactive process.
	• Family should be included in therapy sessions and learn how to safely assist the patient with activities.
	• Re-educate the family about the warning signs of stroke, and advise to seek immediate medical care in the presence of new stroke symptoms
	• Document the education that takes place.
Referral and care coordination with primary care physician within 30 days	• Address stroke risk factors, diet and exercise, hypertension control, risk for depression; recommend community rehabilitation programs as well as community-based activity programs, and stroke support groups, access to support services/community transportation or senior citizen activities.
	• Provide the history of rehabilitation management, expected outcomes, and recommendations for continued care to the primary care physician. Provide the primary care physician the name of J's rehabilitation case manager as a point of contact.

ADLs, activities of daily living; DVT, deep vein thrombosis; IADLs, instrumental activities of daily living; LE, lower extremity; ROM, range of motion; SLP, speech language pathology; UE, upper extremity.

10 improve safety awareness and decrease falls risk;

11 motor recovery of the upper and lower extremity.

The long-term expectation for J is that he will return home with the support of his family. He is not expected to have a full recovery. He will adapt to the consequences of stroke and be independent in ADLs and home ambulation. He will become engaged in community-based physical and social activity programs and return to some leisure activities. J is not likely to be able to drive again or be fully independent in instrumental ADLs (e.g., manage finances, cook, clean, yard work) (Table 8.3).

To optimize recovery, J will require intensive and progressive exercise and training programs. The intensity with which stroke rehabilitation therapies are provided is correlated with the rate of recovery post-stroke. Highly repetitive practice and careful monitoring of direct therapy time are required to ensure that J is continuously engaged in interactive therapy. The use of therapy aides, robotic devices, and assistive technologies could be used to increase exposure to practice. Families and caregivers should be involved in therapy sessions and instructed in methods to encourage practice and utilization of new skills. Endurance for therapies should be increased and determined by heart rate, blood pressure, or Borg exertion scales.

J will require continued outpatient therapies after discharge and engagement in community-based activity programs. In addition to individualized therapy programs with physical therapy, occupational therapy, and speech and language, well-resourced, community-based adaptive exercise programs should be recommended. These programs integrate social support, with physical activity, and training in instrumental ADLs to support continued recovery and to improve quality of life. Collaborating with Area Agency on Aging Programs and Senior Citizen Programs could be a low-cost method to provide ongoing physical activity.

The success of the rehabilitation and recovery programs for J should be periodically assessed using the Stroke Impact Scale. This self-report or proxy report instrument will capture J's recovery of upper extremity and lower extremity function, communication, emotional well-being, mobility, ADLs, and instrument ADLs, as well as participation. The Stroke Impact Scale can be administered within 1 month post-stroke and at follow-up 3, 6, or 1 year post-stroke. Due to the high incidence of falls in stroke survivors living in the community, history of falls and falls risk should be evaluated at each primary care visit and subsequent recommendations made to manage and reduce the risk of falls. Ongoing community-based care must include continued monitoring and management of J's hypertension and screening and management of depressive symptoms.

There are substantial improvements in outcomes from well-organized, intensive acute rehabilitation programs. Stroke is, however, a chronic disease, and there is ever-growing evidence that individuals can continue to experience recovery beyond the initial 3 months. Community-based programs integrated with rehabilitation programs are needed to decrease the probability of functional decline post-recovery and to ensure better fitness and improved quality of life for J. Adherence to post-stroke rehabilitation guidelines will maximize his independence and quality of life.

Acknowledgement

The Duke University Doctor of Physical Therapy Class of 2009 made contributions to the development of recommendations for assessments and interventions for the clinical case.

References available online at www.wiley.com/go/ strokeguidelines.

Part II

Special Topics

Stroke in Women

Cheryl D. Bushnell

EXAMPLE CASE

A 48-year-old right-handed woman was seen in consultation for evaluation of a stroke. Three months earlier, she had the acute onset of unsteadiness, difficulty in walking, vertigo, and vomiting. The patient was initially seen by her cardiologist because of a concern that she was having a heart attack. This evaluation was negative for an acute myocardial infarction, and she was sent home. The symptoms persisted, however, and she was seen by her primary care provider who then ordered a head CT. This revealed a subacute left cerebellar ischemic stroke, and she was subsequently admitted to a local hospital. After a thorough evaluation, no underlying cause for her stroke was identified, and she was referred to a neurologist for a second opinion.

Six years earlier, while feeding her 6-month-old baby, the patient had had an episode of left-sided weakness that resolved after a couple of hours. Three years later, she had an episode of unsteadiness, gait

MAJOR POINTS

- Women have a lifetime risk of stroke of 20% and represent 60% of stroke deaths.
- Recognition of an acute stroke in women may be challenging because they are more likely to present with nontraditional symptoms, such as pain, change in level of consciousness, disorientation, or other nonspecific symptoms.
- Women may be less likely to receive thrombolytic therapy because they are less willing to accept the risks associated with this treatment. Therefore, women require more information about the risks and benefits prior to consenting to receive thrombolytic therapy than men.
- Natural menopause is associated with depletion in estrogen levels and a subsequent worsening of cardiovascular risk factors, such as increased blood pressure, blood glucose, and lipid levels, as well as abdominal obesity.
- Preeclampsia and gestational hypertension are associated with an increased risk of hypertension, stroke, and cardiovascular disease later in life. Therefore, screening for cardiovascular risk factors in these women represents an opportunity to recognize risk earlier and emphasize prevention.
- Following stroke, women are more likely than men to have poor functional status, especially related to quality of life, ability to perform activities of daily living, and depression.
- Physical activity is an important risk factor for initial stroke in women, and exercise nomograms have been developed to guide exercise counseling for women.

A Primer on Stroke Prevention Treatment: An Overview Based on AHA/ASA Guidelines, 1st Edition. Edited by L Goldstein.
© 2009 American Heart Association, ISBN: 9781405186513

imbalance, vertigo, and right-sided weakness. With this episode, she presented to the emergency department, but by the time she was seen, most of the symptoms had resolved. The patient has a past medical history significant for severe preeclampsia during her second pregnancy, which required bed rest for 70 days. She may have had elevated blood pressures during her third pregnancy as well. She also has a history of hypertension and depression. She admitted to frequent hot flashes and an increased frequency of her menstrual cycles, which occur about every 2 weeks.

Her mother had a stroke at age 46, and died of a myocardial infarction at age 71. Her sister has a history of deep venous thrombosis. She does not smoke cigarettes and has only occasional alcohol use. Medications include clopidogrel 75 mg daily, aspirin 81 mg daily, candesartan 8 mg daily, and escitalopram 10 mg daily.

Physical examination

Well-appearing woman who weighs 176.4 lbs, with a blood pressure of 116/77 mm Hg and a regular pulse of 67 bpm. There were no carotid bruits, lungs were clear to auscultation, and heart was regular rate and rhythm. Dorsalis pedis and radial pulses were both 2+.

Neurological examination

The patient was alert and oriented to person, place, time, and situation. She gave a clear history, her speech was fluent, and her language was normal. The remainder of the mental status testing was unremarkable. Cranial nerves were intact with the exception of decreased sensation to pin prick on the left face involving V1, V2, and V3 distributions. Motor exam revealed normal bulk and tone, and intact strength without any pronator drift. Sensory exam showed decreased sensation to all modalities on the left arm and leg compared with the right. On coordination testing, she had mild dysmetria in the left arm and leg, as well as clumsy rapid alternating movements on the left. Gait testing showed a broad-based and unsteady gait, both with casual and tandem walking. Romberg was positive. Her reflexes were 2+, and symmetric and plantar responses were flexor.

Imaging studies

Magnetic resonance imaging of the brain revealed a left cerebellar infarction in the distribution of the posterior inferior cerebellar artery (PICA). CT angiography showed no evidence of vertebral dissection but moderate stenosis of the mid and distal left PICA. Transthoracic echocardiogram with microcavitation showed no evidence of right to left shunting.

Laboratory studies

Complete blood count, electrolytes, glycosylated hemoglobin, and lipid panel were all unremarkable. Thrombophilia screening studies including anticardiolipin antibodies, lupus anticoagulant, anti beta-glycoprotein-I antibodies, homocysteine, lipoprotein (a), and activated protein C resistance were all unremarkable. Polymerase chain reaction testing for heritable thrombophilias revealed a heterozygous prothrombin gene mutation (20210 GA genotype).

Epidemiology of stroke in women

Stroke is a major public health problem. In the year 2005, there were 780,000 new or recurrent strokes in the United States, 420,000 of which were in women [1]. The sex differences in stroke prevalence seem to differ based on age. Black and white women have lower prevalence than men until age 65, as shown by female-to-male prevalence ratios (Figure 9.1) from the Reasons for Geographic and Racial Differences in Stroke Study [2]. However, the burden of stroke in women is most distressing when we examine mortality. Of the 150,000 stroke deaths in 2004, 91,000 were women, or 60% of the total [1].

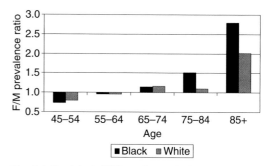

Fig. 9.1 Female/male (F/M) prevalence ratios for stroke by age. From the Reasons for Geographic and Racial Differences in Stroke Study [2]. Previously unpublished and courtesy of personal communication with George Howard, PhD.

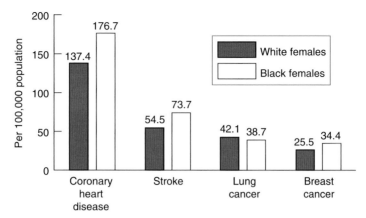

Fig. 9.2 Age-adjusted death rates for coronary heart disease, stroke, and lung and breast cancers for white and black females in the United States: 2001.

This is most probably because women live longer, and the likelihood of dying from stroke increases with age. In addition, it is important to note that twice as many women die from stroke than breast cancer (Figure 9.2). Given that the lifetime risk of stroke is nearly 20% in women [3], reducing the burden of stroke will require an improvement in the processes of evaluation, prevention, and post-stroke care.

Evaluation of stroke in women

In hindsight, the woman described earlier may have been having transient ischemic attacks (TIAs) in the years leading up to her stroke. This would have been an opportunity to perform a full evaluation for possible etiologies, and perhaps improve upon her risk factor management to reduce her risk of stroke. In addition, there was a delay in the diagnosis of her stroke by several days, despite seeking medical attention. This may have been due to a lack of recognition of stroke symptoms on the part of the patient and the initial treating physician.

There are several studies suggesting that women and men with acute stroke can present with different types of symptoms, which could therefore impact the acute stroke evaluation. The TLL Temple Foundation Stroke Project showed that women were 62% more likely than men to present with nontraditional stroke symptoms (pain, change in level of consciousness–disorientation, and unclassifiable neurological and

nonspecific symptoms), even after the adjustment for age (odds ratio [OR] 1.62; 95% confidence interval [CI] 1.2–2.2) [4]. Other cohorts have compared presenting stroke symptoms in men and women and found no differences, but only the traditional stroke symptoms of numbness, weakness, visual deficits, or language were evaluated without specific questions related to nontraditional symptoms. Therefore, it is important to keep in mind that women with nontraditional or nonspecific symptoms may indeed be experiencing a stroke.

Several studies have suggested that women receive fewer diagnostic tests for the evaluation of acute stroke than men. For example, the Brain Attack in Corpus Christi study showed that women were 36% less likely to receive either transthoracic and/or transesophageal echocardiography (OR 0.64; 95% CI 0.42–0.98) and 53% less likely to receive any carotid imaging (OR 0.57; 0.36–0.91) than men [5]. This difference was present even after the adjustment for confounders such as age, ethnicity, stroke risk factors, affiliation with a primary care provider, disability at discharge, and insurance status. Similarly, a multicenter registry from Europe reported that women were less likely than men to receive echocardiography (23% vs. 31% in men), carotid Doppler (33% vs. 44%), and cerebral angiography (5.5% vs. 9.5%), even after the adjustment for age [6]. A separate study of utilization of cerebral angiography and carotid endarterectomy in a US state-wide database revealed that women were less likely to receive either procedure. The best explanation for this disparity, however, was that women were less likely to have strokes attributed to carotid disease, which suggested that biological differences in anatomy and stroke etiology led to the observed patterns of testing and treatment [7].

Women may be less likely than men to receive thrombolytic therapy (tissue-type plasminogen activator [tPA]) for acute stroke. This was shown in a stroke registry from Michigan [8] as well as a very large administrative database (Nationwide Inpatient Sample) [9]. However, an analysis of the Canadian Stroke Network [10], a database of 84 academic medical centers (University Health Systems Consortium) [11], and the National Hospital Discharge Survey [12] showed no difference in tPA administration by sex. A recent single-center study from Canada focused specifically on gender differences in all aspects of the stroke evaluation, and acute treatment showed that 61 of 1149 (5%) women received tPA versus 109 of 1244 (9%) men. This difference remained significant even after adjusting for confounding variables of age, pre-stroke functional status, atrial fibrillation, stroke severity, anatomical stroke location, and presentation within 3 hours of symptom recognition (OR 0.55; 95% CI 0.38–0.80; $P = 0.002$) [13]. Although there is a clear variability in whether gender differences exist, these data indicate that women may be less likely to receive tPA than men.

There are a few possible explanations for this observation. The most important may be related to patient preferences. A survey of patient preferences for stroke treatment was administered to men and women with and without a history of prior stroke residing in Ontario, Canada [14]. The results of the survey demonstrated that women (79%) were less likely to consent to receiving tPA than men (86%; $P = 0.014$) and were less certain about this decision. Women were also more likely to express fear about the risks involved with this treatment and the need for more information about the risks than men. Women, however, were just as likely as men to consent to carotid endarterectomy [14]. Therefore, in some situations, women who are candidates for tPA may be reluctant to consent because of the risks and the lack of reassurance about the benefits of this treatment. Another reason why women may not receive tPA as frequently as men is because they are older and have more comorbidities that may appear to increase the risks of treatment. Whether fewer women are actually eligible for tPA than men because of older age and frailty is not clear, but these factors could influence decision making. Understanding this gender disparity of treatment with tPA is very important because women receive even more benefits from the treatment with tPA than men and, otherwise, have a very poor outcome after stroke compared with men [15].

The guidelines for tPA treatment and other issues pertaining to the management of acute stroke have been clearly outlined in the American Heart Association/American Stroke Association (AHA/ASA) guidelines [16]. Although there are observed gender differences in stroke symptoms and risk factor profiles, these guidelines provide comprehensive tools to effectively manage stroke patients, regardless of gender, in the acute setting.

Secondary prevention of stroke in women

Long-term treatment for stroke prevention is frequently guided by an understanding of stroke etiology. Because the example patient had no cardioembolic or large-vessel source for her stroke, she underwent extensive hematological testing to evaluate for a thrombophilia. In this patient's case, she was tested for inherited prothrombotic conditions and was found to be heterozygous for the prothrombin gene mutation (20210 GA genotype). Although these mutations are more commonly uncovered in patients with venous thrombosis, there appears to be no association with arterial thromboembolism in unselected patients [17]. A systematic review found a significant association between this mutation and stroke only in patients with strokes that occur before the age of 50 [18]. Therefore, there were no clear data to suggest that the presence of this mutation contributed to the etiology of this patient's stroke; but the combination of hypertension and a strong family history in addition to this mutation may have synergistically increased her risk.

There is uncertainty about the choice of antithrombotic therapy for preventing recurrent stroke following the diagnosis of a thromobophilia such as the prothrombin gene mutation. Assessing the risk of recurrent stroke in a patient with thrombophilia requires an echocardiogram with microcavitation to evaluate for a patent foramen ovale (PFO). If a patient has a deep vein thrombosis (DVT), a PFO with right-to-left shunting (i.e., paradoxical embolism), then the treatment should include anticoagulation according to the guidelines for treatment of an acute DVT [19]. Studies have shown, however, that the risk of recurrent DVT in patients with prothrombin gene mutation is the same as in patients without the mutation, and therefore that lifelong anticoagulation is not recommended [20]. Lifelong treatment with warfarin post-stroke in a patient who possesses the prothrombin gene mutation is not likely to be necessary, but this decision should be individualized.

Detailed and evidence-based approaches to secondary prevention of stroke and TIA were comprehensively reviewed in the most recent update of the AHA/ASA secondary prevention guidelines [21]. These recommendations are generalizable to men and women. Pertinent to the topic at hand, the most recent update on cardiovascular prevention in women outlines the evidence and strategies that are specific to women. Secondary prevention with antiplatelet therapy is recommended for high-risk patients (as in our case) in both sets of guidelines. Treatment for specific risk factors will be covered individually later.

Risk factors for stroke in women

This case highlights several risk factors that are unique to women, and others that may be more common in women than men. The epidemiology of stroke prevalence has shown that women in our patient's age group (under age 50) are generally considered to have a lower incidence and prevalence of stroke than men [1]. Recent data from the National Health and Nutrition Examination Survey, however, has shown that women are having a more substantial increase in the prevalence of stroke in midlife versus men. In this analysis, women aged 45–54 had a higher odds of stroke compared with men of the same age (OR 2.39; 95% CI: 1.32–4.32) [22]. Consistent with the surge in stroke events, there was also a surge in cardiovascular risk in women greater than in men. For instance, systolic blood pressure increased at a steeper rate in women with each decade from 35 to 44 years (average SBP 113.9 mm Hg),

45–54 years (average SBP 123.5 mm Hg), and 55–64 years (average SBP 132.0 mm Hg) [22]. Men, however, initially had a higher SBP between the ages of 35 and 44 (average SBP 120.0 mm Hg), but there was a more gradual increase to the ages of 55–64 (average SBP 128.6 mm Hg). In addition, women had a substantial increase in total cholesterol, triglycerides, waist circumference, homocysteine, and glycosylated hemoglobin, and a lowering of the ankle brachial pulsatility index, between the cohort aged 45–54 and those aged 55–64 [22]. These data suggest that there is an acceleration of multiple risk parameters in women a decade or more before cardiovascular and stroke events traditionally occur. Assuming these data are valid, there is a significant opportunity to increase the efforts to recognize the risk factors in women during midlife and improve prevention strategies.

Menopause

The midlife prevalence of stroke in women may be related to the menopausal transition that occurs naturally in women with at least one intact and functioning ovary. During perimenopause, estradiol levels decline by about 60% [23]. After menopause, estradiol levels continue to decline but then plateau after 1–3 years. Overall, there is a 7- to 10-fold decrease in estradiol levels between pre- and postmenopause [24]. In contrast to the rapid decline in estradiol, circulating testosterone levels are decreasing more gradually during this period [25], leading to a relative androgen excess [25]. Postmenopause, circulating androgens aromatized to estrogens may be the only source of estradiol, and thus, variations in estrogens parallel that of androgens [25,26].

The menopausal shifts in hormonal levels and ratios of estrogens to androgens are important because these sex steroids appear to have opposite effects on vascular risk. Estrogens have multiple beneficial effects on the cardiovascular system, including improving vasodilation and arterial compliance [27] by decreasing cerebral vascular tone and increasing cerebral blood flow [28]. The physiological basis for this is that estrogen facilitates production and sensitivity to vasodilatory factors, most importantly, endothelial nitric oxide synthase (eNOS). Interestingly, progestins and testosterone have no effect on levels of cerebrovascular eNOS protein [29]. In addition, estrogen has protective effects on cerebral endothelial cells by increasing the efficiency of mitochondrial energy production while decreasing free radical production, and enhancing endothelial cell survival [29,30].

In addition to anti-inflammatory and antioxidant effects, estrogen may also reduce atherosclerotic risk through its impact on lipids. Exogenous estrogen replacement improves lipid profiles by lowering total and low-density lipoprotein (LDL) cholesterol, lipoprotein (a), and raising high-density lipoprotein (HDL) cholesterol [31,32].

Conversely, androgens have a detrimental effect on cerebral blood vessels by increasing arterial tone. They also lead to a pro-atherogenic profile by decreasing HDL and by increasing triglycerides, LDL, and total cholesterol [25].

Concurrent with the decline in sex steroids, women develop changes in cardiovascular risk factors during menopause. Lipid measurements in women across the menopausal transition in the Healthy Women Study showed that LDL cholesterol and triglycerides increased and HDL cholesterol decreased during perimenopause, whereas fasting glucose and blood pressure levels increased during postmenopause [33]. Along with a change in body fat distribution toward abdominal obesity, the lipid, blood pressure, and glucose changes are consistent with metabolic syndrome. Some menopausal experts have argued that the changes that occur from estrogen deficiency during menopause justifies the use of the term "menopausal metabolic syndrome" [34]. In addition to the metabolic changes, estrogen deficiency during menopause also leads to a shift from anti-inflammatory to pro-inflammatory cytokines such as IL-1β, IL-6, and TNF-α [35]. These cytokines are important because they have been associated with an increased risk of heart disease and stroke [36].

To determine the significance of the increased cardiovascular risk profile associated with the menopausal transition, subclinical vascular disease has been measured and compared between pre- and postmenopausal women. For example, carotid intimal medial thickness was increased and plaque prevalence was higher in postmenopausal women compared with premenopausal women [37]. There are also changes in cerebrovascular blood flow. One study of cerebral vasomotor reserve assessed the use of transcranial Doppler measurement of blood flow

velocity in the setting of breath holding to induce hypercapnia [38]. Compared with premenopausal women and men at all ages, postmenopausal women had a large reduction in vasomotor reactivity, suggesting a poorer response to cerebrovascular stress [38]. Whether this observed difference between men and women is due to estradiol levels is unknown.

Although decreased vasomotor reserve has been associated with an increased risk of stroke in patients with carotid stenosis, it is unknown whether this is associated with stroke risk in the absence of extracranial or intracranial vessel stenosis. The evidence for cardiovascular risk increasing during and after menopause, however, suggests that it is during this transition that women should be followed most closely in order to recognize and optimally treat these risk factors to prevent stroke.

Hormone therapy

Replacing the depletion of endogenous estradiol with replacement hormone therapy was widely believed to be an effective method to reduce cardiovascular disease in women. Randomized trials of hormone therapy (specifically, conjugated equine estrogens [CEEs], CEE with medroxyprogesterone acetate, and 17-beta estradiol), however, showed no benefit for the secondary prevention of heart disease [39] and stroke [40], as well as an increased risk of both types of events in healthy women (Women's Health Initiative [WHI]) [41]. In an attempt to investigate why hormone therapy increased the risk for cardiovascular disease in the WHI, events were analyzed based on the time of initiation following menopause. This post hoc analysis showed that there was a trend toward a reduction in the risk for heart disease among women who initiated HT within 5 years of menopause [42]. In contrast, the risk of stroke with HT was increased regardless of the timing of initiation [42]. The importance of the timing of initiation of HT has been demonstrated in animal studies of atherosclerosis. In monkeys, the administration of CEE at the time of oophorectomy was associated with a 50–70% reduction in coronary plaque, but if CEEs were started years later, there was no benefit [43]. Once atherosclerosis has reached the stage of fibrous plaque, exogenous estrogens may actually exacerbate thrombosis and hematoma formation (Figure 9.3) [44].

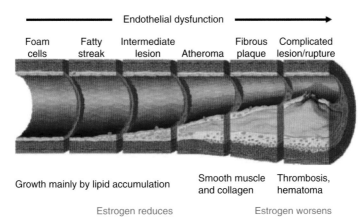

Fig. 9.3 The impact of the timing of initiation of estrogen replacement on the timeline of atherosclerosis and endothelial dysfunction [44]. From The ESHRE Capri Workshop Group. Hum Reprod Update. 2006;12:483–497.

Based on the strong evidence from these trials, and the supporting physiological data suggesting harm at the later stages of atherosclerosis, the only recommended use for hormone therapy is for the treatment of vasomotor symptoms (i.e., hot flashes) and osteoporosis [45]. The cardiovascular disease prevention guidelines for women state that both hormone therapy and selective estrogen receptor modulators should not be used for primary or secondary prevention (Class III, Level A) [46].

Preeclampsia and maternal placental syndrome

This patient's second pregnancy was complicated by moderate to severe preeclampsia. Preeclampsia, one of the hypertensive disorders of pregnancy, occurs in approximately 5% of pregnancies. The diagnostic criteria includes the de novo appearance of hypertension (systolic blood pressures ≥ 140 or diastolic pressures ≥ 90 mm Hg) and new onset proteinuria (≥ 300 mg per 24 hours) [47]. This pregnancy complication is being increasingly recognized as the initial occurrence of hypertension in women who then develop chronic hypertension following the childbearing years, particularly women who have more than one preeclamptic pregnancy [48]. Chronic hypertension is one of the leading risk factors for ischemic and hemorrhagic stroke. Therefore, it is not surprising that preeclampsia is also associated with stroke following childbearing. In a study from Scotland, women with preeclampsia/eclampsia were four times more likely to have hyper-

tension (OR 3.98; 95% CI 2.8–5.6) and three times more likely to have had a self-reported stroke (OR 3.4; 95% CI 0.95–12.2) [49]. The Stroke Prevention in Young Women Study, a case-control study of women with ischemic stroke between ages 15 and 44, showed a 50% higher prevalence of self-reported preeclampsia versus controls, although the association was diminished when adjusted for hypertension [50]. In addition, women with maternal placental syndrome, which includes gestational hypertension, preeclampsia/eclampsia, placental abruption, and placental infarction, have an increased risk of heart disease later in life [51].

One of the major pathophysiological consequences of preeclampsia is endothelial dysfunction. This prevents the normal dilatation of the uterine spiral artery, leading to reduced placental blood flow [47]. In addition to endothelial dysfunction, there are other manifestations that overlap with atherosclerosis, including hemostatic abnormalities, dyslipidemia, elevated insulin levels, and evidence of acute atherosclerosis with lipid-laden foam cells in the placental vascular bed of women with preeclampsia [52]. Based on these metabolic abnormalities, some experts have argued that preeclampsia may represent an early manifestation of identifiable risk factors for vascular disease, and that women with preeclampsia maintain a higher risk of vascular disease throughout life than women who have normotensive pregnancies (Figure 9.4) [53]. Therefore, at a minimum, women with a history of preeclamp-

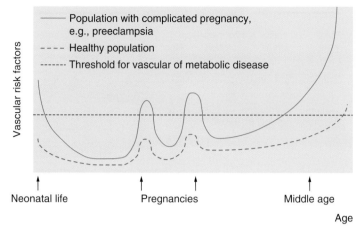

Fig. 9.4 Preeclampsia represents the metabolic disease of pregnancy and a time when vascular risk factors become evident [52]. From Sattar N, Greer, I. BMJ. 2002;325:157–160.

sia should be carefully screened for the early onset of hypertension and other vascular risk factors early after childbearing. One of the major research gaps includes how we can identify women with pre-eclampsia who are at high risk of a developing hypertension or having stroke at a relatively young age.

Hypertension

Hypertension, one of the most common risk factors for stroke, is especially common in women. In fact, compared with men with stroke, women are consistently more likely to have hypertension. Unfortunately, hypertension in women with a history of stroke may go unrecognized and therefore untreated. A secondary analysis of the Women Estrogen Stroke Trial, a trial of 17-beta estradiol versus placebo in women with stroke or TIA [40], showed that, about 1 month after stroke, only 44% of women had blood pressure values within national guidelines (Joint National Committee on Prevention VI at the time this analysis was published) [54]. Of those outside of the guideline measurements, 55% were still beyond the guideline at follow-up [54]. This analysis demonstrated that even women participating in a stroke secondary prevention trial had poorly controlled blood pressure, in part because hypertension was undiagnosed.

A study of blood pressure management in ambulatory care clinics reported that women were less likely than men to have adequate blood pressure control (54% for women versus 58.7% for men; $P < 0.02$). In addition, women aged 65–80 years had inadequate blood pressure control compared with men of the same age [55]. With regard to specific blood pressure treatments, men were more likely to be prescribed angiotensin-converting enzyme inhibitors (28.7% vs. 20.9% in women; $P < 0.0001$), whereas women were more likely to be prescribed diuretics (20.9% vs. 16.9% in men [$P = 0.05$]) [55]. In those patients with cardiovascular disease, women were less likely to be taking beta-blockers and aspirin than men. The reasons for this disparity are unknown but may be related to the misperception of cardiovascular risk in women, or less adherence by providers to the guidelines for female patients.

Women are less likely than men to develop hypertension until after menopause, when the incidence of hypertension in women equals that of men [56]. The mechanism may involve the positive influence of estrogens on the renin-angiotensin system, thereby protecting females from vascular injury more than males [57]. Further research is needed to determine whether specific blood pressure-lowering therapies should be prescribed differently for men and women. For now, guidelines for blood pressure treatment and targets [58] and the recommendations contained in the AHA/ASA primary and secondary prevention guidelines provide evidence-based approaches to managing blood pressures in both men and women [21,59].

Family history

Our patient had a significant family history for two reasons. First, her mother had a stroke at the age of 46. The importance of maternal family history of stroke was shown recently with a systematic review of the literature and a meta-analysis that included unpublished data [60]. This analysis of 18 studies involving 7941 patients showed that women with stroke (probands) were about 50% more likely to have a maternal than a paternal history of stroke (OR 1.47; 95% CI: 1.27–1.70) [60]. Interestingly, the excess of maternal versus paternal history of stroke did not exist for male probands. In addition to stroke, there may be a higher maternal transmission for other conditions that increase vascular risk, including diabetes, hypertension, and low HDL cholesterol [60]. The other important aspect of family history was that her sister had had a DVT. Uncovering this information prompted more aggressive screening for an inherited thrombophilia and led to the diagnosis of prothrombin gene mutation.

Guidelines for cardiovascular disease prevention in women

The most recent AHA Guidelines for Cardiovascular Disease Prevention in Women contain updated clinical information relevant to the care of women at risk of stroke. Although these guidelines are not specific for stroke, the majority of the risk factors for stroke and heart disease overlap, and the prevention strategies are relevant for both conditions.

Listed in Table 9.1, the new classification of risk in the updated guidelines includes high risk, at risk, and optimal risk. The rationale for reclassifying women is related to their very high lifetime risk of cardiovascular disease. In fact, the lifetime risk of stroke is about 20% [3], and for all cardiovascular disease, this approaches 40% [61]. The traditional Framingham risk score limits the prediction to 10 years or less, but it may underestimate the future risk of CVD in women who are found to have subclinical disease, measured with coronary artery calcium or carotid intimal medial thickness [46]. In addition, because women are frequently misclassified by physicians as having lower than actual risk [62], this redefinition was intended to guide and ultimately to improve recognition and appropriate

Table 9.1 Definitions of risk categories for cardiovascular disease (CVD) prevention in women [46]

Risk status	Criteria
High Risk	Established coronary heart disease
	Cerebrovascular disease
	Peripheral arterial disease
	Abdominal aortic aneurysm
	End-stage or chronic renal disease
	Diabetes mellitus
	10-year Framingham global risk >20%
At risk	>1 major risk factors for CVD, including:
	Cigarette smoking
	Poor diet
	Physical inactivity
	Obesity, especially central adiposity
	Family history of premature CVD (CVD at <55 years of age in male relative and <65 years of age in female relative)
	Hypertension
	Dyslipidemia
	Evidence of subclinical vascular disease (e.g., coronary calcification or carotid intimal–medial thickness)
	Metabolic syndrome
	Poor exercise capacity on treadmill test and/or abnormal heart rate recovery after stopping exercise
Optimal risk	Framingham global risk <10% and a healthy lifestyle with no risk factors

From Mosca L, *et al.* Circulation. 2007;115:1481–1501.

prevention strategies for women based on a simpler risk classification [46].

The guidelines also included a very useful algorithm for the evaluation and implementation of various prevention strategies (Figure 9.5). All women, regardless of risk, should be counseled on class I lifestyle recommendations (smoking cessation, heart-healthy eating patterns, regular physical activity, and weight management). Blood pressure control, LDL goal <100 mg/dL, aspirin/antiplatelet agents, glycemic control in diabetic women, and aldosterone blocker in selected women are recommended for high-risk women who have not had a recent cardiovascular event and do not meet the

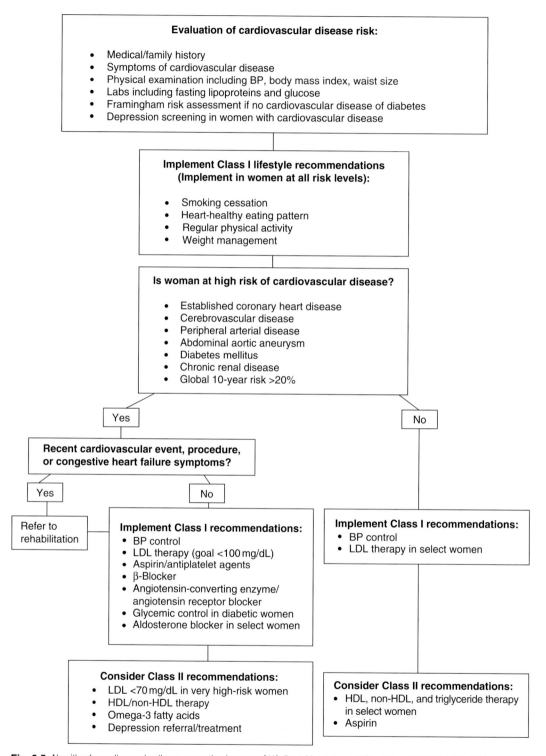

Fig. 9.5 Algorithm for cardiovascular disease prevention in women [46]. From Mosca L, *et al.* Circulation. 2007;115:1481–1501. BP, blood pressure; HDL, high-density lipoprotein; LDL, low-density lipoprotein.

requirements for rehabilitation. At risk women (Table 9.1) should have blood pressure control and LDL therapy in select women [46].

The guideline recommendations for weight maintenance/reduction is to work to a goal body mass index of 18.5–24.9 kg/m² and a waist circumference of ≤35 inches through a balance of physical activity, caloric intake, and formal behavioral programs when indicated [46]. Recommended diets are those rich in fruits and vegetables, whole-grain, high-fiber foods, fish (especially oily fish) at least twice a week, as well as very limited proportions of saturated fats and trans-fatty acids. Physical activity recommendations for women include an accumulated total of at least 30 minutes of moderate-intensity physical exercise (for example, brisk walking) on most days of the week. Women who are working to lose weight or sustain weight should increase to 60–90 minutes of moderate-intensity activity on most, if not all, days of the week [46].

Gender differences in post-stroke recovery and treatment

Although there is no clear evidence of a gender difference in initial stroke severity, there is a growing literature suggesting that women tend to have less favorable outcomes than men after stroke. Examples of unfavorable outcomes include disability (modified Rankin Score [mRS] >3) and limitations of activities of daily living (ADLs) (Barthel Index [BI] <95). The Canadian Stroke Registry reported that a higher percentage of women (30%) had moderate to severe disability (mRS ≥4) compared with men (26%) [14]. A statewide registry in Michigan reported similar results (33% of women vs. 27% of men had mRS ≥4) [63]. In Europe, a multicenter registry reported that women were more likely to be disabled at 3 months (BI <70), even after adjusting for age [6]. The Swedish Riks-Stroke Registry showed that 54% of women were independent in primary ADLs at 3 months post-stroke versus 67% of men [64]. Similarly, in 108 subjects with stroke in the Framingham Study, 34% of women were disabled at 6 months (BI <60) compared with 16% of men [65].

Age and sex are related in complex ways in outcome studies, and cross-sectional studies may not provide the full picture. For example, a longitudinal study of predictors of recovery and a post hoc analysis of the Management of Atherothrombosis with Clopidogrel in High-risk Patients trial showed that women age <65 years (vs. women aged ≥75 years) was independently associated with good recovery, defined as mRS <3 [66]. Other factors that were associated with recovery included less disability early post-stroke, no prior history of stroke, the presence of peripheral artery disease, and diabetes [66]. Therefore, this analysis confirmed the importance of age as a bimodal factor related to outcome, especially related to recovery in women.

One possible reason for women's poor outcomes could be related to disparities in the access to rehabilitation services. There do not, however, appear to be any differences in rehabilitation referrals by gender [67,68]. Despite equal access to rehabilitation, women have poorer physical functioning than men. In the Kansas Stroke Registry, women were older and had worse pre-stroke physical function than men. In the functional measurements of interest, women were less likely to achieve a score of >95 on the BI than men (hazard ratio [HR] 0.68; 95% CI 0.52–0.90), less likely to perform eight of nine instrumental ADLs without assistance (HR 0.46; 0.30–0.68), and less likely to score >90 on the Short Form 36 (SF-36) Health Survey physical functioning scale (HR 0.54; 0.28–1.01). These poor functional status scores were still present even after adjusting for age, pre-stroke physical function, and depression status at baseline [69]. Poorer pre-stroke disability in women has also been observed in at least two studies [6,64]. One study showed that 32% of women had a pre-stroke mRS of 2–5 versus 23% of men [6]. This is a very important but poorly understood factor in the gender differences in outcome.

One possible explanation for the greater pre-stroke disability in women is that this represents the presence of one or more comorbidities. In a study of women admitted with acute stroke, disability (measured with mRS) at 90 days or more was associated with atrial fibrillation, diabetes, history of coronary heart disease (CHD), and a higher score on the Charlson Index (a measure of comorbidities that impact 1-year survival), shown in Figure 9.6. In the multivariable analysis adjusted for initial stroke severity, diabetes and CHD were each independently associated with worse disability at 90 days or more after stroke [70]. Although this is one of

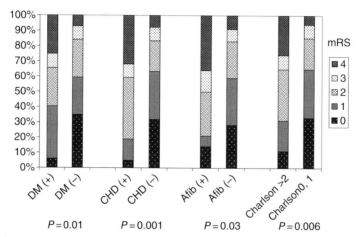

Fig. 9.6 Association between disability measured with the modified Rankin Score (0 = no disability and 4 = moderate to severe disability) and various comorbidities [70]. The Charlson Index is a score based on the presence of one or more comorbidities that impact 1-year mortality. From Bushnell C, *et al.* Stroke. 2008;39:2138–2140.
Afib, atrial fibrillation; CHD, coronary heart disease; DM, diabetes mellitus; mRS, modified Rankin Score.

the few detailed outcomes studies of women after stroke, there were no men included; so whether these comorbidities are unique to women is unknown.

These data address two major research gaps in outcome studies. First, stroke outcome studies need to take into account comorbidities in their assessments of outcomes. In addition, these studies need to include men and women concomitantly, and be inclusive of the age ranges likely to influence outcomes in order to determine gender-specific patterns in these outcomes.

Quality of life (QOL)

QOL has been quantified for stroke with the Stroke Impact Scale (SIS) [71] and the Stroke-Specific QOL (SS-QOL) Scale [72], and these scales have been used in various cohorts of stroke subjects. QOL has also been the focus of gender comparison studies. In the Canadian Stroke Registry, women were significantly more likely to score lower than men on the SIS-16, which represents the physical function domain of the SIS [14]. In addition, the Michigan statewide registry found that women scored lower on the physical domain scores of the SS-QOL than men [63]. More research is needed to better understand the gender differences related to QOL and how to improve QOL for stroke subjects in general, and women in particular.

Depression

Women are not only more prone to have depression than men throughout the life, but women are also more likely to experience depressive symptoms following stroke. This was shown in 301 consecutive stroke patients admitted to the University of Maryland Hospital who were evaluated for depression using the Hamilton Rating Scale for Depression and the modified Present State Examination (PSE), in addition to other measures of cognition and ADLs [73]. Women were twice as likely to have major depressive disorder as men (23.6% vs. 12.3% in men; $P = 0.01$). Depression was also associated with left hemisphere lesion location, but only among women. In addition, the factors associated with major depressive disorder were different for men and women. For example, for women, younger age, personal history of psychiatric disorder, and cognitive impairment were associated with major depressive disorder, whereas in men, it was younger age and impairment in ADLs and social functioning [73]. Another study from Sweden, the Risk-Stroke Registry, found that 12.4% of men and 16.4% of women reported that they always or often felt depressed [74]. In the multiple regression analysis, women were 30% more likely to have self-reported depression (OR 1.30; 95% CI 1.17–1.44). Other factors included age <65, history of recurrent stroke, and living at home alone, or in an institution. The study also assessed reported use of antidepressant drugs, and this was again more common in women than men [74]. The Sunnybrook Stroke Study evaluated depression using the objective, observer-rated scale (Montgomery Asberg Depression Rating Scale) and a subjective scale (Zung Self-Rating Depression Scale) in 436 patients with stroke [75]. The prevalence of self-reported depression at 3 months post-stroke was 21%, whereas the objective measure was 27%, the majority of which was due to mild depression. These rates of depression were similar at 1 year post-stroke. Consistent with other cited studies, female sex was associated with depression measured with both scales. The other important finding was that depression was associated with worse functional status, quantified with the Functional Independence Measure, and disability, measured with the Oxford Handicap Scale (same as the mRS) [75]. In summary, these studies have demonstrated that depression is more common in women and is associated with poorer functional status after stroke.

Another important reason to recognize depressive symptoms following stroke is because its presence is associated with increased mortality. A randomized trial of treatment strategies for depression post-stroke screened for the presence of self-reported mood symptoms within the PSE and the General Health Questionnaire (GHQ)-28 (a measure of general psychological distress) at 1 month and then followed the cohort for 24 months. The investigators found that subjects in the highest quartile of the GHQ-28 (signifying increased psychological distress) were at a 3-fold risk of death by 12 months (OR 3.1; 95% CI 1.1–8.8; $P = 0.037$) and 2-fold risk of death by 24 months (OR 2.2; 1.0–4.8; $P = 0.048$). Interestingly, an International Classification of Diseases-10 diagnosis of major depression was not associated with mortality.

Depression and psychological stress have also been investigated as risk factors for incident stroke. In a large study from the United Kingdom, there was no significant relationship between major depressive disorder and incident stroke, but there was a significant and positive association with psychological stress [76]. Therefore, screening for psychological distress may become an important aspect of risk factor modification.

A major knowledge gap in stroke outcomes is how depression and psychological distress affect stroke risk. Is this because it leads to reduced physical activity, or weight gain and thus a worsening cardiovascular risk profile? This is especially important for women because they are at risk of having depression prior to having a stroke, and for having more depressive symptoms following the stroke.

Physical activity

The patient described in the case study had a cerebellar stroke, which limited her mobility for several months. Patients who have disability from ischemic stroke should be considered for a supervised exercise regimen. Not only have exercise programs been shown to improve outcomes in physical functioning, but they have also been associated with improved measures of QOL (higher ADL scores, improved social function, and physical role function) [77] and fewer depressive symptoms [78]. Specific recommendations for physical activity for stroke survivors are summarized in an AHA guidelines statement [79]. These guidelines provide recommendations for aerobic, strength training, flexibility, and neuromuscular aspects of potential exercise programs, depending on the goals and needs of the stroke survivor [79].

With regards to sex differences, a recent randomized controlled trial of supervised versus unsupervised exercise program reported that both men and women improved in the 6-minute walking speed and the SF-36 Physical Component summary score, regardless of treatment assignment. However, women made greater gains in the supervised programs, whereas men had greater gains in the unsupervised programs (interaction term of gender by treatment $P = 0.01$) [80]. The reasons for this outcome are unclear but may relate to social interactions.

Measuring exercise capacity is an opportunity to optimize primary and secondary cardiovascular prevention. This is important because poor exercise capacity has been associated with cardiac death in women [81]. This was shown in a study in which women with and without coronary disease symptoms underwent symptom-limited treadmill tests and were followed for cardiac outcomes. The percent of predicted exercise capacity was measured with exercise nomograms developed for women who were active and those who were sedentary (Figure

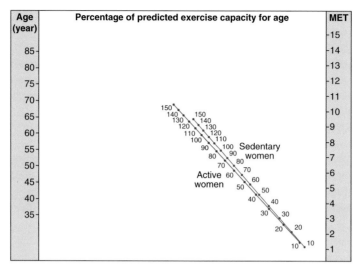

Fig. 9.7 Exercise nomogram for determining exercise capacity in active and sedentary women [81]. From Gulati M, *et al*. N Engl J Med. 2005;353:246–475.

MET, metabolic equivalent.

9.7) [81]. Regardless of the presence of symptoms, women with an exercise capacity less than 85% of the age-appropriate predicted value had a 2-fold increased risk of death from any cause and a 2.4-fold risk of cardiac death [81]. Although not specifically developed for stroke, this type of exercise nomogram is useful for general cardiovascular prevention screening and would help identify women who would benefit from exercise programs. A major research gap related to physical activity for women is how to motivate women who are at risk for stroke to become active. In addition, given the evidence that women are more likely to have worse functional status and QOL than men post-stroke, various exercise programs could be utilized to improve function and QOL for women after stroke

and concomitantly reduce the risk of recurrent stroke.

In summary, women have a greater lifetime risk of stroke than men, and therefore we have many opportunities and challenges to provide high-quality preventive care. In addition, women may present with unorthodox stroke symptoms, which requires astute history taking to recognize a stroke and direct treatment. During the acute stroke hospitalization, we have an opportunity to improve outcomes by recognizing and treating depression, providing appropriate rehabilitation and exercise programs, and initiating secondary prevention strategies.

References available online at www.wiley.com/go/ strokeguidelines.

Stroke in Black Patients

Fernando D. Testai and Philip B. Gorelick

EXAMPLE CASE

A 68-year-old African-American woman with a history of hypertension and hypercholesterolemia awakens in the morning with new onset of slurred speech and right-sided face, arm, and leg weakness. She had quit smoking cigarettes about 2 months previously. The patient was taken to a local hospital for evaluation. On arrival, her temperature was 36°C, her pulse was 75 bpm, and her blood pressure was 175/105 mm Hg. Her height was 5 feet and her weight was 325 lbs. In the general physical examination, her neck was supple and no carotid bruits were appreciated. The pulmonary exam was normal, and her heart rate was regular with no murmurs or gallops. The peripheral pulses were unremarkable. The fundoscopic exam disclosed grade II hypertensive changes. Other pertinent neurological findings included slurred speech, flattening of the right nasolabial fold, and right-sided hemiparesis. Deep tendon reflexes were brisk in the right arm and the right patella; the ankle jerks could not be elicited and the plantar responses were flexor bilaterally. A metabolic profile, complete blood count, coagulation studies, and cardiac enzymes were obtained and were remarkable only for a glucose level of 175 mg/dL. Other laboratory tests included erythrosedimentation rate (ESR) (42 mm/h), triglycerides (350 mg/dL), low-density lipoprotein cholesterol (124 mg/dL), and glycosylated hemoglobin A1c (9.2%). The urinalysis showed proteinuria. The electrocardiogram revealed a

MAJOR POINTS

- The incidence and prevalence of stroke in African Americans is significantly higher than in Caucasians; this disparity is inversely related to age.
- Black patients are about twice as likely to die from stroke than are whites.
- Blacks may have more severe and disabling strokes than whites.
- The reasons for an excess burden of stroke in African Americans have not been clearly defined yet; explanations may include a higher rate of cardiovascular risk factors such as hypertension, diabetes, obesity, smoking, and end stage renal disease, socioeconomic factors, and the influence of geography.

- Stroke mechanism may differ among race-ethnic groups; white patients may have a higher proportion of cardioembolic stroke and symptomatic large artery extracranial occlusive disease, and black patients more small-vessel (lacunar) strokes and symptomatic intracranial occlusive disease.
- Age, lower educational level, history of myocardial infarction, recent smoking, and left cortical infarction may be predictors of dementia with stroke in black patients.
- Cardiovascular risk factors may be risk factors for vascular cognitive impairment and also, possibly, for Alzheimer's disease.

A Primer on Stroke Prevention Treatment: An Overview Based on AHA/ASA Guidelines, 1st Edition. Edited by L Goldstein.
© 2009 American Heart Association, ISBN: 9781405186513

normal sinus rhythm and left ventricular hypertrophy (LVH) by voltage criteria. The brain CT scan showed old lacunar strokes but no evidence of acute ischemic changes or bleeds. The brain magnetic resonance imaging (MRI) revealed the presence of a small, acute left-sided capsular stroke, chronic ischemic changes, and evidence of prior brain hemorrhage. Whereas echocardiography showed LVH, magnetic resonance angiography (MRA) showed high-grade occlusive disease of the horizontal portion of the middle cerebral artery.

Case vignette discussion

The patient described illustrates key features that may occur in African-Americans with stroke. These include a high prevalence of hypertension and other cardiovascular risk factors, which may include dyslipidemia, obesity, diabetes mellitus, and cigarette smoking; nonoptimally controlled risk factors; history of cerebral hemorrhage; and lacunar stroke subtype and intracranial occlusive disease. These and other topics germane to stroke in blacks are discussed.

Introduction

Blacks and other racial and ethnic minorities may be disproportionately affected by stroke. Disparities in their level of general health and access to health care in the United States continue to exist [1–6]. African-Americans have approximately two times the stroke risk as compared with their white counterparts, as well as lower life expectancy, poorer health care, and discrimination in the medical care system [3]. Of the three leading causes of mortality, the black-to-white ratio of death is greatest for stroke [1]. The US Institute of Medicine concluded that racial and ethnic minorities receive lower quality of health care than others even after access to healthcare-related factors are taken into account [5]. Furthermore, medical care for minorities may be poorly matched to their needs based on language barriers, geography, cultural issues, stereotyping, biases inherent to the healthcare system, and uncertainty on the part of healthcare providers [5]. These gaps may be overcome by comprehensive, multilevel healthcare system strategies.

In this chapter, we discuss the prevention, diagnosis, and treatment of stroke in blacks. Although blacks traditionally have been underrepresented in clinical trials, more recent focused trials have helped us to better understand stroke prevention and treatment in this important group. A theme of barriers to participation in clinical trials and the healthcare system has emerged for blacks, and we recommend means to overcome these challenges.

Descriptive epidemiology

Mortality

Stroke is the third leading cause of death in the United States, and it is estimated that one person dies of a stroke approximately every 3 minutes. Over the years, a decrease in the rates of strokes has been noted. Blacks and men, however, consistently have had higher stroke mortality rates than whites and women, respectively (Figure 10.1). In 2004, the stroke death rate in the United States was 50.0 per 100,000, with race and sex subgroup mortality rates of 48.1 for white men, 73.9 for black men, 47.4 for white women, and 64.9 for black women [7]. The 2008 US National Vital Statistics Report indicates that since 1999, the age-adjusted stroke death rate decreased by 24.4%, almost reaching the 25% national goal set by the American Heart Association for 2010. This drop was not uniform, however, among different race–ethnic groups: the stroke death rate decrease, for example, was 20.3% for blacks and 25% for whites [8,9]. The overall excess in stroke mortality in the African-American community decreases with age. In younger and midlife groups (<64 years of age), the death rate for stroke is three to four times higher for blacks than whites, whereas those differences fall substantially for individuals older than 75 (Figure 10.2) [3,10,11].

Stroke mortality is not uniformly distributed across the United States. Death rates for blacks and whites have been documented to be 1.5 times higher than the national average in the *stroke belt*, a geographic area that includes primarily the southeast

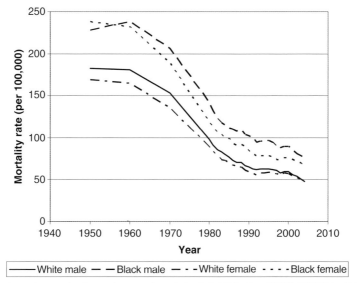

Fig. 10.1 Death rates for cerebrovascular diseases by sex and race in the United States from 1950 to 2004 (data obtained from the National Center for Health Statistics [8]).

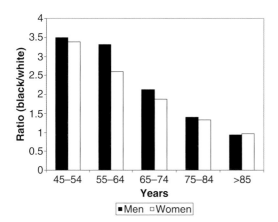

Fig. 10.2 Stroke mortality ratios by sex and age for the year 2004 (data obtained from the National Center for Health Statistics [8]).

United States (North Carolina, South Carolina, Georgia, Tennessee, Mississippi, Alabama, Louisiana, and Arkansas) [12]. Within the stroke belt, mortality rates reach the absolute highest level in the *stroke buckle*, a region that includes the coastal plains of North Carolina, South Carolina, and Georgia (Figure 10.3) [12]. The excess in stroke mortality for blacks is substantially greater in southern than in nonsouthern states, and this difference

is more pronounced in younger patients. The black-to-white stroke mortality ratios for men (southern vs. nonsouthern states) are 3.24 versus 2.76 at age 55–64, 2.19 versus 1.81 at age 65–74, and 1.45 versus 1.22 at age 75–84. Similar results have been observed in women [14].

A National Institutes of Health (NIH)-funded study, Reasons for Geographic and Racial Differences in Stroke Study (REGARDS), is being conducted in an attempt to understand the causes for excess stroke mortality in the southeast United States and among blacks [12]. It is hypothesized that geographic and racial differences in the awareness, treatment, and control of hypertension, which is considered the major risk factor for stroke, may be the main underlying factors contributing to the reported disparities in stroke mortality. Data from REGARDS suggest that blacks have higher awareness and treatment but poorer control of hypertension than whites [15]. Therefore, the improvement of blood pressure control may provide a window of opportunity to reduce the racial disparity in stroke mortality. REGARDS, however, found no geographic differences in awareness and treatment of hypertension [15]. In fact, a trend toward better control of this risk factor within the stroke belt was noted. This implies that a regional difference in

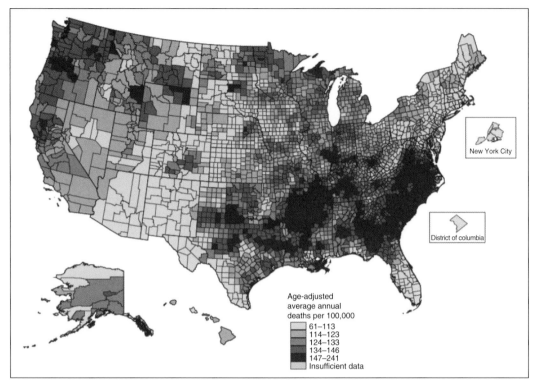

Fig. 10.3 County age-adjusted annual stroke death rates for individuals aged 35 years or older. Increasing intensity represents higher death rates (see insert) (modified from Casper *et al.* [13]).

hypertension management may not be a major contributor to excess in stroke mortality in the southeast United States.

An interesting observation from the Health and Retirement Study is that residence in the stroke belt during childhood increases the risk of stroke in adulthood, even for those who leave the region [16]. If the stroke belt is primarily caused by a higher prevalence of artherosclerotic risk factors, it might not explain the high risk of stroke for those who migrate from the area. Similar to adults, children who live in the southeastern United States have a higher stroke mortality rate compared with non-southeastern US children (relative risk [RR] 1.21; 95% confidence interval [CI] 1.12–1.29) [17]. This suggests that factors other than cardiovascular risks could be active in the stroke belt.

There has been a trend toward a slowdown in the decline of national death rates for cerebrovascular diseases in whites and blacks since the 1980s (Figure 10.1). Important findings from the Greater Cincinnati/Northern Kentucky Stroke Study (GCNKSS)

are illustrative. In the GCNKSS, the 30-day case-fatality rates after the first ischemic stroke, intracerebral hemorrhage (ICH), and subarachnoid hemorrhage (SAH) for whites and blacks did not change significantly during the 1990s despite the increased use of medications to modify stroke risk factors (e.g., aspirin, antihypertensive medications, oral hypoglycemics, and lipid-lowering agents) [18]. The nature of the failure to translate risk-factor management into substantial decreases of stroke-related mortality is a source of debate. This finding may be explained, at least in part, by taking into account stroke incidence rates. Data from the GCNKSS suggest that the higher stroke-related mortality in blacks for all categories (ischemic, ICH, and SAH) is attributable to higher stroke incidence rates rather than to increased case fatality [10]. Other plausible causes to explain the higher mortality in blacks beyond hypertension include suboptimal risk factor control, stroke severity and/or subtype, increased prevalence and severity of comorbidities, differences in stroke evaluation and treatment, limited access to medical care, and race–ethnic differences in response to stroke therapies.

Prevalence

The Behavioral Risk Factor Surveillance System (BRFSS) is a state-based, random-digit dialed telephone survey of the noninstitutionalized US civilian population aged ≥18 years. BRFSS is administered by state health departments in collaboration with the Centers for Disease Control. According to the 2005 BRFSS, 2.6% of the adults surveyed had a history of stroke [19]. Stroke prevalence was similar between men and women and increased with age: 0.8% between ages 18 and 44, 2.7% between ages 45 and 64, and 8.1% above the age of 65. Substantial differences were observed among race–ethnic groups, with an overall stroke prevalence of 4% in blacks and 2.3% in whites. Middle-aged women have about 2.5 times the prevalence of stroke than men in the United States with stroke prevalence being higher in the United States as compared with the corresponding rates in representative European countries [20,21]. The higher stroke prevalence rates in the United States are driven by higher prevalence rates among African-Americans, though white Americans have higher stroke prevalence rates than Europeans [21]. Furthermore, according to the 2003 BRFSS, the prevalence of stroke was higher in the 10 southeastern states than in the other states surveyed. The highest age-adjusted prevalence of stroke was found in southeastern blacks (3.4%), followed by nonsoutheastern blacks (2.8%), southeastern whites (2.5%), and nonsoutheastern whites (1.8%) [22].

The Atherosclerosis Risk in Communities (ARIC) Study is an NIH-funded initiative to investigate the cause, natural course, and clinical consequences of atherosclerosis. In this study, the overall prevalence of silent cerebral infarction (SBI) in subjects aged 55–70 years – diagnosed with brain MRI – was 11% [23]. After adjusting for risk factors (hypertension, elevated triglycerides, low HDL, and diabetes) and lifestyle choices (dietary fat intake, reported leisure-time physical activity, alcohol intake, and body mass index [BMI]), SBI was more prevalent among black participants than in whites (odds ratio [OR] 1.64; 95% CI 1.12–2.41). Recently, the tri-racial Northern Manhattan Stroke Study (NOMASS) reported the overall prevalence of SBI to be almost 18%. In this cohort, age, male sex, and hypertension were inde-pendently associated with SBI. Significant racial disparities were noted as blacks had an age-adjusted SBI prevalence of 24.5%, whereas whites had one of 17.6% [24].

Incidence

About 780,000 Americans experience a stroke each year. Of these, 600,000 are first attacks, and 180,000 are recurrent attacks. Furthermore, it is estimated that a new stroke occurs in the United States every 40 seconds [7].

Data from large population-based stroke studies, such as GCNKSS, ARIC, and NOMASS, indicate that stroke incidence is not uniformly distributed among different race–ethnic groups, with blacks having a disproportionate burden compared with whites [10,25–27]. NOMASS found the overall annual age-adjusted incidence of stroke in blacks aged ≥20 to be 2.4 times higher than in whites. The incidence of ischemic stroke in blacks was two times higher for men and three times higher for women compared with their white counterparts. A similar disparity was noted in ICH. Also, blacks had an excess incidence of SAH, but the small number of events prevents definitive conclusions [27]. A similar trend was noted in the GCNKSS, in which the adjusted incidence rates for all stroke categories (either ischemic, ICH, or SAH) were almost two times higher for African-Americans. Similar to stroke mortality, the disparity between stroke incidence in blacks and whites is a phenomenon inversely related to age (RR 5.0, 95% CI 3.9–6.1 for ages 35–44; RR 2.2, 95% CI 1.6–2.8 for ages 55–64; RR 1.3, 95% CI 1.4–1.8 for ages ≥85) [10].

The estimated stroke/transient ischemic attack incidence rates (per 10,000) for ages 45–54, 55–64, and 65–74 years are 24, 61, and 122 for white men, 97, 131, and 162 for black men, 24, 48, and 98 for white women, and 72, 100, and 150 for black women, respectively [28].

Epidemiology of stroke in young adults

Several large population-based studies, such as the GCNKSS, the NOMASS, and the Baltimore-Washington Cooperative Young Stroke Study (BWCYSS) have shown that young black adults have a significantly higher risk of stroke than their white counterparts. In NOMASS, the 30-day stroke mortality rate in the 25–44 year age strata was 33% in blacks, whereas no cases were documented in whites. In this age group, the annual stroke incidence was 25 (per 100,000) for blacks and 10 for whites, conferring a relative risk of stroke in blacks of 2.4 [11]. In the GCNKSS, the stroke incidence in the 35–44 year age group was 96 (per 100,000) in blacks and 19 in whites, and in the BWCYSS, the annual stroke rate for persons aged 15–44 years was 23 (per 100,000) in blacks and 10.3 in whites [10,29]. The excess burden of stroke in young African-Americans may have a substantial public heath impact based on associated direct (e.g., inpatient care, rehabilitation, follow-up care) and indirect (e.g., long-term disability, lost years of productivity) costs of stroke.

Risk factors

Hypotheses have been proposed to explain the excess burden of stroke in blacks [1]. These have included differences in the prevalence of cardiovascular risk factors, socioeconomic factors and limitations in access to medical care, and genetic factors. Stroke disparities by race–ethnic group, however, may be a complex phenomenon that is difficult to explain by a single factor.

Blacks are known to have a higher prevalence of cardiovascular risk factors such as hypertension, diabetes mellitus, smoking, obesity, end-stage renal disease, LVH, and congestive heart failure than their white counterparts [3,30]. According to the 2003 BRFSS, stroke risk factors are highly prevalent in the US population: 25.6% for high blood pressure, 25.3% for elevated blood cholesterol, 25.0% for obesity, 24.1% for physically inactivity, 22.6% for smoking, and 7.4% for diabetes. Overall, 29.8% of the responders reported having no risk factors; 33.1% reported one risk factor; and 37.2% reported two or more risk factors. The prevalence of having two or more risk factors was 48.7% in blacks and 35.5% in whites, indicating a significant excess of potentially modifiable stroke risk factors in African-Americans [31].

The prevalence of hypertension in US blacks is among the highest in the world, and it continues to increase. The frequency of hypertension in the African-American community was 35.8% in 1988–1994 (24.3% in whites), 35.8% in 1995–1998 (24.3% in whites), and 41.7% in 1999–2002 (28.1% in whites) [7]. Compared with whites, blacks have a

2.6-fold excess of hypertension. Furthermore, blacks develop hypertension earlier in life, and their average blood pressures are higher [7,9,32]. In REGARDS, African-Americans had higher awareness (OR 1.31; 95% CI 1.07–1.59) and treatment (OR 1.69; 95% CI 1.40–2.05) but were less likely (OR 0.73; 95% CI 0.64–0.83) than whites to have their blood pressures controlled [15].

NOMASS noted several race–ethnic differences in the prevalence of stroke risk factors. African-Americans had higher rates of hypertension (62% vs. 43%), diabetes (21% vs. 11%), and physical inactivity (27% vs. 23%) as compared with whites. Compared with whites, however, blacks had lower rates of coronary artery disease (22% vs. 36%) and atrial fibrillation (5% vs. 8%) [30]. The etiological fraction (i.e., the proportion of a condition in a population group attributed to a particular factor) for hypertension, diabetes mellitus, and physical inactivity in blacks was 37%, 14%, and 29%, respectively.

There is an obesity epidemic in the United States. The prevalence of overweight and obesity has increased between 1980 and 2004 from 47% to 66% [33]. According to the National Health and Nutrition Examination Survey (NHANES) 2001–2004, the prevalence of obesity in adults is 30.8% in black men (30.2% in white men) and 51.1% in black women (30.7% in white women) [7]. Obesity and metabolic syndrome are known cardiovascular and stroke risk factors considered "potentially modifiable." NOMASS found abdominal obesity (measured as waist-to-hip ratio) to be an independent and potent stroke risk factor, especially in subjects aged ≤65 years [34]. Furthermore, as many as 76% of stroke survivors (70% of men and 81% of women) in the African-American Antiplatelet Stroke Prevention Study (AAASPS) were overweight or obese. In addition, in AAASPS, increasing weight was associated with hypertension, diabetes, dyslipidemia, and metabolic syndrome, underscoring the relationship between body habitus and stroke risk factors [35].

Socioeconomic status (SES) has also been associated with stroke, and different mechanisms have been proposed to explain this relationship. Low SES has been linked to poor control of comorbid conditions, decreased access to medical care, cultural disparities and mistrust in the medical community, lifestyle factors (e.g., smoking, physical inactivity, and poor diet), communication barriers, and other factors [36]. In the GCNKSS, the relative risk of first stroke in blacks versus non-blacks was 1.69 (95% CI 1.46–1.96) before and 1.42 (95% CI 1.19–1.71) after adjusting for SES, suggesting that 39% of the disparity in stroke risk among blacks was accounted by SES [37]. The effect of SES on stroke risk was similar for blacks and whites. African-Americans, however, may have lower SES than whites [38,39].

In the ARIC Study, echocardiographically determined left ventricular mass index (LVMI) was an independent predictor of stroke. The age-adjusted incidence of stroke in blacks (per 10,000) was 43 for LVMI in the range of 16.2–38.9 g/m^2 and 123 for LVMI of 58.2–140.7 g/m^2 ($P = 0.004$) [39].

Stroke may be a powerful predictor of subsequent stroke risk. In AAASPS, for example, previous stroke and residual disability predicted recurrent stroke. Stroke could lead to disability, thereby limiting the access of subjects to medical care and resulting in subsequent suboptimal control of medical risk factors [40]. AAASPS also found that black women have higher frequency of hypertension, diabetes, family history of stroke, and no reported leisure exercise, and lower rates of smoking and heavy alcohol use, than black men [41].

In younger persons, nontraditional cardiovascular risk factors may contribute to stroke disparities. In the BWCYSS study, 17% of black subjects aged 15–44 years tested positive for illicit drugs compared with 7% of whites [42]. The prevalence of other stroke risk factors such as patent foramen ovale, homocysteine level, antiphospholipid antibody syndrome, and thrombophilias was similar between blacks and whites [43–46].

Pregnancy as a risk factor for stroke

According to the BWCYSS, the risk of ischemic stroke and ICH is 2.4 times higher during pregnancy and the first 6 weeks postpartum than for nonpregnant women of similar age and race [47]. Black women, in particular, have higher risk of stroke during pregnancy than white women (52.5 per 100,000 deliveries vs. 31.7 per 100,000, respectively). This disparity is more pronounced in older persons. Compared with white women <35 years, the OR of stroke for white women ≥35 years is 2.2 (95% CI 1.6–2.9), for black women <35 years is 1.5 (95% CI 1.1–2.0), and for black women ≥35 years is 4.5 (95%

CI 2.9–6.8) [48]. Different medical conditions were associated with stroke during pregnancy. These included migraine headache (OR 16.9; CI 9.7–29.5), thrombophilia (OR 16.0; CI 9.4–27.2), systemic lupus erythematosus (OR 15.2; CI 7.4–31.2), heart disease (OR 13.2; CI 10.2–17.0), sickle-cell disease (OR 9.1; CI 3.7–22.2), hypertension (OR 6.1; CI 4.5–8.1), thrombocytopenia (OR 6.0; CI 1.5–24.1), postpartum hemorrhage (OR 1.8; CI 1.2–2.8), preeclampsia and gestational hypertension (OR 4.4; CI 3.6–5.4), transfusion (OR 10.3; CI 7.1–15.1), and postpartum infection (OR 25.0; CI 18.3–34.0) [49].

Stroke subtypes

Ischemic stroke

In the GCNKSS and the NOMASS, blacks had a higher incidence of ischemic stroke than whites across the different ischemic stroke subtypes (cardioembolic, large vessel, small vessel, and cryptogenic) [26,49]. Stroke mechanism, however, may differ within race–ethnic groups. Whites have been reported to have a higher proportion of cardioembolic stroke [26,49], and blacks have more small-vessel (lacunar) stroke [50,51]. These race–ethnic differences may be a reflection of the increased prevalence of atrial fibrillation in whites and higher rates of hypertension, diabetes, tobacco use, and obesity in blacks.

Furthermore, previous studies suggested that whites had more extracranial occlusive disease, and blacks have more intracranial occlusive disease [52–57]. These observations, however, were challenged in the GCNKSS and the NOMASS, where the difference in extracranial and intracranial occlusive disease prevalence in blacks and whites did not reach statistical significance [26,49]. The intracranial vasculature, however, was evaluated in a relatively small number of patients in these studies. For example, in the GCNKSS, only 5% of the patients underwent conventional cerebral angiography (CCA), and 8% underwent MRA. In the NOMASS, only 3% of the patients underwent CCA, and 61% underwent MRA, transcranial Doppler (TCD) ultrasound, or CCA. Burke and Howard provided a thoughtful review of the controversies concerning propensity for intracranial and extracranial occlusive disease by race [58].

Hemorrhagic stroke

As with ischemic stroke, blacks have an excess burden of ICH and SAH [10,11]. In the GCNKSS, African-Americans had an age- and sex-adjusted incidence (per 100,000) of first ICH of 37 and of first SAH of 10.4. Compared with whites, the risk ratios of blacks having a first ICH or a first SAH were 2.0 and 1.8, respectively [10]. The predominant risk factor for ICH is hypertension, which may also be a risk for SAH. In this regard, the disparity of hemorrhagic strokes observed in African-Americans may be related, at least in part, to the higher prevalence of hypertension in blacks.

Vascular cognitive impairment (VCI)

Background

VCI represents the spectrum of mild, moderate, or severe cognitive impairment related to stroke [59,60]. The presence of VCI is based on a history of cognitive impairment, which is temporally related to stroke, and the involvement of at least one cognitive domain. In the milder forms, the term *cognitive impairment, no dementia* (CIND or vascular CIND) is used to indicate what is believed to be a milder transitional stage, which may lead to a more severe form of VCI or vascular dementia (VaD). Clinical and neuropathological evidence of Alzheimer's disease (AD) may coexist with VCI and provide a challenge in terms of accurate diagnosis of dementia subtype [61,62]. Most of the epidemiological research in cognition of later life has focused on AD. VCI is an important construct, however, as it is estimated that up to about one-third of stroke patients have significant cognitive impairment at 3 months after stroke.

Risk factors

The risk factors for stroke are also risk factors for VCI [63,64]. In the mid- to late 1980s, we carried out an NIH-funded case-control study of consecutive ischemic stroke patients who were predominantly African-American and who had VCI with dementia (i.e., the cases referred to as "multi-infarct dementia" or "MID" at the time) or stroke without dementia (SWD) (i.e., the control group) [65]. We found that age, lower educational level, history of myocardial infarction, and recent cigarette smoking were predictors of dementia with stroke, but systolic blood pressure was inversely associated with dementia risk. When cranial CT findings were analyzed, we found that left cortical infarction was the best imaging predictor of dementia associated with stroke [66].

Our next series of companion NIH-funded studies explored cardiovascular, neuroimaging, and other risk factor relationships exclusively among African-American hospital-based referral patients with AD, stroke with dementia, and SWD. Baseline observations suggested that African-American patients had traditional cardiovascular risk factors, yet might have concomitant AD [67]. This finding was a somewhat radical departure from conventional thinking at the time, since for many years, based on standard AD criteria, cardiovascular risk factors were not considered to be risks for AD or might exclude one from the diagnosis. In our study, however, we found that factors such as hypertension and diabetes mellitus were common among this black patient group, yet they still carried a diagnosis of AD. When we accrued and reported brain neuropathological findings [68], we were able to validate our clinical diagnoses pathologically, which further supported the concept that traditional cardiovascular risk factors could be associated with AD. Based on subsequent comprehensive epidemiological studies, cardiovascular risk factors such as hypertension, diabetes mellitus, and atrial fibrillation were shown to be possible risk factors for AD [63,64].

The key results of our three-group comparison studies referred to previously were (a) black VaD patients had a higher frequency of traditional cardiovascular risk factors, focal neurological findings, and medication use versus black AD patients who were more likely to have a family history of AD, Parkinson's disease, and dementia, and a history of head injury with loss of consciousness [67]; (b) on cranial CT, there were more white-matter lesions, nonlacunar infarcts, and left subcortical infarcts distinguishing VaD from AD patients, although atrophy of the third ventricle and equal distribution of white-matter lesions distinguished VaD from SWD [69]; and (c) finally, based on brain MRI, atrophy of the temporal sulci, temporal horns, and third ventricle and right hemisphere infarcts were predictors of AD versus VaD, but atrophy of the third ventricle predicted VaD versus SWD [69]. Overall, we noted that our cranial CT and MRI brain

Table 10.1 Possible risk factors of vascular cognitive impairment [63]

1 Demographic factors: age, male sex, lower educational attainment
2 Traditional cardiovascular factors: hypertension, cigarette smoking, myocardial infarction, diabetes mellitus, and hyperlipidemia
3 Genetic factors: familial vascular encephalopathies (e.g., cerebral autosomal dominant arteriopathy with subcortical infarct and leukoencephalopathy), apolipoprotein epsilon 4 allele
4 Stroke-related factors: volume of brain tissue loss, bilateral cerebral infarction, strategic infarction (e.g., thalamus, angular gyrus), white-matter disease, silent cerebral infarcts, cerebral atrophy, and ventricular size

Table 10.2 Four key elements for a diagnosis of vascular cognitive impairment [70]

1 Presence and severity of acquired cognitive impairment
2 Presence of cerebrovascular disease
3 Temporal relationship between cerebrovascular disease and cognitive impairment
4 Presence or absence of other potential sources of cognitive impairment (e.g., Alzheimer's disease)

findings were similar to the expected findings in AD and VaD observed in other studies, especially in regard to atrophy as a predictor of AD and infarcts and white-matter lesions as predictors of VaD [66].

We have been carrying out additional studies in patients with stroke with and without VCI to collect comprehensive epidemiological and neuropsychological variables and diffusion tensor imaging (DTI) and voxel-based morphometry (VBM) data, and to determine brain and stroke volumes. The preliminary findings suggest that whole-brain DTI and focused VBM (thalamic region) plus left hemisphere strokes and lower education attainment may be predictors of VCI without dementia [70].

Possible risk factors for VCI are listed in Table 10.1 [63].

Diagnosis

A number of nosological systems have been proposed to characterize and diagnose cognitive impairments in conjunction with stroke and cerebrovascular disease [71]. A detailed review of these classification systems is beyond on the scope of this chapter but are referenced and detailed by Nyenhuis and Gorelick in another citation [71]. The possible neuropsychological domains involved in VCI are variable and may reflect the diverse pathophysiology of stroke (e.g., ischemia vs. hemorrhage) and size and location of stroke (small and strategically located subcortical strokes and white-matter disease vs. large cortical strokes). Subcortical VCI is considered the most prevalent form of this disorder.

The four key requirements for a diagnosis of VCI are listed in Table 10.2. Clinical and neuroimaging validation of the elements for a diagnosis of VCI has been recommended [72] and is now being studied in a research setting [71]. To optimize knowledge acquisition and application in stroke and VCI, transdisciplinary, translational, and transactional interchanges are recommended [73] as are the development of harmonization criteria [74].

Prevention and treatment

Treatment of cardiovascular risk factors may form the foundation for prevention and treatment of VCI [62]. This may be the case as treatment of stroke risk factors may prevent recurrent cerebral ischemia and may also be beneficial for the prevention of AD [64]. Nonprimary analyses from a number of cardiovascular disease prevention trials, which have administered blood pressure-lowering agent(s), for example, suggest a rather consistent signal for the reduction of dementia including AD and VaD [61,64]. These findings need to be validated by large-scale, appropriately statistically powered studies as such study has been lacking [59]. Randomized clinical trials such as the Systolic Hypertension in Europe (Syst-Eur) and the Perindopril Protection against Recurrent Stroke Study (PROGRESS) found the maintenance of cognitive vitality associated with blood pressure-lowering therapy. It remains to be shown whether a specific class of blood pressure-lowering agent (e.g., angiotensin-converting enzyme inhibitor, angiotensin receptor blocker, long-acting calcium channel agent, thiazide-type diuretic) is superior to another or whether blood pressure lowering is the key factor to maintain cognitive vitality with these agents [71].

There remains controversy about lowering blood pressure in persons with VCI. Specifically, it has been argued that persons with the VaD form of VCI may need a higher level of blood pressure to maintain cognition, whereas those without cognitive impairment or those with vascular CIND may benefit from blood pressure lowering [65,71].

Finally, the use of acetylcholinesterase inhibitors and the NMDA-receptor antagonist, memamtine, have been approved for use in AD but have *not* been approved by the US Federal Drug Administration for treatment of VCI or VaD [71]. The details of clinical trial results relating to these agents in VCI treatment are reviewed elsewhere [71]. Neuropsychiatric symptoms such as agitation, aggression, depression, delusions, hallucinations, and wandering may be common in VCI. Pharmacological and nonpharmacological treatments for these and associated symptoms are reviewed by Sink *et al.* [75]. Clinicians should familiarize themselves with possible side effects associated with psychopharmacological agents that may be used to treat VCI patients as some may be associated with risk of myocardial infarction, stroke, hypertension, and metabolic syndrome.

Stroke severity and recovery from stroke

In addition to the higher incidence, prevalence, and mortality of stroke, there is evidence suggesting that blacks have more severe strokes and, among the stroke survivors, worse residual physical deficits than whites. In a small cohort of 146 ischemic stroke patients (28% blacks and 72% whites), Horner *et al.* showed that race is an important predictor of physical impairment at 180 days, and that blacks have a trend toward recovering from stroke more slowly [76]. Compared with whites, the excess of physical impairment among blacks (measured using the Fugl-Meyer Scale) was 30% at 30 days and almost 9% at 90 and 180 days. These observations, however, could have been confounded by an increased severity of stroke in blacks, evidenced by the trend toward a lower level of consciousness on admission noted in this group. In the Veterans Administration Acute Stroke Study, blacks had a small but significant increase in stroke severity even after controlling for potential confounders, such as atrial fibrillation, stroke type, and previous history of stroke [77]. In the same cohort, there was no racial difference in the proportion of patients referred to rehabilitation or in the intensity of therapy offered. Low-income black patients had delays in the initiation of stroke rehabilitation, probably due to lack of supportive social resources, and had poorer physical functional recovery [78]. Similarly, a trend toward increased stroke severity and less favorable outcome at 7 days and 3 months was found for blacks in the Trial of Org 10172 in Acute Stroke Treatment (TOAST) [79].

Blacks have been historically underrepresented in clinical trials, and more research is necessary to determine with certainty if they have more severe strokes and poorer recovery than whites. Blacks, however, have a tendency to higher prevalence of comorbid conditions such as hypertension, diabetes mellitus, congestive heart failure, obesity, and lower SES than whites [7,30,37,38,79]. Diabetes mellitus [80,81] and cardiac failure [82] are predictors of worse outcome after stroke, and a higher BMI has been associated with a lower likelihood of being discharged directly home and a longer hospital stay [83]. Furthermore, recurrent stroke is a predictor of disability [40], and persons with lower SES may have a decreased likelihood of achieving a maximum rehabilitation potential owing to limited transportation to rehabilitation centers and less access to supplemental home therapy.

These data suggest that regardless of a possible intrinsic racial vulnerability to stroke, blacks are more likely to be exposed to potentially modifiable risk factors that may put them at risk of having worse outcomes after stroke than whites.

Clinical trials and barriers to participation

Background disparities in health and health care

US blacks have had a survival disadvantage for some time. Recent data from the National Center of Health Statistics show that a child born in the United States in 2005 can expect to live to almost 78 years of age [84]. The increase in life expectancy represents an improvement from 1955 when the statistic was 69.6 years and from 1995 when it was 75.8 years. Life expectancy for the black population has increased over time; however, in 2005 it was only 73.2 years, about 5 years behind the white population. Overall, the black–white life expectancy gap in the United States widened during the 1980s but has declined more recently due to relative mortality improvements in homicide, HIV, unintentional injuries, and, among women, heart disease [85].

Explanations for disparities in life expectancy and stroke risk in US blacks have been linked to higher prevalence of risk factors, greater severity or sensitivity to risk factors, and lack of access to medical care [1]. Whereas behavioral and psychosocial factors remain important in conferring risk of disease, new avenues of study such as genomics and proteomics are being explored. Results of a recently published study utilizing NHANES 1999–2002 continues to show that US blacks have a higher prevalence of blood pressure exceeding 140/90 mm Hg than other racial and ethnic subgroups and that treated blacks and Mexican-Americans have the lowest rates of blood pressure control [86]. Severity or sensitivity to risk factors may also play a role in conferring risk. Such mechanisms, however, are less well understood. For example, some blacks may have a propensity for salt sensitivity and a volume-type hypertension, which is hypothesized to have deleterious effects in certain vascular beds including the brain.

Black patients have generally had less access to medical care as reflected in the distribution of health insurance, the discrimination against minorities, and the utilization of procedures, treatments, and surgery [1]. Blacks are less likely to have private medical insurance, and a recent study shows that compared with privately insured patients, uninsured patients have higher levels of neurological impairment, longer average length of hospital stay, and higher mortality risk for stroke [87]. In another example in relation to access to care, US blacks with acute myocardial infarction continue to be less likely to receive coronary revascularization intervention whether they are admitted to hospitals with or without such services [88]. Even in medical care systems that provide a more universal type of access to care, blacks may be less likely to have cerebral angiography and carotid endarterectomy [89]. This raises the questions as to whether such patients are risk aversive and why this may be the case. There has been a long history of mistrust of the medical care system in the black community, which could certainly be an important factor in risk-aversive behavior [90]. The Society of General Internal Medicine Health Disparities Task Force has recommended comprehensive education of healthcare providers and administrators geared toward better understanding of racial and ethnic disparities in health and health care as a possible solution to help bridge gaps in minority health care [91].

We now discuss novel stroke clinical trials targeted to the African-American community. These studies have helped to shape our modern approach to stroke prevention and treatment in the US blacks.

AAASPS

AAASPS was a recurrent stroke prevention clinical trial targeted to African-American patients [2]. The study design included provisions to engage the community in development, recruitment, safety monitoring, and dissemination of information in relation to the study [92]. In addition, AAASPS serves as a model for recruitment and retention of minority study subjects who traditionally have been underrepresented in clinical trials [90,93,94].

AAASPS was a landmark National Institute of Neurological Disorder and Stroke/NIH-funded double-masked, randomized, controlled clinical trial, which was designed to assess the efficacy and safety of aspirin and ticlopidine to prevent recurrent stroke among African-American noncardioembolic ischemic stroke patients [2]. A main study tenet was the establishment of grassroots community support and conceptual acceptance of the potential importance of such a trial during the pretrial planning phase, and community involvement during the main field phases to assure adequate recruitment and retention of study subjects [92]. How were we able to successfully recruit and retain over 1,800 African-American stroke patients from over 60 academic and community hospitals across the United States? A key component of the study design was careful preplanning to meet the needs of the African-American community during each phase of the trial. We carried out surveys to better understand African-American sensitivities in relation to the medical care system, given the legacy of past healthcare abuses that were incurred by this community [90,93]. These types of studies led to the identification of barriers to entry into clinical trials, such as lack of awareness of trials, mistrust, economic factors, and basic communication issues (Table 10.3). When we identified such barriers, steps were taken to systematically resolve them across all of the study sites. Cultural

Table 10.3 Key barriers to entry into clinical trials as identified in the African-American Antiplatelet Stroke Prevention Study [90]

1 Lack of awareness of clinical trials
2 Mistrust of the medical care system
3 Economic disadvantages
4 Social isolation and communication challenges

Table 10.4 Key efficacy and safety findings from the African-American Antiplatelet Stroke Prevention Study [2]

Efficacy
1 Primary outcome end point of recurrent stroke, myocardial infarction, or vascular death: reached by 14.7% of ticlopidine patients ($n = 902$) and 12.3% of aspirin patients ($n = 907$) for a hazard ratio = 1.22 (95% confidence interval: 0.94, 1.57).
2 Secondary outcome of fatal or nonfatal stroke approached a statistically significant reduction favoring aspirin over ticlopidine, $P = 0.08$.
3 Nine myocardial infarctions and 18 vascular deaths occurred in the ticlopidine treatment group versus eight myocardial infarctions and 18 vascular deaths in the aspirin treatment, none of which was statistically significant.

Safety
1 Laboratory-determined serious neutropenia occurred in 3.4% ticlopidine-treated patients versus 2.2% aspirin-treated patients ($P = 0.12$) and 0.3% versus 0.2%, respectively, for thrombocytopenia ($P = 0.69$).
2 There was one possible case of ticlopidine-induced thrombotic thrombocytopenia purpura.
3 Other serious adverse events did not differ significantly between treatment groups.
4 For study subjects prematurely discontinuing the blind phase of the intervention, rash was more common in the ticlopidine versus aspirin groups (1.7% vs. 0.6%; $P = 0.02$).

sensitivity training programs were developed and carried out by the AAASPS management staff and shared with the local study staff at the site investigator meetings. Local study staff were educated about the importance of spending adequate time and developing a trustful relationship with potential study participants, and serving as their study advocates. Furthermore, the involvement of a study staff from the African-American community was recommended, as was the development of an overall study community advisory panel for the main study management site. The same concept was to be embraced locally as satellite community advisory panels were encouraged at local study sites. Attempts to enhance community awareness were achieved by a community service coordinator, Internet postings about the study, involvement of church healthcare coordinators, a community volunteer corps to promote the study, involvement of minority health professionals to identify potential study subjects, a speaker's bureau, and the use of the media. Church support was sought as was the recognition of the study by major black legislative groups [94].

We also developed a recruitment and retention triangle model, which consisted of three arms: the study patient, his or her family members, and the study subject's healthcare professionals [93]. Conceptually, if any one of the components of the triangle weakened, recruitment and retention could be endangered. We emphasized engagement and communication with the patient, family members, and the patient's community physician and healthcare team in an attempt to strengthen study recruitment and retention.

We showed that by careful pretrial planning and thoughtful study measures, our research team could successfully recruit and retain minority subjects in a large-scale, national, clinical trial by breaking down study barriers and being culturally sensitive. Although we were convinced based on the preliminary trial data from the Ticlopidine Aspirin Stroke

Study (TASS) that ticlopidine would be safe and substantially more effective than aspirin for recurrent stroke prevention in African-Americans, an efficacy advantage of ticlopidine over aspirin therapy was not found [2]. In fact, the study was stopped early by the NIH-appointed Data and Safety Monitoring Board for reasons of futility, and we could not support the use of ticlopidine for stroke prevention in African-Americans. Had the study been continued, there was a 40–50% likelihood that *aspirin* would be more efficacious than ticlopidine for recurrent stroke prevention. The AAASPS efficacy findings are a reminder that subgroup and other nonprimary analyses (e.g., from TASS in this case) may be useful for hypothesis generation but not necessarily for making patient management decisions as there may be uncontrolled confounding in such analyses [95,96]. The safety profile of the two study interventions was similar [2]. Key efficacy and safety findings from AAASPS are listed in Table 10.4.

Sickle disease trials in stroke

The Stroke Prevention Trial in Sickle Cell Anemia (STOP) was another landmark study funded by the NIH and conducted in the United States and Canada during the time period 1995–2000 [97–100]. Close to 2,000 children or young adults aged 2–16 years were screened using TCD, and those with two TCD ultrasounds showing middle cerebral artery or internal carotid artery velocity of ≥200 cm/s could be randomized. The trial was halted prematurely when it became apparent that 11 of 67 subjects randomized to standard treatment (episodic transfusions for symptoms such as pain) had stroke compared with only one study subject in the long-term transfusion group. Therefore, with regular transfusion there was a more than 90% reduction in stroke over and above the 10% per year stroke risk in the other treatment group [100].

STOP II was then designed to determine whether transfusion could be safely withdrawn [99]. About 53% of the STOP subjects undergoing transfusion had their TCD ultrasound velocities revert to lower risk levels (e.g., <170 cm/s). Conceptually, STOP II was designed to enroll 100 children who had high-risk TCD velocities that had reverted to <170 cm/s after at least 30 months of transfusion and MRA did not show higher grades of stenosis or occlusion. Half of the subjects would have continuation of transfusion, and half would have transfusion discontinued [100]. Again, the study was stopped early when it was noted that there was rapid reversion of TCD velocities to higher risk levels in those who had stopped transfusion therapy. There were two strokes in the latter group.

Other studies including one testing screening approaches in children with sickle-cell disease and one testing hydroxyurea with transfusion for sec-

Table 10.5 Stroke prevention in children with sickle-cell disease: American Heart Association/American Stroke Association Guideline Recommendations [100,101]

---

1 Screen children with sickle-cell disease with TCD starting at age 2 years.
2 Consider transfusion therapy for those with elevated stroke risk.
3 Continued TCD is recommended for younger children and those with TCD velocities in the conditional range to detect high-risk TCD indications for intervention.
4 Pending additional study, it is reasonable to continue transfusion therapy even if TCD velocities revert to normal.
5 Adults with sickle-cell disease should be screened for cardiovascular risk factors and managed according to general guidelines.
6 Adults with sickle-cell disease and ischemic stroke or TIA should receive general treatment recommendations for control of risk factors and use of antiplatelet agents. Regular transfusion therapy should be considered to reduce hemoglobin S to <30 to 50% of total hemoglobin as should hydroxyurea or extracranial to intracranial bypass surgery when there is advanced occlusive brain disease.

TIA, transient ischemic attack; TCD, transcranial Doppler.

ondary stroke prevention are ongoing [99]. Long-term transfusion therapy may pose a risk of iron load, which has become easier to treat with the availability of an oral iron chelator agent. Recommendations from current guideline statements for the management of children with sickle-cell disease are listed in Table 10.5 [101,102].

References available online at www.wiley.com/go/strokeguidelines.

Stroke in Children

Gabrielle A. deVeber

EXAMPLE CASE

Four-year-old Adam was brought to the emergency room by his mother. He had been irritable for the prior 24 hours – having what seemed like temper tantrum after temper tantrum. Between the tantrums, he fell backwards on a couple of occasions, as though "limp." He complained of a headache after his last tantrum. He was put to bed early, irritable and cried himself to sleep. He awakened his mother at 5:00 AM, wanting to be escorted to the bathroom and was noted to be unstable on his feet. After going to the bathroom, he returned to bed with an obvious right-sided facial droop. By 9:00 AM, his facial droop was worse, and he was unable to speak. His mother rushed Adam to the closest local community hospital.

At the local community hospital ER, he was found to have a left hemiparesis (facial droop and arm and leg weakness). An urgent brain CT scan was normal, and he was transferred to the local pediatric hospital.

Adam's past history included that he was born at term, weighing 5 lbs, 6 oz, one of fraternal twin boys. He had normal development and was usually a healthy and happy child who attended junior kindergarten. He had no past history of seizures or migraine headache. He had a supracondylar right arm fracture 2 weeks earlier when he fell from the monkey bars in the school playground. Immunizations were current including a varicella vaccination 16 months previously. He had no allergies and was not receiving any medications. His family history was negative for hyperlipidemia, stroke, coronary heart disease, or thrombosis in relatives at ages younger than 55 years.

MAJOR POINTS

- Computed tomography or magnetic resonance imaging diagnosis is necessary, given nonspecific presentations.
- Data supporting the use of tissue-type plasminogen activator in children are limited to case series and reports.
- Although clinical trials are lacking, antithrombotic therapy is commonly used to prevent early recurrence.
- Although clinical trials are lacking, initial anticoagulation is commonly used in the setting of suspected dissection or cardiogenic stroke.
- Aspirin is used as part of the secondary preventive therapy in most cases in which anticoagulants are not used.
- Etiological diagnosis is critical to guide treatment.
- Rehabilitation is important with an evidence base developing.
- Functional deficits often become apparent with maturation.

A Primer on Stroke Prevention Treatment: An Overview Based on AHA/ASA Guidelines, 1st Edition. Edited by L Goldstein.
© 2009 American Heart Association, ISBN: 9781405186513

Physical and neurological exam

His blood pressure was 110/46 mm Hg, pulse was 80 and regular, and respiratory rate was 22, and he was afebrile. He was healthy, appearing with no rashes, a normal cardiac examination, and no carotid or cranial bruits. He was lethargic and irritable, unable to vocalize, but able to follow simple commands. Fundoscopy, pupillary reactions, and extraocular movements were normal, including no gaze deviation. There was an obvious right-sided facial droop; however, tongue protrusion and uvula were midline. He was unable to lift his right arm off the bed (casted for prior fracture) and had only slight movement of the fingers of his right hand. His right leg was weak; he was able to move on the bed but not against gravity when stimulated. His deep tendon reflexes were difficult to elicit. His right plantar response was extensor. Sensory testing was not completely reliable, but his response to cold was intact bilaterally. There was no limb ataxia. Gait could not be tested due to inability to bear weight on the right leg.

Initial laboratory results

On arrival, Adam's complete blood count, electrolytes, blood glucose, and routine coagulation studies (prothrombin and activated partial thromboplastin times) were normal.

Radiographic results (for stroke diagnosis and arteriopathy)

1 Day 1 initial head CT scan normal
2 Day 1 magnetic resonance imaging (MRI) at 7 hours post-onset
   • Fluid-attenuated inversion recovery (FLAIR) and diffusion-weighted imaging showed infarction in the left basal ganglia, adjacent white-matter and peri-insular cortex conforming to lenticulostriate vascular territory (Figure 11.1).
   • Magnetic resonance angiography (MRA) of intracranial vessels showed minimal irregularity of proximal segments of the left middle cerebral artery (MCA) (M1 and M2) (Figure 11.2).
   • MRA of neck vessels showed no evidence of occlusion or dissection.

Acute management

Elapsed time from the onset of facial droop to arrival at a pediatric hospital was 5 hours, and to MRI scan

was 7 hours. From arrival, oxygen saturation, blood pressure, temperature, and blood glucose were monitored. Low molecular weight heparin (LMWH) was initiated 8 hours after admission after the diagnostic MRI scan, at a treatment dose of 1 mg/kg/d subcutaneously every 12 hours. LMWH was titrated to a 4-hour post-dose anti-Xa level of 0.5–1.0 units. At 24 hours post-onset, Adam was mute and had severe hemiparesis.

Further studies

Over a period of 7 days, he had the following investigations, all of which were normal:

1 Hematological investigations – normal complete blood count (CBC) including platelets (for infection, anemia)
2 Prothrombotic investigations: protein C, protein S, antithrombin, plasminogen, homocysteine, lipoprotein (a), factor V Leiden, prothrombin gene (for prothrombotic abnormalities)
3 Vasculitis investigations: ESR, CH50, C-reactive protein (for vasculitis); echocardiogram including agitated saline ("bubble") study (for cardiac lesions including congenital heart disease or patent foramen ovale)

Day 3 conventional angiography revealed focal beaded irregularity consistent with the appearance of transient cerebral arteriopathy (TCA) involving the distal left internal carotid, proximal MCA, and proximal anterior cerebral arteries (Figure 11.3).

Chronic management

Antithrombotic treatment was changed to IV unfractionated heparin on the evening of day 2 in preparation for conventional angiography. Following angiography, he was switched to aspirin 5 mg/kg/d. Aspirin was continued through the hospital stay and continued indefinitely at 3–5 mg/kg/d. In the discussion with pediatric rheumatology, IV steroid therapy for possible central nervous system vasculitis was considered but not pursued. Conventional angiography was repeated at 2 months post-onset and revealed smooth stenotic narrowing of the M1 segment at the previously "beaded" segment. MRA at 6 months showed stenosis at sites of the prior abnormalities. Conventional angiography at 1 year showed no change. Follow-up angiography confirmed the diagnosis of TCA.

Neurological course and rehabilitation

During the initial 7 days, Adam had return of some right limb power. While at the acute care pediatric hospital, he and his family were linked with occupational therapy, physiotherapy, speech therapy, and the social worker. The clinical nurse specialist/nurse practitioner was also an ongoing source of support and education about pediatric stroke and the need for multiple investigations as well as treatment planning. Adam was transferred to a specialized pediatric rehabilitation hospital at 7 days for further intensive therapy (occupational, physical, and speech therapy). By discharge, he was able to ambulate with assistance and lift his right arm against gravity, although no wrist or finger movements were present.

Follow-up at 3 months in the Pediatric Stroke Clinic showed moderate weakness with functional slowing in his right arm and a moderate speech deficit. At 5 months, he presented with new onset dystonia in the hemiparetic limbs, which worsened over the subsequent 6 months. With the emergence of dystonia, he was started on an anticholinergic with only minor improvement. When dystonia persisted despite oral medications, botulinum toxin injections of selected upper limb muscles was provided with modest improvement. This was repeated every 3 months.

At 4 years post-stroke, Adam's speech was mildly abnormal, he had learning difficulties, and his right arm dystonia remained severe. He ambulated with an ankle-foot orthosis. He has, however, learned to water ski and participates in most activities typical for a boy his age. Adam has had neuropsychological testing showing several areas of learning difficulty related to his basal stroke. He has in-school assistance to complete his schoolwork.

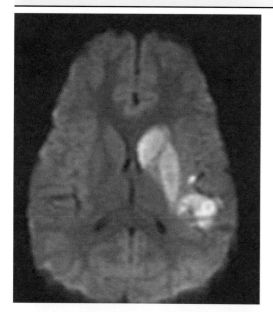

Fig. 11.1 Initial magnetic resonance imaging.

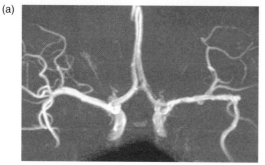
(a)

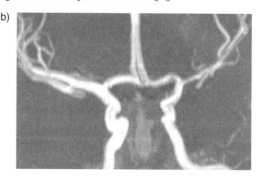
(b)

Fig. 11.2 Initial and follow-up magnetic resonance angiography (MRA). (a) Initial MRA; (b) MRA at 3 months.

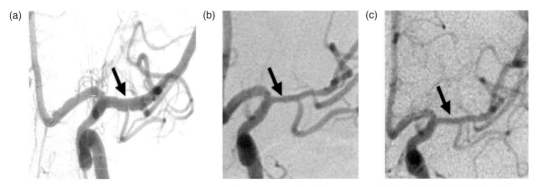

Fig. 11.3 Initial and follow-up conventional angiography. Cerebral angiography (CA) performed at (a) 1 week (initial CA), (b) 2 months, and (c) 6 months post-stroke showing unilateral intracranial arteriopathy characteristic of "transient cerebral arteriopathy of childhood" [15].

Discussion

This otherwise healthy boy presents with signs and symptoms of a focal brain lesion with acute onset over hours, consistent with stroke. Investigations confirmed arterial ischemic stroke (AIS). Many physicians are not familiar with stroke in childhood. Pediatric stroke, however, is emerging as an important cause of neurological morbidity in children and ranks in the top 10 causes of death in infants [1,2]. Studies over the past two decades estimate an incidence of 2–8/100,000 children per year and, in neonates, 1 : 4,000 live births [3]. Healthcare costs during the year after stroke were recently estimated at $42,338 per child, excluding out-of-pocket and lost parental productivity costs [4]. Previously, children were thought to have better outcomes after focal brain injury, including stroke, than adults. This historical impression has been refuted in recent outcome studies that document a high rate of morbidity [5–7]. Thus, despite being relatively uncommon, disabling long-term sequelae from childhood stroke are likely to result in a larger burden on society than previously estimated. The impact per affected individual is greater for children, since with full life expectancy, the burden of illness is expected to manifest over many more decades than in a comparably affected adult.

Initial stroke diagnosis

Adam was diagnosed with stroke 7 hours after onset when MRI was performed. Urgent diagnosis of AIS in children presents major challenges. A lack of public and physician awareness of pediatric stroke probably accounts for the delays in arrival to the hospital, which averages to 1.7 hours [8]. At pediatric hospitals, acute stroke systems with provision of around-the-clock MRI imaging for suspected stroke are rarely available. Consequently, delays from arrival to initial neuroimaging average to 12.7 hours for children [8].

Adam presented with a rapidly progressive hemiparesis starting in the face and accompanied by mutism. This same presentation in an adult would lead to a presumptive diagnosis of stroke. His initial CT was normal. A normal head CT in an adult at this early stage following stroke onset would then lead to diagnosis of ischemic stroke, hemorrhage and other stroke mimics having been ruled out as the cause. Treatment with tissue-type plasminogen activator might be provided. Although such a presentation in children should also be considered as due to stroke until proven otherwise, the differential diagnosis for acute focal neurological deficits in children is much wider and includes unwitnessed seizures with Todd's paralysis, complicated migraine, demyelinating disorders, and meningoencephalitis [9]. When CT is normal, MRI with diffusion is necessary to confirm the diagnosis of AIS. Further confounding early diagnosis is that in young infants and newborns, clinical presentations of AIS are usually very nonspecific, frequently including only mental status change or seizures alone [10]. This is because focal lesions in the immature, unmyelinated brain occur in areas not yet functioning. Instead, as the affected brain area becomes important with development, the child will "grow into" deficits. Thus, family doctors, pediatricians, and emergency physicians need to have a high index of suspicion for stroke in children with an acute focal neurological deficit. Although Adam had no preceding transient ischemic attacks, these occur often in children in the days and weeks preceding ischemic stroke and frequently represent missed opportunities to initiate preventive treatment.

Etiological diagnosis

The search for an etiology begins once a diagnosis of stroke is established in a child. Childhood AIS is not due to atherosclerosis, the predominant cause for stroke in adults. Common conditions causing childhood stroke include congenital cardiac malformations, acquired cardiac conditions, and cerebral arteriopathies. A multitude of additional systemic and head and neck disorders can also cause childhood stroke including conditions both acute (dehydration, head trauma) and chronic (iron deficiency anemia, brain tumor). Prothrombotic disorders are frequent additional risk factors reported in 30–50% [11]. Cardiac disorders are usually evident prior to stroke, and stroke may be a complication of cardiac catheterization or surgery [12].

Overall, arteriopathy is the most common mechanism for pediatric AIS [13]. In most children, arteriopathy is unsuspected at the time of stroke presentation, and detection requires vascular imaging. Arteriopathies range from mild, reversible disorders to severe and progressive types and include migraine, dissection, TCA or post-varicella arteriopathy, vasculitis, Moyamoya, and others [14] (Table 11.1). In contrast to the extracranial distribution of atherosclerosis, childhood arteriopathies tend to be intracranial. Intracranial arteriopathies can be bilateral, including progressive vasculitis or the Moyamoya syndrome (either sickle or non-sickle related) or unilateral, including TCA and post-varicella angiopathy. Progressive vasculitis usually involves multiple caliber anterior and posterior circulation arteries at onset. Aggressive treatment with steroids and cyclophosphamide is frequently used. Arterial dissection is frequently extracranial and, along with migraine, favors the posterior circulation in children. Close monitoring of unilateral intracranial arteriopathy over at least 1 year is warranted to ensure it does not evolve into bilateral Moyamoya or progressive vasculitis.

Table 11.1 Cerebral vasculopathies in children

Cervicocephalic arterial dissections
Moyamoya disease and Moyamoya syndrome
Fibromuscular dysplasia
Vasculitis
Transient cerebral arteriopathy
Post-varicella angiopathy
Migrainous infarction
Ergotism
Traumatic cerebrovascular disease
Radiation-induced arteriopathy
Tumoral encasement of cervicocephalic vessels
Hypoplasia and agenesis of cervicocephalic vessels
Congenital arterial fenestration

Cerebral Vasculopathies in Children from AHA Pediatric Stroke Guidelines from [17].
Adapted from Biller J, Mathews KD, Love BB. Stroke in Children and Young Adults. Boston: Butterworth-Heinemann, 1994, with permission from Elsevier.

Adam was a previously well child, and only upon vascular imaging was the mechanism of his stroke clarified – a focal unilateral intracranial arteriopathy. Initial vascular imaging suggested, and follow-up imaging confirmed, that he had TCA, a disorder that has been recognized in recent years among children with AIS [15]. This unilateral, intracranial, anterior circulation disorder is limited to the distal internal carotid artery and proximal middle and anterior cerebral arteries, and is associated with a large, deep AIS involving basal ganglia. TCA is a presumed inflammatory disorder, and is self-limited with some initial stenosis during the acute period (several weeks to months), then stabilization or regression of the arteriopathic lesions after 6 months (Figures 11.2 and 11.3). Post-varicella angiopathy is radiographically indistinguishable from TCA but is preceded by a varicella infection by several weeks to months. The inflammatory nature of post-varicella angiopathy has been established by postmortem histopathology on multiple adult cases and one childhood case. Vascular imaging shows stabilization from several months to 1 year – characteristic of TCA.

The series of investigations that were conducted in Adam are generally performed in children presenting with AIS. Frequently, multiple risk factors are discovered in individual children, with some, including prothrombotic disorders, playing a predisposing role and others, including head or neck trauma and dissection, playing a triggering role. In particular, prothrombotic laboratory testing should be considered even if other stroke mechanisms are found, as they play an important additive role in initial and recurrent stroke [16]. The recent American Heart Association (AHA) Guidelines on Pediatric Stroke indicate that "it is reasonable to evaluate for the more common prothrombotic states even when another stroke risk factor has been identified (Class IIa, Level of Evidence C) [17]. Other hematological disorders that are common in children with stroke require consideration including sickle-cell disease, and iron deficiency anemia which is associated with stroke through as yet unclear mechanisms [18]. The AHA Pediatric Stroke Guidelines provide comprehensive lists of possible causes of childhood stroke and a discussion of investigations in addition to treatment guidelines [17].

Management

Age-specific considerations underlying pediatric stroke treatment

As in adult stroke, the treatment of pediatric AIS is largely etiology-driven. Antithrombotic treatment aims to prevent initial or recurrent stroke. Although randomized trials in children are lacking, antithrombotic drugs during the acute stroke period are frequently used due to the high risk of early recurrent stroke. Up to 50% of children not treated with aspirin or anticoagulants have recurrent strokes [19]. The risk of recurrent stroke in children is maximal in the first days and weeks after index stroke [19]. Antithrombotic treatment generally consists of either antiplatelet (aspirin) or anticoagulant (heparin or LMWH) medication. The challenge facing clinicians is whether to select an antiplatelet drug or an anticoagulant. In adults, anticoagulants have not been shown to be of any benefit in the acute period. Treatment decisions in children are based on the likelihood of recurrence and the presumed biological basis of the thrombus in an individual child. The etiology largely determines whether thrombus is predominantly fibrin based or platelet based, although most clots are apt to be composed of a combination of the two thrombotic systems.

Children clearly differ from adults in the cause for stroke and risks of treatment. Childhood AIS is not due to atherosclerosis; the predominant cause for adult stroke and the etiology is frequently arterial dissection or structural cardiac disease with embolism. Combined, these two etiologies are found in approximately one-third of children with AIS [13]. Prothrombotic risk factors, present in 30–50% of children with AIS, increase the risk of stroke recurrence [11,16].

The first institutional protocols for the management of pediatric stroke were published in 1997 [20]. In the past 4 years, three consensus-based guidelines for pediatric stroke have been published. Each assigns levels of evidence for individual recommendations [20–23]. Tables 11.2 and 11.3 compare the treatment recommendations from these three sources for the acute and chronic treatment of subtypes of childhood AIS. The original guidelines also provide additional recommendations for other stroke subtypes, including neonatal stroke and cerebral sinovenous thrombosis. The participation of hematologists in clinical management decisions, pediatric stroke research, and clinical guideline developments has played critical roles in expanding our understanding of non-atherogenic cerebral artery thrombosis. Experience gleaned from the management of children with systemic arterial thrombosis and expertise in the safe use of aspirin and anticoagulants has benefited pediatric neurologists, the primary treating physicians for children with acute stroke.

The "UK" guidelines published in 2004 by the Royal College of Physicians of London are comprehensive consensus guidelines including general care, medicinal and nonmedical treatment, and rehabilitation [22]. They also provide an educational handbook for children with stroke and their parents. For the first time in 2004, the American College of Chest Physicians Antithrombotic Guidelines included a chapter devoted to pediatric stroke. These were updated in 2008 [21]. Most recently, the "Management of stroke in infants and children, a scientific statement from a Special Writing Group of the AHA Stroke Council and the Council on Cardiovascular Disease in the Young" was published [18]. These are very comprehensive guidelines encompassing diagnosis and medical, surgical, and rehabilitative treatments for all subtypes of pediatric stroke. Given the absence of randomized controlled trials in pediatric stroke, the evidence supporting individual recom-

Table 11.2 Comparison of the American Heart Association (AHA) and other childhood stroke guidelines: acute treatment

Acute treatment of childhood arterial ischemic stroke by subtype

Subtype	UK guidelines 2004 Recommendation	G	S	Chest guidelines 2008 Recommendation	G	S	AHA 2008 Recommendation	G	S
Acute supportive measures	Maintain normal temperature and oxygen saturation	D	4	Not addressed			Control fever, maintain normal oxygenation, control systemic hypertension, and normalize serum glucose	1-C	1
General	ASA 5 mg/kg	WPC	1	UFH or LMWH or ASA 1–5 mg/kg/d until cardioembolic and dissection excluded	1B	1	UFH or LMWH (1 mg/kg/12 hours) up to 1 week until cause determined	2b-C	3
Sickle-cell disease	Exchange transfusion to HbS ≤30%	WPC	1	IV hydration and exchange transfusion to HbS <30%	1B	1	Exchange transfusion to HbS <30%	2a-B	2
Cardiac	Anticoagulation should be discussed by senior pediatric neurologist and pediatric cardiologist	WPC	1	LMWH 6+ weeks	2C	3	For cardiac embolism unrelated to patent foramen ovale, and judged to have high recurrence risk:		
							UFH or LMWH as a bridge to oral anticoagulation	2a-B	
							Alternative: UFH or LMWH as a bridge to maintenance LMWH	2a-C	2
Dissection	Anticoagulation for extracranial dissection with no hemorrhage	WPC	1	LMWH 6+ weeks	2C	3	UFH or LMWH as a bridge to oral anticoagulation	2a-C	2
tPA	Not recommended		1	Not recommended	1B	1	Not recommended	3-C	1
tPA in teens	Not addressed			Not addressed			No consensus on use		

Childhood defined as 28 days to 18 years (Chest), 1 month to 16 years (UK).

ASA, aspirin; G, grade of evidence/recommendation; HbS, sickle hemoglobin; LMWH, low molecular weight heparin; S, strength of evidence/recommendation; tPA, tissue-type plasminogen activator; UFH, unfractionated heparin; WPC, working-party consensus.

mendations in all three sets of guidelines is sparse. They represent consensus opinions, based primarily on experience or intuition, or, in some cases, case-control or cohort study data, rather than random-ized controlled trials. In many cases, evidence from adult treatment trials has been selectively extrapo-lated, keeping in mind that the major mechanism in adults, atherosclerosis, does not play a role in the causation of pediatric stroke.

Primary prevention was not an option in Adam. But treatment aimed at preventing a first stroke is highly desirable, and is available in certain subgroups of children at significant risk for AIS. For children with sickle-cell disease, regular transfusions can prevent a first stroke based on a randomized con-trolled trial [24]. Vaso-occlusive stroke complicates 1 in 185 cardiac surgeries in children, and reopera-tion is a risk factor for stroke. It should therefore be

Chronic treatment of childhood arterial ischemic stroke

Subtype	UK guidelines 2004 Recommendation	G	S	Chest guidelines 2008 Recommendation	G	S	AHA 2008 Recommendation	G	S
General	ASA 1–5 mg/kg/d	WPC	1	Once dissection and cardioembolism are excluded, ASA 1–5 mg/kg/d, 2+ years	1B	1	ASA 3–5 mg/kg/d	2a-C	3
Dissection	Consider anticoagulation until evidence of vessel healing or up to 6 months	WPC	1	LMWH ongoing depending on radiographic results	2C	3	Intracranial dissection or associated subarachnoid hemorrhage: anticoagulation not recommended	3-C	1
							Extracranial dissection: LMWH or warfarin 3–6 months ASA may be substituted	2a-C	
Cardiogenic embolism	Consider anticoagulation after discussion with the cardiologist managing the patient	WPC	1	LMWH ongoing depending on radiographic results	2C	3	ASA beyond 6 months	2a-C	
							LMWH or warfarin ≥1 year	2a-B	2
Prothrombotic states	Refer patient to a hematologist	WPC	1	Not addressed			Warfarin long term for selected hypercoagulable states	2a-C	2
Vasculopathy	ASA 1–3 mg/kg/d	WPC	1	Not addressed			Not addressed		
Moyamoya	Revascularization surgery	D	3	Revascularization surgery	1B	1	Revascularization surgery	1-B	1
Sickle-cell disease	Blood transfusion every 3–6 weeks to HbS 30%	C	3	Long-term transfusion program	1B	1	Regular transfusion program	1-B	1
	After 3 years, aim for HbS <50%	C	3	Not addressed			Not addressed		
	If no transfusion, hydroxyurea	C	3	Not addressed			If no transfusion, hydroxyurea	2b-B	2
	Consider bone-marrow transplant	B	2	Not addressed			Consider bone-marrow transplant	2b-C	3
Recurrent stroke on ASA	Consider anticoagulation	WPC	1	Change to clopidogrel or anticoagulation	2C	3	Not addressed		
Rehabilitation	Rehabilitation developmentally relevant and appropriate to home, community, and school environment	D	4	Not addressed			Age-appropriate rehabilitation and psychological assessment of cognitive and language deficits	1-C	
Preventing atherosclerosis	Advise re: preventable risk factors, smoking, exercise, and diet	D	4	Not addressed			Advise re: diet, exercise, and tobacco	2a-C	

Child defined as 28 days to 18 years (Chest), 1 month to 16 years (UK).

ASA, aspirin; G, grade of evidence/recommendation; LMWH, low molecular weight heparin; S, strength of evidence/recommendation; WPC, working-party consensus.

feasible to develop strategies to prevent this [12]. A high rate of thromboemboli and stroke occurs after Fontan cardiac surgery, and a primary prevention trial comparing antiplatelet to anticoagulation is pending [25].

Other situations conferring increased risk for AIS in children include intracardiac thrombus and systemic venous thrombosis with intracardiac shunt. The identification and treatment of these conditions may offer the opportunity to prevent initial AIS, although this has not been studied in randomized trials (now in progress in adults).

Finally, the prevention of atherosclerosis and adult stroke through the reduction of reversible risk factors for atherosclerosis should start in childhood. Measures geared to initiation of low-fat diet, exercise, prevention of smoking and exposure to second-hand tobacco smoke, and screening for hypertension are all target treatments currently being emphasized in the pediatric population and are recommended in the AHA guidelines [18].

Measures to protect the brain from undergoing progressive acute infarction, including optimization of oxygen, blood pressure, glucose and temperature, are recommended in the UK and AHA pediatric guidelines [18,22]. When Adam presented with acute suspected stroke, he was urgently managed with these general measures. Seizures, though not present in Adam, are common at onset of childhood stroke and require aggressive treatment since they place major increases in metabolic demands on the brain. In the early days following stroke, progressive edema with impending herniation can occur and be fatal. Although not required for Adam, early decompressive hemicarniectomy is advocated at some centers for children with evidence on imaging of impending herniation. Availability and decision making around this treatment option require that children with acute stroke are managed in pediatric centers with specialized care including neurosurgery.

Adam was a healthy child at the time of his stroke, and the initial urgent treatment with LMWH was selected based upon the suspicion of occult dissection or cardiogenic embolism. This medication has been shown to be safe with no major drug-related complications in a large multicenter cohort study of childhood AIS [26]. In Adam, once the diagnosis of TCA was established by conventional angiography,

he was switched to aspirin therapy. The use of anticoagulation as an initial treatment for children with acute AIS of unclear etiology is standard at some centers and is recommended in the ACCP and AHA pediatric stroke guidelines [21] (Table 11.2). Children with unknown stroke etiology are also sometimes treated with aspirin as initial therapy, an approach recommended by the UK guidelines [22]. There are no treatment trials to guide this decision in children. This lack of data and consensus should spur the development of clinical trials [23].

Chronic medical treatment in Adam consisted of long-term aspirin to prevent recurrent stroke. Aspirin was selected because his principle stroke mechanism was arteriopathy. In children with dissection, cardiogenic stroke, or prothrombotic states, anticoagulation is given for several months up to lifelong, depending on perceived pathophysiology of thrombus and risk of recurrence (Table 11.2). The duration of long-term aspirin therapy in general childhood stroke is debated and is often continued for at least 2 years. Aspirin at the treatment doses of 2–5 mg/kg/d is not associated with Reye's syndrome or significant bleeding risk in children [26].

Adam later developed dystonia that was refractory to medical treatment and persisted as a disabling consequence of his stroke. He required ongoing rehabilitation focused on his motor and speech deficits and learning challenges. Both the UK and AHA guidelines emphasize the need for age-appropriate rehabilitative therapy. Randomized controlled trials demonstrate that children with hemiparesis after stroke benefit from constraint-induced therapy and under experimental conditions from transcranial magnetic stimulation, even years after stroke in infancy or childhood [27,28]. Adam was not a candidate for constraint-induced therapy due to risk of increasing his dystonia.

Gaps in current knowledge

There exist major gaps in knowledge in childhood stroke reflected in a high proportion of children with adverse outcomes. Pediatric stroke expertise is required to make management decisions regarding investigations and treatment. In adults, multidisciplinary stroke units save lives largely owing to their provision of expert stroke care supported by evidence-based best-practice guidelines (see Chapter 2). In children with stroke, no such similar care is yet available for two reasons. First, there is a need for the training and development of pediatric stroke specialists in neurology and related specialties. In pediatric rehabilitation, very few therapists specializing in the area of childhood stroke are available. Second, evidence-based best-practice treatment guidelines in adults are based mainly upon randomized controlled trials, the ultimate research study design with which to determine best clinical treatment. In contrast, in pediatric stroke, only two randomized controlled trials have been conducted [24,28]. Because the evidence upon which treatment guidelines are based is scanty, specialized care in decision making is paramount and current consensus-based recommendations are likely to change as better data become available.

Future directions

Within children's hospitals, standardized pediatric stroke protocols and programs are developing, including rapid access to neuroimaging for the diagnosis of stroke. These programs are based in "pediatric stroke teams" comprised of pediatric neurologists, hematologists, neuroradiologists, neurosurgeons, and other specialists. This trend will increase as awareness and research publications in this field increase. In the rehabilitation sector, functional MRI and other research tools are providing a better understanding of brain plasticity and repair relevant to the developing brain after pediatric stroke. The field of pediatric stroke rehabilitation will grow. Ideally, developmental therapists with their understanding of the developing brain will collaborate with adult stroke rehabilitation specialists who understand the phases of recovery from stroke. The development of expertise in pediatric stroke rehabilitation will enable the development and application of effective treatments.

Clinical trials to support management guidelines in pediatric stroke are becoming increasingly feasible. A growing body of researchers focused on pediatric stroke have linked together in the International Pediatric Stroke Study to design and conduct clinical studies to reduce adverse outcomes from pediatric stroke [29]. This collaboration is enrolling patients in a large multicenter observational study with a centralized database, and initial analyses are becoming available [30,31]. Subsequent data on larger numbers of children with stroke sufficient to study etiological subtypes will enable the design of clinical and laboratory studies to increase our understanding of childhood stroke, together with clinical trials to inform treatment approaches. Discrepancies in guideline recommendations from various sources provide an urgent focus for comparison of treatment approaches in these trials.

References available online at www.wiley.com/go/ strokeguidelines.

Coagulopathy and Stroke

Mark Chan, Richard C. Becker, Svati H. Shah, and Steven R. Levine

EXAMPLE CASE

A 37-year-old right hand dominant African-American woman was admitted to the hospital for evaluation of sudden onset of speech disturbance accompanied by weakness of the right upper extremity. Her symptoms began while giving a seminar at a nearby college. Her past medical history is remarkable for two miscarriages – the first occurring in the second trimester of pregnancy, while the second occurred in the third trimester. There is no family history of stroke or venous thromboembolic disease. Her social history is noted for second-hand smoke exposure. She denied alcohol, illicit drug, or over-the-counter stimulant medications. She takes a multiple vitamin daily.

The patient's blood pressure was 140/80 mm Hg in both arms, with a regular pulse of 86 bpm. Her respirations were 20 per minute and nonlabored. She was afebrile. Her skin was moist without rashes. The patient's peripheral pulses were 2+ and symmetric; neither carotid nor subclavain artery bruits were heard. Her lungs were clear to auscultation. Her first and second heart sounds were normal. There were no murmurs, rubs, or gallops. Her abdomen was soft and nontender with normal bowel sounds. Organomegaly was not detected. There were no palpable masses. Peripheral edema was not present, nor were warmth, swelling, or deformity of the joints.

Neurological examination found her to be alert, attentive, and able to follow simple verbal commands. She spoke with difficulty, making frequent paraphasic errors. There was a left-gaze preference and right homonymous visual field deficit. Motor examination revealed 3/5 proximal and 3/5 distal strength in the right upper extremity. There was 4/5 strength in the right lower extremity. Full strength was present in both the left upper and

MAJOR POINTS

- Hypercoagulable states, currently referred to as thrombophilias, as traditionally defined, are an uncommon cause of stroke.
- Acquired hypercoagulable states represent an important treatable cause of stroke.
- Young patients with a first arterial thrombotic event should be screened for antiphospholipid antibodies and the presence of a circulating lupus anticoagulant.
- Patients with an ischemic stroke or TIA with an established inherited thrombophilia should be evaluated for deep venous thrombosis, as a potential cause or nidus of a paradoxical embolism, which is an indication for short- or long-term anticoagulant therapy.

A Primer on Stroke Prevention Treatment: An Overview Based on AHA/ASA Guidelines, 1st Edition. Edited by L Goldstein.
© 2009 American Heart Association, ISBN: 9781405186513

lower extremities. Deep tendon reflexes were diminished on the right with a right plantar extensor response.

A complete blood count showed thrombocytopenia with a platelet count of 110×10^9 per liter. The other cell lines were within normal limits, as were the red blood cell indices. Renal, hepatic, and electrolyte laboratory studies were unremarkable. A 12-lead ECG revealed normal sinus rhythm with normal intervals and nonspecific T-wave abnormalities. A brain CT scan was also unremarkable.

Discussion

The acute onset of symptoms, coupled with focal neurological findings on physical examination, supports a diagnosis of acute ischemic stroke in an otherwise healthy woman. While the initial management must focus on therapies to reduce brain injury and its clinical sequelae, consideration must be given to potential etiologies of acute ischemic stroke, namely the "ABCs": Arterial, Blood, and Cardiac. These range from arterial and venous cerebrovascular disease to primary thrombosis in situ, cardioembolic stroke, and paradoxical embolism. A carefully crafted diagnostic approach to ischemic stroke that includes the consideration of inherited and acquired thrombophilias has important implications for treatment and the prevention of future events [1].

The evolution of coagulation

In mammalian coagulation, the complex network of integrated biochemical events is composed primarily of five proteases (factor II or prothrombin, factor VII, factor IX, factor X, and protein C), which interact with five cofactors (tissue factor, factor VIII, factor V, thrombomodulin, and membrane proteins) to generate fibrin [2]. Data from protein structure and gene and sequence analysis suggest that coagulation regulatory proteins probably emerged earlier than 400 million years ago from duplication and diversification of two gene structures: a vitamin K-dependent serine protease with an epidermal growth factor (EGF)-like domain (common to factors VII, IX, and X, and protein C) and a second domain structure common to factors V and VIII.

Prothrombin, also a vitamin K-dependent serine protease, contains kringle domains rather than EGF domains, which suggests a replacement during gene duplication and exon shuffling. Thrombin has active-site amino acid residues that distinguish it from other serine proteases, supporting its position as the ancestral blood enzyme [3]. Furthermore, there is evidence that local duplication and/or translocation may have contributed to the evolution of multigene families residing on disparate chromosomal regions [4]. The mammalian coagulation genome itself probably evolved from invertebrate or early vertebrate species, where the corresponding genes (i.e., orthologs) for the primary coagulant and fibrinolytic proteins exhibit homology to mammalian sequences [5].

In evolutionary terms, however, hemostasis is a more recent phenomenon [6], arising first in vertebrates along with a closed, high-pressure circulatory system [7]. Concomitantly, there was a need for a hemostatic system that could respond rapidly, since even a minor injury could cause lethal bleeding, but that would be tightly regulated, to avoid a potentially lethal excessive response [6]. Evolutionary forces fostered a highly integrated hemostatic system that is characterized by many points of interface with an underlying architecture of numerous functional genes. In fact, genetic mutations have been identified in nearly every component of the human hemostatic system [6].

Cellular model of arterial thrombosis

The complexity and interdependence of coagulation proteins, platelets, hemodynamic forces, and the vessel wall in acute thrombosis are best understood by employing a "biological systems" approach – highlighted by distinct individual components within a dynamic yet highly orchestrated network [8]. Landmark studies employing a cell-based model of coagulation demonstrated a pivotal role for tissue factor-bearing cells as the primary site of *initiation*, and platelets as the *primed* template for thrombus growth or *propagation* [8]. Coagulation protein

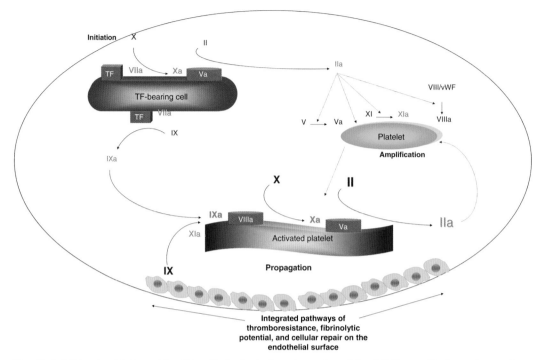

Fig. 12.1 Cell-based model of coagulation. Schematic showing the three phases of coagulation: initiation, amplification, and propagation. TF, tissue factor; vWF, von Willebrand factor.

complexes are assembled on these cellular surfaces, providing an effective means for localizing proco-agulant substrates to the site of vascular injury [8]. Coagulation is highly regulated by stoichiometric and dynamic reactions that operate on these surfaces, and the proteome of blood coagulation can now be studied in biochemically quantifiable terms [9,10] (Figure 12.1).

Paradigm of atherothrombosis

The vast majority of acute occlusive diseases in the arterial circulatory system require the participation of two conditions – atherosclerosis and thrombosis. It has become increasingly clear that each process affects the other substantially, and the pathobiologi-cal interface of atheroma formation and thrombosis, beginning with endothelial cell injury, occurs long before the phenotypic expression of atherothrom-bosis is clinically manifested [11]. The vascular endothelium is vital for thromboresistance and inflammoresistance, producing nitric oxide, throm-bomodulin, tissue factor pathway inhibitor, and heparan sulfate proteoglycans that augment the

inhibition of serine proteases by antithrombin [12].

In some cases, however, endothelial injury may be less dependent on traditional atherogenic risk factors, and a heightened state of coagulation may be sufficient for thrombosis to occur [13]. Seem-ingly "normal" endothelium has been shown to produce substantial amounts of a biologically active, alternatively spliced soluble tissue factor isoform upon stimulation with inflammatory cytokines [14]. The potential for undisrupted endothelium to par-ticipate actively in arterial thrombosis is further sup-ported by observations that cytokine-stimulated endothelium from human internal mammary arter-ies is sufficient to initiate thrombin generation [15].

Vascular bed specificity of thrombotic disorders

Despite the assumption that inherited or acquired thrombophilias should affect all vascular beds equally, this is often not the case [16]. For instance, congenital deficiencies of antithrombin III, protein C, and protein S are associated with a heightened

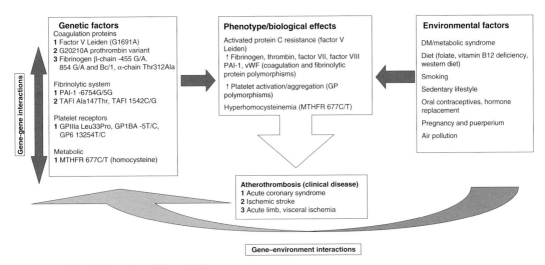

Fig. 12.2 Pathophysiology of arterial thrombophilias.
DM, diabetes mellitus; GP, glycoprotein; MTHFR, methyltetrahydrofolate reductase; PAI, plasminogen activator inhibitor; TAFI, thrombin-activatable fibrinolysis inhibitor; vWF, von Willebrand factor.

risk of deep vein thrombosis of the lower extremities, whereas a clear and consistent link with arterial thrombosis is uncertain [17]. This may be the result of several distinctions between venous and arterial thrombogenesis, creating a permissive environment within the venous but not the arterial circulation. In particular, high shear stress within the arteries governs the expression of profibrinolytic and platelet-regulating endothelial cell-derived genes, including tissue-type plasminogen activator (tPA) and nitric oxide synthase [18]. In contrast, thrombosis in the lower shear stress environment of the venous system predominantly involves tissue factor/tissue factor pathway inhibitor and thrombin-regulating (thrombomodulin, activated protein C [APC], protein S) local systems [19].

Vascular-bed specificity for thrombosis may apply not only to differences between the arterial and venous circulation but also to organ-specific vessels [16]. Inherited and acquired thrombophilias are discussed in greater detail in subsequent sections. The genetics of stroke is highlighted in Chapter 13.

Inherited thrombophilias and stroke risk
Coagulation proteins
The pathobiology of inherited thrombophilias with potential, of varying degrees, to cause arterial throm-

bosis falls into three major categories: factors governing thrombotic potential (coagulation proteins and platelets), thromboresistance (fibrinolytic proteins and intrinsic regulatory pathways), and response to vascular injury (endothelial progenitor cells and associated mechanisms of vascular repair). The focus of our chapter will be on the first two categories and the important influence of environmental factors on the phenotypic expression of disease (Figure 12.2).

Fibrinogen
Fibrinogen is the precursor of fibrin and also serves as a linker protein in platelet aggregation. Elevated fibrinogen levels have been associated with both stroke and myocardial infarction (MI) [20]. Genetic factors contribute to nearly 50% of variability in fibrinogen levels [21]. Polymorphisms in the genes encoding the three pairs of fibrinogen polypeptide chains (α, β, and γ) have been studied in relation to arterial thrombotic risk, with most studies focusing on variants within the gene encoding β-fibrinogen. The –455G/A and BclI variants are in linkage disequilibrium with one another. The AA genotype of the –455G/A single nucleotide polymorphism (SNP) has been associated with 10% higher fibrinogen levels when compared with the GG genotype [21]. Studies have also shown that the A allele binds less

well to a putative repressor protein complex, resulting in increased fibrinogen-β chain transcription [22]. However, the relationship between this particular fibrinogen gene variant and the risk of arterial thrombosis, including ischemic stroke, remains unclear, with some studies showing an association and others showing none [23–29]. In one study, the –455 allele was associated with a 2.5-fold increase in risk of multiple cerebral lacunar infarcts but not with large-artery strokes [30]. A variant in the α-fibrinogen gene Thr312Ala produces extensive α-chain cross-linking [31] and has been shown to be associated with increased stroke-related mortality [32].

Factor V Leiden (FVL) and prothrombin G20210A

The FVL and prothrombin G20210A SNPs have been investigated for their potential association with arterial thrombotic disorders (reviewed by Kim and Becker) [33,34]. The prevalence of the FVL mutation among both ischemic stroke patients and controls is approximately 7% [33,34]. Most large case-control and cohort studies have failed to establish FVL as an independent risk factor for arterial ischemic stroke in the general population and suggest that FVL may be seen as relevant in the same settings as proteins S, C, and AT. A few studies reported a positive association of FVL with ischemic stroke, especially in women [35] and in children [36] and one of prothrombin 20210 with stroke in children [36]. In a meta-analysis of greater than 17,000 patients, the association between these inherited gene mutations and arterial ischemic events was modest (FVL odds ratio [OR] 1.21 [95% confidence interval {CI} 0.99–1.49]) – prothrombin G20210A OR 1.32 (95% CI 1.03–1.69), with subgroup analyses of patients less than 55 years old and of women showing slightly stronger association overall (see gain-of-function gene variants) [33,37]. Additionally, cigarette smoking may induce arterial thrombosis in patients with FVL [17].

Prothrombin 20210A, in individual studies, has not been independently associated with ischemic stroke specifically, although a meta-analysis by Bushnell and Goldstein has suggested a modest increased risk conferred by the presence of the mutation – an OR of 1.4 with a 95% CI of 1.03–1.9 [38].

Antithrombin III, protein C, and protein S deficiencies

The association between intrinsic thromboresistence proteins, antithrombin III, protein C, and protein S deficiencies and venous thromboembolism is incontrovertible; however, there is no clear and consistent association with ischemic stroke [39]. The only exception to this generally accepted principle is in homozygous mutations characterized by early onset and recurrent venous, and still less commonly, arterial thrombotic events to include stroke.

Factor VII

Given the role of factor VII in the initiation of coagulation, the *factor VII* gene and the alterations of plasma levels have been a topic of interest in arterial thrombogenesis. Factor VII levels have been inconsistently associated with coronary artery disease (CAD) and polymorphisms in the *factor VII* gene account for less than 30% of the variability in factor VII plasma levels [21]. The relationship, if any, with ischemic stroke is poorly defined.

Factor XIII

Factor XIII stabilizes fibrin clot through covalent linkage. Studies have reported an association between a polymorphism in the A subunit of factor XIII (Val34Leu) and arterial thrombotic risk, with the 34Leu allele being protective against stroke (reviewed by Ariens and colleagues [40]). This SNP influences the transglutaminase activity of FXIII, and the homozygosity for the mutation is associated with increased enzyme activity [41].

Thrombomodulin

Plasma thrombomodulin levels have been associated with increased risk of MI [42]. Two polymorphisms in the thrombomodulin gene are associated with MI (Ala455Val [43] and Ala25Thr [44]). The association between thrombomodulin mutations and ischemic stroke remains poorly defined.

Tissue factor

Tissue factor, the major initiator of the blood coagulation cascade, has been investigated in relation to the genetic risk of thrombotic disease. Sequencing of the promoter region of the *TF* gene revealed six novel polymorphisms, and the 1208D allele was found to be associated with lower levels of circulating tissue factor and, concomitantly, was [45] protective against VTE, though it did not influence the arterial thrombotic risk [46].

von Willebrand Factor (vWF)

vWF, a large mutimeric protein synthesized predominantly by vascular endothelial cells, participates directly in platelet adhesion to sites of vessel injury and platelet aggregation under high shear conditions. Multimers of vWF can be as large as 20,000 kDa and are highly functional.

Elevated vWF levels have been associated with the occurrence of acute ischemic stroke [1]. In addition, plasma vWF levels may provide an incremental value to clinical risk stratification schemes for stroke and other vascular events among individuals with nonvalvular atrial fibrillation [2,3].

Fibrinolytic system proteins

Increased levels of tPA (the primary endothelium-derived activator of the fibrinolytic system) and plasminogen activator inhibitor-1 ([PAI-1] the major inhibitor of tPA) have both been associated with arterial thrombosis risk [39]. Variants in the genes encoding both of these proteins have also been associated with increased arterial thrombotic risk. The most studied variant in the *PAI-1* gene is the 4G/5G insertion/deletion polymorphism located in the promoter of the gene. The 4G allele has been associated with elevated PAI-1 plasma levels [47] and increased mRNA transcription [48]. Several studies have shown that carriers of the 4G allele have an elevated risk of stroke [49–53]; however, larger studies have failed to confirm an association with arterial thrombotic events [54–56].

There has been no clear relationship between the mutations of the *tPA* gene and circulating levels of tPA antigen [57]. The most studied variant, a 311-basepair Alu insertion/deletion, influences release rates of total tPA [58] and has been associated with a 50% increase in risk of MI in one study [59], though later studies did not validate this finding [60,61]. Further work to identify other variants in the *tPA* gene yielded the discovery of the −7351 promoter polymorphism, which, like the Alu polymorphism, is associated with tPA release after stress [62], suggesting that decreased local release of tPA, but not systemic levels, may increase the risk of arterial thrombosis [57,62].

Thrombin-activatable fibrinolysis inhibitor (TAFI) participates in fibrinolysis regulation; it removes lysine and arginine residues from fibrin, and hence decreases plasminogen binding to its surface [63]. Elevated TAFI levels have been associated with VTE [64] and CAD [65], and several variants within the *TAFI* gene have been associated with plasma TAFI levels. Only one variant, the Ala147Thr SNP, has been associated with arterial thrombotic risk [65].

Lipoprotein (a) (Lp(a))

Lp(a) is a low-density lipoprotein (LDL) particle with structural homology to plasminogen. Its presence in higher than normal concentrations may attenuate intrinsic fibrinolytic activity on the surface of vascular endothelial cells. In addition, Lp(a) facilitates the oxidation of LDL cholesterol – an important step in atheromatous plaque development. While a majority of studies designed to determine the relationship between Lp(a) and ischemic stroke have been retrospective, case-control investigations and several prospective studies have also been undertaken [66–71]. The totality of evidence supports a modestly increased risk.

Other factors associated with stroke risk
Homocysteine

Elevated levels of homocysteine are an independent risk factor for stroke [72]. Studies of the 677 C/T SNP have shown that this variant is associated with a greater than 3-fold increase in risk, although results of other studies have been less robust (reviewed by Fletcher and Kessling [73]). A meta-analysis showed that individuals homozygous for the T allele had higher fasting homocysteine levels than heterozygous or normal individuals; however, of the 12 studies included, only four reported an association between the TT genotype and increased cardiovascular risk [74]. Two larger meta-analyses corroborated these findings, with the overall OR modestly significant at 1.16–1.20 [33,75]. Hence, it appears that this SNP confers only a minor risk of arterial thrombosis.

Gain-of-function gene variants

A meta-analysis of 54 studies and 54,547 patients that employed random effects modeling was undertaken to determine the potential relationship between three common gene mutations that cause gain-of-function intermediate phenotypes and arterial thrombosis. FVL and prothrombin G20201A mutations were modestly associated with an increased risk of ischemic stroke (OR 1.27 [95% CI 0.86–1.87] and OR 1.30 [95% CI 0.91–1.87], respectively). In contrast, the C677T variant of methylenetetrahydrofolate reductase was more robust, with an OR for ischemic stroke of 1.46 (95% CI 1.19–1.79) [76].

Venous thrombotic disorders

The pathobiology of venous thrombosis is best understood as representing the interface of acquired factors such as age, obesity, prolonged immobilization, surgery, pregnancy, oral contraceptives, and cancer, in the setting of a genetic predisposition to disease. In fact, one or more predisposing factors are identified in approximately 80% of patients, with inherited thrombophilia being identified in 24–37% of unselected patients with VTE [77–79] and in the majority of patients with familial thrombosis [77]. In the context of stroke, venous thrombophilia is postulated to have a pathophysiological role among selected patients experiencing paradoxical embolism [80] or dural venous thrombosis [81], a hypothesis that will require testing in future larger case-control studies.

Antithrombin III deficiency

In 1965, Egeberg discovered the first genetic predisposition to VTE, namely that of antithrombin III deficiency [82]. Egeberg described low antithrombin and low heparin cofactor activity in a family heavily burdened with VTE, and identified the genetic predisposition as transmitted in an autosomal dominant fashion. Antithrombin III deficiency has since been shown to be a heterogeneous disorder and as such is currently subclassified into two categories. Type I antithrombin deficiency is characterized by reduced function of immunological and functional antithrombin. Type II is characterized by a variant antithrombin molecule with a defect in its reactive site (type II RS), in the heparin binding site (type II

HBS), or multiple functional defects (type II PE [pleiotrophic effects]) [83,84] (Table 12.1). There is also heterogeneity in clinical presentation by subtype, with type II HBS having the lowest risk for VTE [84]. Conversely, type I defects are more prevalent among thrombophilic families.

In patients with antithrombin III deficiency, 80% of patients have their first thrombotic event prior to age 40, and 32–62% of thrombotic events occur in the presence of other risk factors such as surgery, immobilization, or pregnancy [84].

Protein S deficiency

Protein C and S deficiencies were first discovered in the 1980s [85]. Protein S is a vitamin K-dependent plasma glycoprotein that functions as a nonenzymatic cofactor to APC in the degradation of factors Va and VIIIa. Protein S deficiency is predominantly inherited as an autosomal dominant trait, and heterozygous individuals are at risk of recurrent VTE [85]. There are three subtypes of protein S deficiency as defined by total and free protein S concentrations and APC cofactor activity. In type I protein S deficiency, the genetic defect results in a reduction of total protein S antigen as well as protein S activity. In the more rare type II protein S deficiency, there is a normal protein S antigen but a functionally abnormal protein S molecule with reduced protein S functional activity. In type III protein S deficiency, there is a normal total protein S antigen but reduced free protein S antigen and activity [86].

Protein C deficiency

Protein C, a vitamin K-dependent plasma glycoprotein is the precursor of the serine proteinase APC, which subsequently inactivates coagulation factors Va and VIIIa, an effect enhanced by protein S. Protein C deficiency is a heterogeneous disorder inherited in an autosomal dominant fashion, and two subtypes have been identified [86]. In the more common type I protein C deficiency, there is reduction both in protein C activity and in protein C antigen, and is characterized by marked phenotypic variability. In type II protein C deficiency, there is evidence of an abnormal protein C molecule but with normal protein C antigen. The gene for protein C is located on chromosome 2 and is closely related to the gene for factor IX [87].

Table 12.1 Inherited thrombophilias

Gene	Variant	Function	Phenotype
Factor V	Factor V Leiden (R506Q)	Increased factor V coagulant activity	Venous thromboembolism [147,148], miscarriages [149], obstetrical complications [150]
	Factor V R2 (H1299R)	Incompletely characterized [146]	
Prothrombin	G20210A	Increased thrombin	DVT, PE [151–155]
Plasminogen activator inhibitor-1	4G/5G promoter	Reduced fibrinolysis	Portal vein thrombosis [156]
Estrogen receptor beta	1730A > G	Unknown	DVT [157]
JAK-2	V617F	Unknown	Budd-Chiari, portal, splanchnic and mesenteric vein thrombosis, catastrophic intra-abdominal thrombosis (reports inconsistent) [158–160]
Endothelial protein C receptor	Haplotype 1 (H1, tagged by rs9574)	Impaired activation protein C functionality	VTE; VTE in carriers of factor V Leiden [161–165]
	Haplotype 3 (H3)		
	Haplotype 4 (H4) 4600AG, 4678CC		
Factor XIIIA	Val34Leu	Changes FXIII activation rate and fibrin structure/function	DVT, MI, CVA [40,166,167]
Fibrinogen Aα	Thr312Ala	Changes fibrin structure/function and FXIII cross-linking	Pulmonary embolism [168]
Thrombomodulin	Several missense mutations	Various	VTE [169–172]
Tissue-factor pathway inhibitor	Pro151Leu	Unknown	VTE (contradictory reports) [173,174]

CVA, cerebrovascular accident; DVT, deep vein thrombosis; JAK-2, janus kinase-2; MI, myocardial infarction; PE, pulmonary embolism; VTE, venous thromboembolism.

Greater than a hundred different genetic mutations have been associated with the two subtypes [88].

Activated protein C resistance (APCR) and prothrombin gene mutation

Dahlbäck and colleagues discovered APCR in 1993 [89], and it is responsible for 20–30% of cases of VTE. Approximately 90% of cases of venous thromboembolism due to APCR are due to an SNP in the *factor V* gene (G to A at position 1691 in exon 10), resulting in an arginine to glutamine in amino acid 506, also known as FVL [90]. FVL is the most common inherited cause of VTE, accounting for 40–50% of cases. Factor Va Leiden has been shown to be inactivated more slowly by APC than normal factor Va, resulting in increased coagulation [91].

APCR can also occur in the absence of a genetic mutation in factor V in, for example, patients with cancer, which may contribute to the increased thrombotic incidence in these patients [92]; however, the clinical utility of diagnosing this type of APCR is unclear. APCR can also be acquired in those using oral contraceptives or hormone replacement therapy [93].

Prothrombin G20210A has also been shown to be a risk factor for cerebral venous thrombosis with a gene–environment effect concentrated in patients using oral contraceptives [81].

Relationship between arterial and venous thrombosis risk

Increased attention has been paid recently to the possible relationship between arterial thrombosis and VTE risk [94]. Observational studies have found associations between arterial thrombotic risk factors, such as metabolic syndrome [95], diabetes [96], waist circumference, and smoking [97], and the development of VTE, and between statin use and lower incidence of VTE [98]. VTE has also been associated with subclinical atherosclerosis: one study found that patients with a prior history of VTE had a higher risk of carotid plaque on ultrasound imaging [99], and another found a higher incidence of coronary artery calcium in patients with idiopathic VTE than in matched controls without VTE [100].

Studies have also suggested an increased risk of development of subsequent arterial thrombotic events after VTE [94,101,102]. One prospective study of 1,919 consecutive patients followed for a median of 4 years after a first episode of VTE found that patients with idiopathic VTE had a 60% higher risk of experiencing at least one arterial thrombotic event [99], suggesting the presence of a common risk factor contributing to a shared prothrombotic state. While FVL, prothrombin G20210A, and APCR have been associated with both VTE and, much less commonly, arterial thrombosis, further studies are necessary to better understand this relationship.

Acquired thrombophilias and stroke risk

The acquired thrombophilic disorders include uncommon but not rare conditions such as drug-induced thrombocytopenia, autoimmune diseases, and myeloproliferative disorders (Table 12.2). Each contributes to the risk of venous and arterial thrombosis to varying degrees. In some cases, familial clustering and genetic influences are discernible [103] (Figures 12.3 and 12.4). Pregnancy, estrogens and estrogen receptor antagonists intake, smoking, drugs of abuse including cocaine and methamphetamines, and fine particulate air pollution can cause profound changes in coagulation [104–106].

Thrombotic disorders associated with thrombocytopenia

Heparin-induced thrombocytopenia (HIT) occurs in 1–3% of patients receiving unfractionated heparin for 5 or more consecutive days [107]. Recent hospital-based registries suggest that the true incidence has been underestimated due to under-recognition in clinical practice [108].

Many patients with platelet factor (PF)4/heparin antibodies remain asymptomatic, implying that host-specific factors influence the development of clinical thrombosis in HIT [107]. When it does occur, thrombosis most often involves the venous circulatory system; however, arterial thrombosis to include stroke is not a rare occurrence.

Thrombotic thrombocytopenic purpura (TTP) is a severe thrombotic microangiopathy characterized by profound thrombocytopenia, systemic platelet aggregation, erythrocyte fragmentation, and multiorgan ischemia [109]. The mental status changes inherent to the diagnosis of TTP may represent microvascular thrombosis of the brain; while fixed neurological deficits are not common, ischemic strokes can occur. TTP must be considered in any patient receiving ticlopidine (or rarely clopidogrel) who develops a platelet count $<100 \times 10^9$ per liter, and either MI or stroke. Most cases of TTP are caused by a severe functional defect of the plasma metalloprotease ADAMTS13, which fails to degrade unusually large vWF multimers. ADAMTS13 regulates platelet adhesion and aggregation through cleavage of vWF multimers. Two recent studies have demonstrated the prognostic value of inhibitory ADAMTS13 antibodies in adult-acquired TTP [110,111]. Patients with TTP and detectable inhibitory anti-ADAMTS13 antibodies had delayed platelet count recovery, higher plasma exchange volume requirements, and a trend toward more frequent flare-ups [110]. High levels of inhibitory ADAMTS13 IgG at presentation were associated with the persistence of an undetectable ADAMTS13 activity in remission, the latter being predictive for relapses within an 18-month period [111].

Autoimmune disorders, myeloproliferative disorders, and malignancy

The *antiphospholipid syndrome* (APS) is strongly associated with atherothrombosis, with several studies indicating that patients with APS experience an increased incidence of atherosclerosis and its complications compared with the general population [112]; however, a major concern is the increased risk of venous and arterial thrombotic events, including stroke. This was, in fact, the diagnosis for the example patient. The overall risk of arterial thrombosis among patients with systemic lupus erythematosus and APS may be heightened in those

Table 12.2 Association of hypercoagulable states with arterial disease

Inherited hypercoagulable states	Association with arterial disease
Coagulation proteins	
Fibrinogen level	CAD [175], stroke [175]
β-chain – 455 G/A	CAD [176] stroke [177]
β-chain – 854 G/A	CAD [178]
β-chain – 1420 G/A	CAD [179]
β-chain Bcl1	CAD [178] PAD [179]
β-chain C448	Stroke [180]
α-chain Thr312Ala	Stroke [181]
Prothrombin G20210A variant	CAD [176], stroke [182], PAD [183]
Factor V Leiden (G1691A)	CAD [176], stroke [184]
Tissue factor Ag level	CAD [185]
Tissue factor pathway inhibitor	CAD [186]
Factor VII level	CAD [185]
FVII Arg353Gln, FVII HRV4, FVII-401G/T, FVII-402G/A	CAD [187]
Factor VIII level	CAD [187], stroke [187]
Factor IX level	CAD [188]
Factor XI level (paradoxical)	CAD [188]
Factor XII level (paradoxical)	CAD [189]
FXII C46T	CAD [189]
FXIII Val34Leu	CAD [190], stroke [191]
von Willebrand factor (vWF) Ag level	CAD [192]
vWF Thr789Ala	CAD [192]
vWF SmaI polymorphism in intron 2	CAD [192], stroke [192]
Thrombomodulin Ag level	CAD [193]
Thrombomodulin Ala455Val, Ala25Thr	CAD [193]
Fibrinolytic system	
Plasminogen activator inhibitor level	Stroke [194]
PAI-1 -6754G/5G	CAD [195]
Thrombin-activatable fibrinolysis inhibitor (TAFI)level	CAD [196]
TAFI Ala147Thr, 1542C/G	CAD [196]
Tissue-type plasminogen activator (tPA)	CAD [197], stroke [198]
tPA Alu insertion/deletion	CAD [196]
tPA – 7351C/T	CAD [196], stroke [199]
Platelets	
Platelet hyperreactivity	CAD [200]
GPIIIa Leu33Pro	CAD [176]
GP1BA – 5C/T	CAD [201]
GP1a C807T	CAD [200]
GP6 T13254C	CAD [61,201]
Biochemical	
Hyperhomocysteinemia§	CAD [72], stroke [72,202]
MTHFR C677T	CAD [203], Stroke [204]

Table 12.2 *Continued*

Inherited hypercoagulable states	Association with arterial disease
Acquired hypercoagulable states	
Thrombotic thrombocytopenic purpura	MI [103], stroke [103]
Heparin-induced thrombocytopenia	MI [107], stroke [107]
Antiphospholipid syndrome	CAD [112], stroke [112]
Rheumatoid arthritis	CAD [113,114], stroke [113]
Nephrotic syndrome	MI [121]
Solid organ malignancy	MI [205], stroke [205]
Myeloproliferative disorders	MI [122], stroke [122]
Essential thrombocytosis, polycythemia vera, chronic myeloid leukemia and myelofibrosis	
Oral contraceptives	MI [106], stroke [106]
Hormone replacement therapy	CAD [125,126], stroke (125,126]
Pregnancy and puerperium	MI [116]
Air pollution	CAD [129], stroke [130]
History of venous thrombosis	CAD [94,99], stroke [94,99]

CAD, coronary artery disease; PAD, peripheral arterial disease; MI, myocardial infarction; MTHFR, methyltetrahydrofolate reductase.

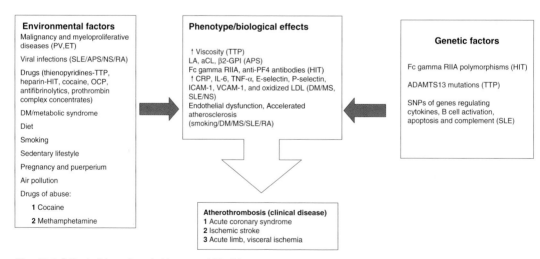

Fig. 12.3 Pathophysiology of acquired hypercoagulable states.
anti-PF4, antiplatelet factor 4; APS, antiphospholipid syndrome; CRP, C reactive protein; DM, diabetes mellitus; ET, essential thrombocythemia; GP, glycoprotein; HIT, heparin- induced thrombocytopenia; ICAM, intercellular adhesion molecule; IL-6, interleukin-6; LDL, low-density lipoprotein; MS, metabolic syndrome; NS, nephritic syndrome; OCP, oral contraceptive pill; PV, polycythemia vera; RA, rheumatoid arthritis; SNP, single nucleotide polymorphism; SLE, systemic lupus erythematosus; TNF, tumor necrosis factor; TTP, thrombotic thrombocytopenic purpura; VCAM, vascular cell adhesion molecule.

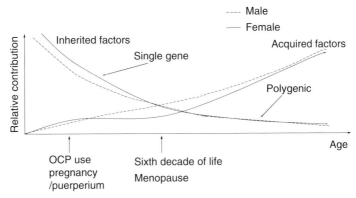

Fig. 12.4 Relative influence of inherited and acquired factors in determining hypercoagulable risk with age. Due to the gendered contribution of pregnancy, puerperium, and menopause, women may have a distinct age-dependent risk profile compared with men. OCP, oral contraceptive pill.

with a circulating lupus anticoagulant, high-titer antibodies to anticardiolipin, particularly if persistently high, and prior thrombotic events [112].

Rheumatoid arthritis (RA) is associated with an increased risk of coronary and cerebrovascular atherosclerotic disease and ischemic stroke. In the Nurses' Health Study, the incidence of the composite end point of MI and stroke was significantly higher among those with RA of more than 10 years' duration compared with normal controls (incidence of 272 vs. 96 per 100,000 person years) [113]. This increased risk of atherothrombosis appears to be the result of heightened inflammation and coagulation rather than concomitant rheumatoid vasculitis [114]. MI as a direct consequence of large- or medium-sized vessel vasculitis is uncommon [115]. There have been isolated reports of acute thrombosis within coronary artery aneurysms in patients with polyarteritis nodosa [116,117] or a history of childhood Kawasaki's disease, but chronic angina due to progressive arterial narrowing is, by far, the more common presentation of coronary or aortic arteritis [118,119].

Patients with the *nephrotic syndrome* (NS), especially membranous nephropathy, have a relatively high incidence of both arterial and venous thrombosis [120]. In an analysis of 142 patients with NS and 142 matched healthy controls, the adjusted relative risk of MI and coronary death with NS was 5.5 and 2.8, respectively [121]. Although the actual mechanism leading to increased coronary thrombosis in NS is unclear, possible pathogenic factors include hyperlipidemia, platelet hyperreactivity, endothelial dysfunction, and functional and quantitative changes in plasma coagulation proteins [120].

Myeloproliferative disorders often elicit unique clinical features such as a tendency toward both hemorrhagic and thrombotic events, including stroke, splenomegaly (which is occasionally massive), and clinical manifestations of microcirculatory disturbances such as ocular migraine, Raynaud's phenomenon, and erythromelalgia [122]. Thrombocytosis (>450,000 platelets/mm^3) is a main feature of essential thrombocytosis and an important diagnostic feature of polycythemia vera, with concomitant increases of both erythrocyte and leukocyte cell lines in the latter disorder [123]. The added presence of the janus kinase-2 mutation may have important diagnostic and management implications [124].

Environmental factors

Estrogen exerts numerous effects on the hemostatic system, including modulation of platelet function and endogenous levels of physiological anticoagulants [125]. Pregnancy and oral contraceptive use are more prevalent in women with acute MI and stroke.

The association between hormone replacement therapy (HRT) and arterial thrombosis is particularly complex. In randomized trials including over 20,000 women followed over 4.9 years, HRT users had a significantly increased incidence of stroke and pulmonary embolism but no significant change in endometrial cancer or coronary heart disease [126]. Psaty and colleagues suggested an interaction with other inherited hypercoagulable states and acquired risk factors [127], while Rossouw *et al.* found that early initiation of HRT in relation to menopause might improve the risk–benefit profile [128]. Currently, however, the weight of the evidence indicates that older women and those with subclinical or overt coronary heart or cerebrovascular disease should not take HRT [126]. Further data on HRT in younger women will come from the ongoing Kronos Early Estrogen Prevention Study (ClinicalTrials.gov identifier: NCT00154180), which is evaluating 5 years of HRT versus placebo in 720 women aged 42–58 years within 36 months of their final menstrual period, using the prevention of progression of carotid intimal medial thickness and accrual of coronary calcium as surrogate clinical end points.

Fine particulate air pollution has been linked to cardiovascular disease. In a study of postmenopausal women without previous cardiovascular disease living in cities exposed to varying levels of air pollution, each increase of 10 $\mu g/m^3$ was associated with a 24% increase in the risk of cardiovascular events and a 76% increase in the risk of death from cardiovascular disease over 6 years [129]. The stroke risk may be increased by as much as 2-fold among individuals exposed to particulate matter and nitrogen dioxide [130].

Diagnostic approach to suspected thrombophilias

Most patients experiencing recurrent arterial thrombotic events, including ischemic stroke, are more likely to have one or more traditional atherosclerotic risk factors than an inherited or acquired thrombophilic disorder [104]. All patients who experience an arterial thrombotic event require a comprehensive history and physical examination, with particular attention given to taking a detailed past, family, and medication history. A recent hospitalization should raise the possibility of heparin exposure and the development of HIT, to include the delayed variant. The following laboratory studies should be performed as they may provide valuable clues to an underlying thrombophilic state: a complete blood count with differential, prothrombin time, activated partial thromboplastin time, blood urea nitrogen/

serum creatinine, and a peripheral blood smear. A urinalysis to determine the presence of proteinuria or features of an "active" sediment is also recommended. Abnormal renal function is an early feature of TTP. Patients with "catastrophic" APS present acutely with thrombotic events involving multiple sites within the venous, arterial, and/or microvascular systems – often in rapid succession.

Acute thrombosis can cause "false-positive" results when testing for inherited thrombophilias: proteins C and S and antithrombin III activity may be spuriously low, and factor VIII antigen or activity may be abnormally high (see Table 12.3). When unfractionated heparin or low molecular weight heparin is used for treatment, certain assays for APCR may be unreliable, and antithrombin activity may appear abnormally low. Vitamin K antagonists (VKAs) suppress protein C and S levels and factor IX activity or antigen levels, while antithrombin levels may appear abnormally high [131]. These observations serve as the basis for diagnostic testing to be performed at a minimum of 6 weeks after the acute thrombotic event, or for subjects prescribed VKA, a minimum of 6 weeks after cessation of therapy [131]. In contrast, a majority of laboratory studies employed in the evaluation of arterial thrombophilias are much less susceptible to the effects of acute thrombosis and can therefore be performed early in the clinical course. Because of the highly variable effect of antiphospholipid antibodies on test reagents used to perform an evaluation of activated partial thromboplastin time (aPTT), young patients with a first arterial thrombotic event should be screened for antiphospholipid antibodies and the presence of a circulating lupus anticoagulant even in the absence of a prolonged aPTT [131]. If these antibodies are present on initial testing, tests should be repeated at a 6-week interval to ascertain persistence of elevated antibody titers. If patients are being treated with anticoagulants during testing for lupus anticoagulant, test kits containing neutralizers that inactivate heparin or low molecular weight heparin should be used [131].

The generally modest link between thrombophilic disorders affecting the venous circulatory system and arterial thrombosis, the marginal effect that individual genetic polymorphisms, at least those described to date, have in predicting clinical phenotypes, and an overall low yield in the detection of

Table 12.3 Influence of acute thrombosis, heparin, and warfarin on thrombophilia test results

Test	Acute thrombosis	Unfractionated heparin (UF)	Low molecular weight heparin (LMWH)	Vitamin K antagonists
Factor V Leiden genetic test	Reliable	Reliable	Reliable	Reliable
Activated protein C resistance assay	Reliable*	Caveat†	Caveat†	Reliable*
Prothrombin 20210 genetic test	Reliable	Reliable	Reliable	Reliable
Protein C activity or antigen	Caveat‡	Reliable	Reliable	Low
Protein S activity or antigen	May be low	Reliable	Reliable	Low
Antithrombin activity	May be low	May be low	May be low	May be elevated
Lupus anticoagulant	Reliable§	Caveat¶	Caveat¶	Caveat¶
Anticardiolipin antibodies	Reliable§	Reliable	Reliable	Reliable
Homocysteine	Reliable	Reliable	Reliable	Reliable
Factor VIII antigen or activity	High**	Reliable	Reliable	Reliable
Factor IX antigen or activity	Reliable**	Reliable	Reliable	Low
Factor XI antigen or activity	Reliable**	Reliable	Reliable	Reliable

Adapted from Moll J. Thromb Thrombolysis. 2006;21:7–15.

*Reliable if the assay is performed with factor V depleted plasma [206]; thus, the clinician needs to inquire how the individual laboratory performs the assay.

†Depending on the way the assay is performed, results may be unreliable; the healthcare provider needs to contact the laboratory and ask how the specific test performs on heparin.

‡Probably reliable, but limited data in literature.

§Test is often positive or elevated at the time of acute thrombosis, but subsequently negative [207].

¶While many test kits used for lupus anticoagulant testing contain a heparin neutralizer that inactivates UF and possibly LMWH, thus making these tests reliable on UF and LMWH, clinicians needs to inquire with their laboratory how their individual test kit performs in samples with UF and LMWH.

**No indication for testing in the acute setting.

thrombophilias, form the rationale behind taking a highly selected approach to laboratory testing [1,39]. We recommend the algorithm modified from Andreotti and Becker in which patients meeting any one of the five criteria undergo further testing [104] (Figure 12.5).

Therapeutic perspectives

Patients presenting with a first episode of arterial thrombosis, who are subsequently found to have an inherited thrombophilic condition, should receive standard treatment for the acute thrombotic episode (Figure 12.6).

Despite an association between elevated serum homocysteine levels and clinical end points, there is no convincing evidence of a reduction in adverse clinical events with vitamin supplementation in patients with a modest elevation [132–134]. However, it may be reasonable to use vitamin B12,

vitamin B6, and folic acid supplementation among patients with hyperhomocysteinemia (serum homocysteine concentration >10 μmol/L) [1], especially those with markedly elevated homocysteine levels (>100 μmol/L) [135] (Table 12.4).

The importance of recognizing acquired causes of arterial thrombophilia relates directly to the availability of beneficial treatments and management strategies for many of these conditions. Long-term, intermediate-intensity anticoagulation with VKA, such as warfarin (international normalized ratio [INR] of 2.0–3.0), reduces the likelihood of recurrent arterial thrombosis in patients with the APS to the same degree as high-intensity anticoagulation (INR 3–4) [1,136].

In essential thrombocytosis and polycythemia vera, increased platelet biosynthesis of thromboxane A2 is suppressible by low-dose aspirin [137]. A randomized trial in patients with polycythemia vera

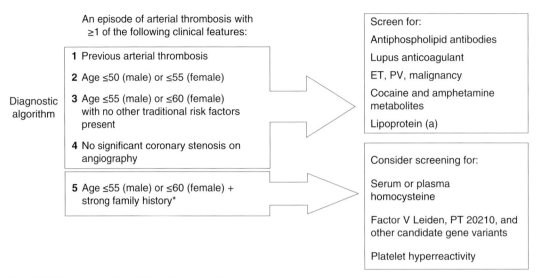

Fig. 12.5 Proposed selection criteria for diagnostic testing.
Adapted from Andreotti F, Becker RC. Circulation. 2005;111:1855–1863.
*May be defined as at least one first-degree relative affected at age ≤50 years if male or ≤55 years if female.
ET, essential thrombocythemia; PV, polycythemia vera.

demonstrated the safety and efficacy of low-dose aspirin in preventing both venous and arterial thromboses over a period of 3 years [138]. Moreover, anagrelide or hydroxyurea added to maintenance antiplatelet therapy reduced the number of thrombotic events, compared with antiplatelet therapy without myelosuppressive therapy, in patients with essential thrombocythemia and high-risk clinical features for thrombosis [139].

Thrombophilia testing influences less than 25% of physicians' treatment of ischemic stroke [140]. Practically, performing these expensive tests is probably not clearly indicated in patients with other reasons to be anticoagulated (i.e., atrial fibrillation) or in patients where anticoagulation is going to be contraindicated anyway. If making a diagnosis is going to affect therapy, then an investigation of a thrombophilia should be performed [1,141].

To improve cardiovascular health and reduce cardiovascular death, it has generally been recommended that patients get regular physical exercise. One specific mechanism by which regular exercise could have beneficial health effects is through reducing prothrombotic factors [1,39,142]. This is in contrast to the known effects of acute strenuous/intense activity linked to acute coronary occlusion/throm-

bosis. While acute exercise has been suggested to be able to induce a prothrombotic state from the activation of platelets (shear-induced platelet aggregation with increased GPIIb/IIIa expression and increased vWF binding to platelets), abnormal fibrinolysis, and increased P-selectin [143], large differences in study methodologies preclude drawing strong conclusions. However, emerging literature suggests that regular exercise (8-week training program at 60% of VO_2 max for 30 minutes a day for 5–7 days per week) can reduce shear-induced platelet aggregation, vWF binding, and P-selectin expression both at rest and during intense exercise [144]. A caveat is that studies have typically been performed in healthy young men. Future studies need to be conducted in a relevant population of older individuals with atherosclerosis disease and atherosclerotic risk factors. Further, given the link between stress and increased cardiovascular disease, stress-reduction strategies may also prove useful in reducing vascular occlusive events.

Triggers for a stroke associated with a thrombophilia are usually unknown, but surgery, trauma, pregnancy, hormone use, and systemic illness have been proposed [1,141]. While avoidance of these triggers is recommended, therapy should be tailored

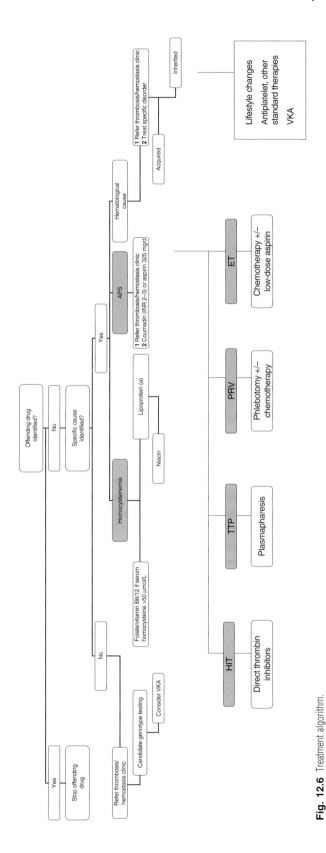

Fig. 12.6 Treatment algorithm.

Adapted from Chan MY, *et al.* Curr Treat Options Cardiovasc Med. 2008;10:3–11.

APS, antiphospholipid syndrome; ET, essential thrombocytosis; HIT, heparin-induced thrombocytopenia; INR, international normalization ratio; PRV, polycythemia rubra vera; TTP, thrombotic thrombocytopenic purpura; VKA, vitamin K antagonist.

Table 12.4 American Heart Association/American Stroke Association guideline recommendations

Hypercoagulable state	Recommendation	Class/Level of Evidence
Inherited thrombophilia	Referral for genetic counseling may be considered for patients with rare genetic causes of stroke (e.g., Fabry's disease, CADASIL syndrome). There remain insufficient data to recommend genetic screening for the prevention of a first stroke.	Class IIb, Level C
	There are insufficient data to support specific recommendations for primary stroke prevention in patients with an inherited thrombophilia (e.g., prothrombin G20210A, factor V Leiden, proteins C and S homozygous state).	
	Patients with an ischemic stroke or TIA with an established inherited thrombophilia should be evaluated for deep venous thrombosis, which is an indication for short- or long-term anticoagulant therapy, depending on the clinical and hematological circumstances.	Class IIa, Level A
	Patients with an established inherited thrombophilia should be fully evaluated for alternative mechanisms of stroke.	Class IIa, Level C
	In the absence of venous thrombosis, long-term anticoagulation or antiplatelet therapy is reasonable.	Class IIb, Level C
	Patients with a history of recurrent thrombotic events may be considered for long-term anticoagulation.	
Hyperhomocysteinemia	Recommendations to meet current guidelines for daily intake of folate (400 µg/d), B6 (1.7 mg/d), and B12 (2.4 µg/d) by consumption of vegetables, fruits, legumes, meats, fish, and fortified grains and cereals (for nonpregnant, nonlactating individuals) may be useful in reducing the risk of stroke.	Class IIb, Level C
	For patients with an ischemic stroke or TIA and hyperhomocysteinemia (levels >10 µmol/L), daily standard multivitamin preparations are reasonable to reduce the level of homocysteine, given their safety and low cost. However, there is no evidence that reducing homocysteine levels will lead to a reduction of stroke occurrence.	Class 1, Level A
Antiphospholipid antibody syndrome	For cases of cryptogenic ischemic stroke or TIA and positive APL antibodies, antiplatelet therapy is reasonable.	Class IIa, Level B
	For patients with ischemic stroke or TIA who meet the criteria for the APL antibody syndrome with venous and arterial occlusive disease in multiple organs, miscarriages, and livedo reticularis, oral anticoagulation with a target INR of 2–3 is reasonable.	Class IIa, Level B
Patent foramen ovale (PFO)	For patients with an ischemic stroke or TIA and a PFO, antiplatelet therapy is reasonable to prevent a recurrent event.	Class IIa, Level B
	Warfarin is reasonable for high-risk patients who have other indications for oral anticoagulation such as those with an underlying hypercoagulable state or evidence of venous thrombosis.	Class IIa, Level C
	Insufficient data exist to make a recommendation about PFO closure in patients with a first stroke and a PFO. PFO closure may be considered for patients with recurrent cryptogenic stroke despite medical therapy.	Class IIb, Level C
Elevated Lp(a)	Although no definitive recommendations about Lp(a) modification can be made because of an absence of outcome studies showing clinical benefit, treatment with niacin (extended-release or immediate-release formulation at a total daily dose of 2,000 mg/d as tolerated) can be considered because it reduces Lp(a) levels by ≈25%.	Class IIb, Level C

Adapted from Goldstein *et al.* [39] and Sacco *et al.* [1].

APL, antiphospholipid; CADASIL, cerebral autosomal dominant arteriopathy with subcortical infarcts and leukoencephalopathy; INR, international normalized ratio; Lp(a), lipoprotein (a); TIA, transient ischemic attack; PFO, patent foramen ovale.

to the individual case. Treating the underlying condition for those with an acquired thrombophilia may reverse the risk. For example, estrogen in women or niacin therapy can reduce Lp(a) [39,145].

In summary, the optimal management of a patient with a hypercoagulable state after a single episode of arterial thrombosis (ischemic stroke) is unknown. In hereditary deficiencies, especially in patients with recurrent ischemic episodes, warfarin is often recommended. There are no randomized control trials comparing long-term anticoagulation to oral antiplatelet therapy or placebo in patients with coagulation disorders. Therefore, the true degree of risk reduction with a specific therapy is not known.

Future therapies

Growing numbers of novel antithrombotics and anticoagulants are becoming available or emerging to consider in the treatment of patients with acute thrombo-occlusive events or prevention of recurrent events. Agents that are oral direct thrombin inhibitors (such as hirudin), factor X inhibitors, low molecular weight heparinoids, platelet surface receptor antagonists, and statins (3-hydroxy-3-methyl-glutaryl coenzyme A reductase inhibitors), among others, are potentially attractive approaches to the problem of thrombophilias.

References available online at www.wiley.com/go/strokeguidelines.

Genetics of Stroke

Natalia Rost and Jonathan Rosand

EXAMPLE CASES

Case 1

A 31-year-old right-handed woman with history of migraines developed paresthesias in her left arm. She had no other vascular risk factors and her history was significant only for diagnosis of depression in her mother (54) and brother (26) and a maternal grandfather who died at 60 years of age in a nursing home with dementia and stroke. Her neurological exam was normal with exception of subjective symptoms reported, and magnetic resonance imaging (MRI) showed several areas of nonspecific T2 white-matter hyperintensity (WMH) foci. A diagnosis of multiple sclerosis was made but no treatment initiated due to minimal symptoms. After 6 years of clinical follow-up, she was admitted to the hospital with a sudden onset of right arm weakness

---

MAJOR POINTS

- Genetic factors can affect an individual's risk of stroke, influence the severity of stroke when it occurs, and modulate the effectiveness of acute and preventative interventions.
- Clinicians are strongly advised to perform genetic counseling prior to obtaining genetic tests in patients with stroke.
- Family history of stroke, evidence of involvement of other systems (eye, skin, kidney, heart), or the presence of cognitive/psychiatric symptoms are suggestive of genetic stroke syndromes.
- Monogenic causes of stroke are exceedingly rare but can be confirmed using commercial laboratory assays.
- Despite being caused by a defined mutation, single-gene stroke disorders have variability in clinical presentation due to the presumed interaction of modifying genetic and environmental factors.

- Dedicated neuroimaging, comprehensive laboratory and clinical testing can provide information about the stroke etiology and point to a potential genetic mechanism of the disease.
- Ongoing genome-wide association studies of cerebrovascular disorders are expected to identify multiple genetic variants with modest effect size that contribute to stroke risk, severity, and outcome.
- The discovery of these new genetic markers holds the promise of novel stroke prevention and treatment strategies, outcome prediction, and clinical risk modeling.
- Currently, clinicians are advised to continue to focus on rigorous treatment of all modifiable risk factors for stroke and to offer thoughtful, competent genetic counseling for patients with suspected genetic syndromes.

A Primer on Stroke Prevention Treatment: An Overview Based on AHA/ASA Guidelines, 1st Edition. Edited by L Goldstein.
© 2009 American Heart Association, ISBN: 9781405186513

associated with dysarthria, for which she received IV methylprednisolone, and her symptoms resolved over a 48-hour period. One month later, she had an episode of right hemiplegia and dysarthria, which resolved with residual deficit. Treatment with interferon-beta was initiated. One year later after this event, she complained of recurrent migraine headaches, difficulties in concentration, generalized weakness, and diurnal somnolence. Paroxetine for a diagnosis of depression was initiated. Seven months later, she experienced paresthesias of the right face, confusion, and urinary incontinence. Pulse treatments with IV methylprednisolone did not improve the course of the disease, and 5 months later, when she was admitted to the intensive care unit (ICU) requiring intubation for poor secretion control and tetraplegia, repeated MRI imaging showed diffuse T2-FLAIR (Fluid Attenuated Inversion Recovery) WMH changes in periventricular as well as bilateral frontal, temporal, and parietal areas, including symmetric signal in external capsule. There was also area of chronic territorial infarct in the left centrum semiovale and six microhemorrhages on T2 Gradient Echo (GRE). During this admission, the diagnosis of cerebral autosomal dominant arteriopathy with subcortical infarcts and leukoencephalopathy (CADASIL) was established by skin biopsy and genetic testing. The patient remained tetraplegic and severely disabled after this episode, requiring tracheostomy and feeding tube. She developed progressive cognitive worsening, generalized seizures, and, after 16 months of nursing home care, developed repeated respiratory and urinary tract infections, deep venous thrombosis, and died in palliative care facility at the age of 42.

Introduction

Genetic variation can influence the pathogenesis of cerebrovascular disease through a variety of mechanisms. At the most basic level, variants in DNA sequence can affect an individual's risk of stroke, influence the severity of stroke when it occurs, and can modulate the effectiveness of acute interventions as well as primary and secondary prevention strategies. Over the past 2 years, the application of genome-wide association methods has yielded over 200 new DNA sequence variants with confirmed roles in the common diseases physicians treat every day, including conditions such as diabetes, myocardial infarction, hyperlipidemia, and dozens more. Whereas these discoveries have brought widespread attention and generated enormous excitement, they represent only the first steps in what can be considered the genetic research cycle [1]. The application of these and other genetic discoveries to bedside decision making will require further, carefully designed studies in patients.

Any effort to apply genetic discoveries to patient decision making must consider the stage of the genetic research cycle in which the state of knowledge currently resides. This cycle begins and ends with patients and their families. Once reliable and valid descriptions of diseases or conditions (phenotype) are assigned, molecular genetic strategies can be applied to identify the underlying DNA sequence variations (genotypes) that confer susceptibility to the disorder or modify its expression. The genes and proteins implicated are then characterized in the laboratory using model systems, from the test tube and cultured cells to genetically modified model organisms. Human genotype–phenotype relationships provide the basis for assessing the clinical relevance of these findings, which together help to define the specific molecular mechanisms producing the disease. Understanding of the fundamental disease mechanism returns benefit to patients through improved diagnostic accuracy, disease management, and the development of rational treatments.

The potency with which a genetic variant influences disease is reflected in the inheritance pattern within families. Highly potent variants, such as those within the *NOTCH3* gene that cause CADASIL, inevitably cause disease in individuals who possess them. The story is very different, however, for those variants that increase susceptibility for disease, such as those on chromosome 9 that contribute to risk of myocardial infarction [2–4]. Here, the culprit DNA variant is present in close to 50% of the population of European descent [5], and many individuals can possess it without ever developing myocardial infarctions or even coronary artery disease. These so-called common variants, which alter the risk of disease only mildly, can revolutionize the biological investigation of a disease process and identify targets for effective drugs. Nonetheless, they present a conundrum for clinicians and their patients, because their application in bedside decision making is by no means clear.

In this chapter, we introduce the fundamental concepts underlying the genetic research cycle in stroke patients and then, through a series of case studies focusing on current questions of genetic testing, illustrate some approaches to bedside decision making in this new era of genetic discovery.

The genetic architecture of cerebrovascular disease

Linkage analysis

Two fundamentally different approaches have been used to identify variants in DNA sequence that contribute to the risk of the disease: linkage analysis and association analysis [6]. In the case of linkage analysis, families in which more than one individual is affected with the disease or trait of interest are assembled and their DNA sampled. Such familial data can be either in the form of extended pedigrees, or, more simply, in the form of pairs of siblings or other relatives of which both or one member has the disease. The ongoing NIH-funded Siblings with Ischemic Stroke Study (SWISS), for example, is utilizing an "affected sib pair" design [7]. DNA from each family member is genotyped with a standard set of markers, creating maps of the genome that allow investigators to track the inheritance of each copy of each chromosome. These maps, in fact, track each chromosome in segments, and the chromosomal segment that carries the disease-causing mutation is identified because it is shared among affected family members more frequently than would be predicted by chance. Although linkage analysis can locate a segment of the genome that influences the disease, the implicated region is typically quite large: millions to tens of millions DNA base pairs, spanning dozens to hundreds of genes.

Linkage analysis has successfully identified the locations of hundreds of genes for rare, monogenic disorders. Indeed, among familial stroke syndromes, for example, the culprit mutations in NOTCH3, APP, and COL4A1 were all discovered through linkage analysis. The application of linkage analysis to complex polygenic diseases, in which strong recognizable patterns of inheritance do not exist, has been more limited [6,8]. PDE4D was originally identified as a candidate gene for common late-onset stroke through linkage analysis using 179 families containing 476 patients with ischemic stroke of any subtype or ICH [9]. The deCODE team located a roughly 16 million base-pair region of DNA where a culprit gene for stroke might be located, and then used association analysis to find the culprit DNA sequence variants in PDE4D that appeared to confer risk of stroke [10].

While data accumulated since the original association of PDE4D variants and stroke suggest this original finding may have been a false-positive one [11,12], the general approach of association analysis has been hugely successful for other common diseases, directly leading to the over 200 novel DNA sequence risk factors mentioned above. Association studies examine the frequency of specific DNA variants (alleles) in groups of unrelated individuals with disease and disease-free controls and use techniques to control for what is called "population stratification." Population stratification results when different ratios of cases and controls are unintentionally included from two or more subgroups with different ethnic or genetic backgrounds. A polymorphism that is associated with ethnicity/genetic heritage (rather than disease) could therefore appear to be associated with disease. Demonstration of association, however, is not by itself sufficient evidence for a causative role of a gene variant. If the pathogenic polymorphism lies very close to the polymorphism studied, it is possible that the studied polymorphism may be associated with the disease simply because it is in "linkage disequilibrium" with the causative gene variant (and is therefore inherited with it). Only studies in the laboratory that confirm the altered function of the identified gene can ultimately confirm a role in the disease.

Until 2007, the main limitation of association studies was that they required the investigators to choose "candidate genes" of interest based on inherently incomplete knowledge of disease biology. The results of this approach were generally not reproducible and yielded very few substantial genetic discoveries [13,14]. The situation changed dramatically, however, with the development of high-throughput techniques for genotyping up to 1 million single-nucleotide polymorphisms (SNPs) per individual. This technology, combined with newly developed statistical techniques for genetic analysis and the application of rigorous statistical thresholds for significance, has revolutionized genetic association methods.

Definition of phenotype

Obviously, any successful search for DNA variants that contribute to disease requires reliable diagnosis of affected and unaffected individuals. This has been a particular challenge for studies of stroke genetics. The heterogeneity of the underlying mechanisms leading to ischemic cerebral infarction and the multiple mechanisms that have a role in determining stroke severity suggest that imprecise or inaccurate characterization of stroke cases could undermine any effort to discover the so-called "stroke genes." Furthermore, symptomatic ischemic and hemorrhagic strokes are not the sole manifestations of cerebrovascular disease. Both clinical syndromes, such as vascular cognitive impairment, and radiographic findings, such as leukoaraiosis and microhemorrhages, are manifestations of cerebrovascular disease. Thus, any attempt to apply association analysis to affected and unaffected individuals will have to take these challenges into account.

Disease susceptibility and the effect size of DNA sequence variants

For diseases that have a predictable familial pattern of inheritance, the responsible gene variants, or alleles, tend to be very rare in the population. The effect of these gene variants is strong, and their presence is both sufficient and necessary to cause disease [15]. These so-called *monogenic (single-gene)*, or *Mendelian*, disorders are often recognized through traditional autosomal dominant or autosomal recessive inheritance patterns.

The overall contribution of monogenic disorders to the population burden of cerebrovascular disease is, however, very small. Common varieties of stroke along with the common manifestations of cerebrovascular disease are much more likely to be deter-mined, at least in part, by large numbers of genes of small effect. This model is emerging for common diseases such as type 2 diabetes, in which as many as 15 individual DNA sequence variants appear to play a role [16], a number that is expected to grow with future study. A common trait for all these variants is that they each individually contribute only a small amount of risk to disease. Both individually and in combination, they only produce disease in a proportion of individuals.

Genetic risk factors/screening

A major goal for genetic discoveries is that they lead to improved methods for identifying individuals who are in the early stages of, or at high risk for, stroke or other diseases of interest [17]. It has become clear, however, that in order for single risk factors to provide a basis for early diagnosis or prediction in the individual patient, the potency of the risk must far exceed those values we have become accustomed to seeing. In other words, the associated odds ratio (OR) for disease in those individuals possessing a culprit genetic risk factor would have to be well above 2.0 [18,19]. For common genetic variants, with their associated ORs or relative risks generally below 2.0, it then becomes clear that it is highly unlikely for a single or even a handful of genetic risk factors to markedly improve prediction of outcomes for an individual patient. For example, when a score combining nine common SNPs known to be associated with blood low-density lipoprotein or high-density lipoprotein cholesterol that modestly affect lipid levels was tested for the prediction of a first cardiovascular event, the use of the genotype score offered little improvement over the established clinical risk prediction model [20]. As increasing numbers of genetic risk factors are identified for each disease, however, this limitation could lessen. Furthermore, it remains to be determined whether the application of genetic risk prediction to individuals at an early age, when clinical risk prediction scores often cannot be assessed, may identify individuals likely to benefit from early intervention.

The remainder of this chapter focuses on the application of current knowledge of genetic risk factors for stroke to bedside decision making. Clearly, the stage of the genetic research cycle in which the most advanced knowledge of stroke genetics lies is far short of novel therapeutics, or even a list of confirmed risk factors comparable to the current state for diabetes. There is a good reason, however, to be optimistic about the progress for cerebrovascular disease. The founding of the International Stroke Genetics Consortium in 2007 brought together major research groups in the field from all over the world in an unprecedented collaboration that has already generated a new discovery (see Case 4) and undertaken large genome-wide association studies (GWASs) in ischemic and hemorrhagic stroke. Furthermore, genome-wide genotyping is currently being completed in several population-based cohorts across the world, each of which is likely to offer insight into the genetic risk factors for stroke.

Case studies

Case 1: Young patient with stroke and family history of stroke

In many aspects, Case 1 stands out from the usual stroke presentation. Young age, family history of stroke, dementia, and depression, as well as absence of traditional vascular risk factors, direct an investigative focus toward "unusual" causes of cerebrovascular disease. CADASIL encompasses a spectrum of cerebrovascular pathology, from asymptomatic progression of leukoaraiosis and evidence of microhemorrhages as detected on MRI to recurrent and debilitating ischemic strokes and, more rarely, ICH [21]. CADASIL results from the systemic involvement of small vessels caused by mutation in NOTCH3 transmitted in an autosomal-dominant pattern [22]. As in the case (Case 1), patients usually present with early-onset cognitive dysfunction, headaches (migraine with aura), psychiatric symptoms, and recurrent strokes and transient ischemic attacks [23,24]. In recent decades, MRI-detectable bilateral WMH in the external capsule and the anterior temporal lobe became recognized as highly characteristic neuroimaging manifestations of CADASIL, allowing its differentiation from much more common sporadic small-vessel disease of the elderly [25–27]. Large territorial ischemic strokes, as well as ICH, are rare; however, microhemorrhages in CADASIL occur commonly and are usually found incidentally on neuroimaging using T2* GRE sequence [28–31]. These features distinguish

CADASIL from a range of other disorders caused by rare and highly potent sequence variants in other genes (Figure 13.1) [32,33].

Differential diagnosis

Other Mendelian (i.e., caused by rare and highly potent mutations) conditions in young patients with stroke and a positive family history may present as part of a broader phenotypic spectrum that includes disease of the eye, skin, heart, and kidneys (Table 13.1) [34]. Stroke mechanisms can include a combination of large-vessel disease (from premature atherosclerosis in homocystinuria, dissection in Marfan and Ehlers–Danlos syndromes, or thrombosis in sickle-cell disease and Fabry's disease), cardioembolic (Marfan syndrome, Fabry's disease, and homocystinuria), or small-vessel disease (CADASIL, mitochondrial myopathy, encephalopathy, lactic acidosis, and stroke syndrome [MELAS], Fabry's disease, and homocystinuria).

Diagnostic approach

This involves a stepwise assessment of (a) clinical presentation, as in any other assessment of stroke [35]; (b) review of family history with evaluation of pedigree for signs of skin, eye, kidney, cardiac, and vascular disease, cognitive decline, headaches, or premature disability (Table 13.1) [34,36]; (c) neuroimaging including MRI with T2* FLAIR (to assess for pattern of white-matter disease and chronic infarctions), T2* GRE (to assess for microhemorrhages), and diffusion-weighted imaging (to assess for evidence of acute infarction) sequences [37]; (d) cerebrospinal fluid evaluation for lactate and pyruvate, if mitochondrial disorders are suspected [38,39]; (e) disease-specific tests based on clinical suspicion (e.g., skin biopsy in CADASIL, enzyme activity in Fabry's disease) [40,41]; and (f) following genetic counseling, selected genetic testing (e.g., Athena Diagnostics, Inc. sequences all known mutations for CADASIL) (Table 13.1).

Role of genetic variation in disease risk, course, and biology

In Mendelian syndromes, a single mutation is necessary and sufficient to cause disease. In conditions in which more than one mutation can cause a similar condition, there can be phenotypic variability depending on which culprit mutation is present. In

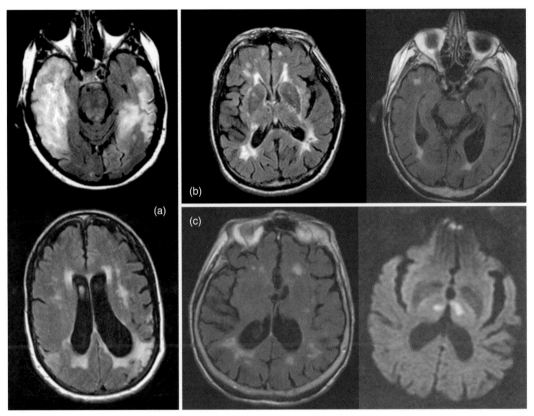

Fig. 13.1 Magnetic resonance imaging (MRI) characteristics in patients with stroke associated with a known single-gene disorder: (a) diffuse involvement in MELAS; (b) white-matter changes in bilateral external capsules and anterior temporal lobe in cerebral autosomal dominant arteriopathy with subcortical infarcts and leukoencephalopathy (CADASIL); (c) multiple white-matter lesions and small-vessel infarcts in Fabry's disease.

homocystinuria and MELAS, different mutations appear to be responsible for responsiveness to vitamin B6 therapy and phenotypic variability, respectively [42–44]. These mutations, however, may be just the beginning of the story. In all familial single-gene cerebrovascular syndromes, there is variation in age of onset and clinical manifestations, pointing to the existence of modifying influences, either environmental or genetic. In fact, accumulating evidence supports a role for other genetic factors in these disorders distinct from the causative mutation. In CADASIL, clinical severity and MRI characteristics including leukoaraiosis volume have been attributed to genetic variation above and beyond that in *NOTCH3* [23,32,45,46]. Modifier genes have been implicated in the extent of white-

matter disease in Fabry's patients through genetic variation in *IL-6, eNOS,* or *factor V* [47], as in the stroke phenotype associated with sickle-cell disease [48].

Genetic counseling and prognosis

In all situations in which a Mendelian stroke syndrome is suspected, professional genetic counseling is advisable prior to obtaining any genetic testing. In patients with single-gene disorders associated with stroke, management is focused on establishing the diagnosis and formulating a plan for disease-specific treatment and delay or prevention of future disease manifestations. For example, in Fabry's disease, enzyme replacement therapy with recombinant alpha-galactosidase is effective in the prevention of

Table 13.1 Single-gene disorders associated with stroke in young patients with family history

Disease	Genetic basis	Clinical spectrum	Diagnostic tools
CADASIL	*NOTCH3* (AD)	Small vessel and territorial strokes, depression, migraine headaches with aura, cognitive decline	MRI, skin biopsy (for granular osmophilic inclusions), mutation screen (*NOTCH3*)
MELAS	Multiple mitochondrial (maternal inheritance)	Mitochondrial myopathy, encephalopathy, lactic acidosis, strokes; developmental delay, sensorineural hearing loss, seizures	MRI and MR spectroscopy, muscle biopsy, CSF for lactate-to-pyruvate ratio; mutation screen of mtDNA
Fabry's disease	*GAL* (X-linked)	Cataracts, small fiber neuropathy, stroke, angiokeratomas, renal and cardiac failure	Alpha-galactosidase activity, mutation screen
Sickle-cell disease	*HBB* (AR)	Vaso-occlusive crisis, stroke, anemia, infection, pain crisis, seizure disorder	Complete blood count and smear, protein electrophoresis, mutation screen
Homocystinuria	*CBS* (AR)	Premature atherosclerosis, lens dislocation, Marfan-like features, stroke, mental retardation	Plasma and urine levels of homocysteine and methionine, mutation screen
Marfan syndrome	*FBN1* (AD)	Skeletal and soft tissue abnormalities, cardioembolic stroke, aortic/cervical vessel dissection, ectopic lens	Morphometric and mutation screen
Ehlers–Danlos type IV syndrome	*COL3A1* (AD)	Excessive soft tissue flexibility, spontaneous arterial dissection/rupture	Clinical and mutation screen

AD, autosomal dominant; AR, autosomal recessive; CADASIL, cerebral autosomal dominant arteriopathy with subcortical infarcts and leukoencephalopathy; CSF, cerebrospinal fluid; MR, magnetic resonance.

glycosphingolipids deposition [42]. The application of transcranial Doppler ultrasonography (TCD) in children with sickle-cell disease can identify those children at highest risk for stroke by using measurements of mean blood flow velocity in the internal carotid and middle cerebral arteries. In these high-risk children, chronic transfusions are 90% effective in preventing stroke risk [39,49]. Most recent guidelines from the American Heart Association [50] recommend referral for genetic counseling in patients with rare genetic causes of stroke, while data are considered insufficient to recommend genetic screening for primary prevention (Class II evidence). On the other hand, the same guidelines strongly recommend an individual stroke risk assessment (Class I, Level A evidence), because nonmodifiable risk factors, including hereditary predisposition, are considered to identify those patients who are at highest risk of stroke and who may benefit from rigorous prevention and treatment of modifiable

stroke risk factors [51]. Professional genetic counseling should address disease characteristics, genetic etiology, available testing, as well as psychosocial counseling with a follow-up medical and support plan.

Case 2: Familial ICH

Rare mutations in a number of genes are known to cause ICH. Mutations in *KRIT1* and *malcavernin*, the proteins encoded by the genes at the CCM1 and CCM2 loci, respectively, are responsible for the majority of familial cerebral cavernous malformations in which macroscopic malformed vessels develop and can cause ICH [52]. Familial disorders of the cerebral small vessels such as cerebral amyloid angiopathy (CAA) (Case 2), CADASIL, and COL4A1-related cerebrovascular disease share many manifestations in common with the common sporadic small-vessel pathologies that lead to spontaneous ICH.

Case 2

A 47-year-old engineer presented with an 18-month history of progressive unsteadiness and a 6-month history of slurred speech. His family history was significant for Alzheimer dementia in his paternal grandfather and cognitive changes in his 51-year-old brother who subsequently died of intracerebral hemorrhage (ICH). The patient complained of vertigo, headache, and inability to concentrate at work. On examination, he was found to have gait ataxia, a cerebellar type of dysarthria, gaze-evoked nystagmus on horizontal versions gaze, and impaired (saccadic) pursuit eye movements but no signs of upper-motor neuron signs. He had no evidence of hypertension or generalized vascular disease, and his neuropsychological testing revealed a mild degree of intellectual deterioration with weak verbal memory for his age. A CT scan showed extensive white-matter hypodensities with white-matter ischemic change. Spinal fluid was normal. Six months later, he was readmitted for new intermittent diplopia, choking, and overall deterioration in the mentioned problems. MRI few years later showed marked white-matter ischemic change and some evidence of cortical atrophy. By age 52, he was wheelchair-bound due to marked cerebellar signs, increased tone in all extremities, blurred vision, and profound memory impairment. In the last year of his life, he was incontinent of urine, unable to speak, and totally dependent. At the age of 54, he died suddenly of a massive cerebral hemorrhage.

Differential diagnosis

CAA-related ICH may occur both as spontaneous ICH in the elderly or a rare familial syndrome in which manifestations generally develop earlier in life as a result of mutations within the gene for the β-amyloid precursor protein (*APP*) and accumulation of β-amyloid peptide (Aβ) within the vessels. In addition to *APP*, mutations in other genes (*cystatin C*, *BRI*, *transthyretin*) can cause familial ICH with autosomal dominant transmission identical to what is seen in APP-related familial ICH,

although the abnormal protein deposited in the cerebral small vessels will differ. Recently described mutations in *COL4A1* have been found to underlie ICH-associated autosomal dominant familial ICH (Figure 13.2) with a pathology that differs from CAA [53,54], whereas CADASIL itself can also rarely cause ICH. Although there are differences among the various familial ICH syndromes that can allow the identification of some general distinctions (Table 13.2), the overlap is sufficiently broad to require genetic testing or histopathological tissue examination to confirm any suspected diagnosis [55].

Diagnostic approach

In patients with familial ICH, a thorough pedigree evaluation must be undertaken including history of ICH/hemorrhagic stroke and cognitive changes/dementia as well as considerations of other available phenotypic data (MRI characteristics including severity of leukoaraiosis, evidence of microhemorrhages and chronic and/or subclinical macrohemorrhages, and stroke), serial neuropsychological testing, and if available, results of neuropathological testing (biopsy vs. autopsy). Disease-specific genetic testing is recommended based on phenotypic considerations.

Role of genetic variation in disease risk, course, and biology

All *APP* mutations associated with CAA cluster within the Aβ-coding region of the gene (exons 16 and 17) [55]. In addition to point mutations within these exons, duplication of the locus on chromosome 21 that contains APP has also been identified in families with familial early-onset Alzheimer's disease (AD) and CAA [56]. A striking observation is that clinical presentations can vary dramatically among different kindreds with the same mutation, suggesting that there are additional genetic factors that modify the strong effect of these mutations [57]. Multiple rare mutations have also been identified in *COL4A1*-related cerebrovascular disease, as in the case of *APP*-related CAA and *NOTCH3* in CADASIL.

COL4A1 and COL4A2, the most abundant universal type IV collagens of basement membrane (BM), contribute to microscopic BM changes consistent with structural disruption in mice har-

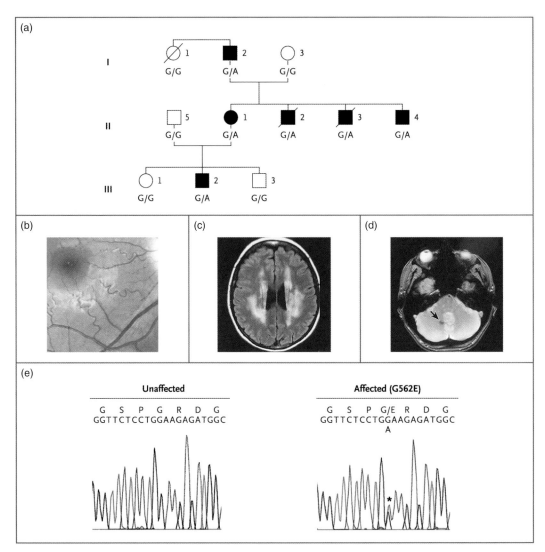

Fig. 13.2 *COL4A1* mutation in a family with retinal arteriolar tortuosity, white-matter abnormalities, and cerebral hemorrhage. (Reprinted with permission from Gould D, *et al.* NEJM. 2006;354:1489–1496. Copyright © 2006 Massachusetts Medical Society. All rights reserved.) Panel (a) shows the pedigree of a French family with small-vessel disease. All affected members of the family (solid symbols) had retinal vascular tortuosity and leukoencephalopathy. The genotype (normal [G/G] or mutant [G/A]) is indicated for each family member. Patients II-2 and II-3 died of cerebral hemorrhage after anticlotting therapy at 40 years of age and head trauma at 33 years of age, respectively. The square symbols represent males, the circles females, and the symbols with a slash a deceased person. Panel (b), a red-free photograph of the right eye of patient III-2 (at 20 years of age), shows marked tortuosity of the medium and small arterioles, particularly in the macula. No changes were apparent in the veins or capillaries, and no microaneurysms were observed. Cerebral magnetic resonance imaging (MRI) in patient II-1 (at 40 years of age) revealed diffuse periventricular white-matter abnormalities on fluid-attenuated inversion recovery (panel (c), bright signal) and silent microbleeding in the deep cerebellum on gradient echo-weighted imaging (panel (d), arrow). No MRI or retinal abnormalities were detected in the absence of a mutant genotype. As shown in panel (e), genomic-sequence analysis of COL4A1 revealed a G1769A transition in exon 25, leading to a change from glycine to glutamic acid at position 562 (G562E) in affected family members; this change was not observed in the chromosomes of unaffected family members or in 196 population-matched control chromosomes. The asterisk indicates heterozygosity for the mutant nucleotide.

Table 13.2 Single-gene disorders associated with intracerebral hemorrhage

	COL4A1	Familial CAA	CADASIL
Age of onset	0–40 s	30–70 s	20–50 s
Neonatal stroke	Reported	Not reported	Not reported
Hemorrhagic stroke	Yes (spontaneous and warfarin-related)	Yes	Rare
Ischemic stroke	Not reported	Rare	Yes
Leukoaraiosis	Yes	Yes	Yes
Microhemorrhages	Yes	Yes	Yes
Dementia	Not reported	Yes	Yes
Other CNS findings	Porenchephaly, birth trauma, traumatic brain injury	Cortical atrophy, diffuse plaque and tangle formation	Migraine with aura, psychiatric disturbances
Other systems involved	Eye, kidney	Not reported	Diffuse vascular wall deposits

CAA, cerebral amyloid angiopathy; CADASIL, cerebral autosomal dominant arteriopathy with subcortical infarcts and leukoencephalopathy; CNS, central nervous system.

boring *COL4A1* mutations [53,58,59]. The majority of the COL4A1 protein forms a triple helical domain, consisting of Gly-X-Y residue repeats, which is essential for its association with other proteins in the formation of extracellular BMs. All of the mutations identified thus far in humans are either missense mutations involving one of the Gly residues or result in the deletion of an exon within the triple helical domain [54]. Mutations in *COL4A1* have been linked to a spectrum of cerebrovascular disease in humans, consistent with a fundamental role for *COL4A1* in the strength of basement membranes. These include perinatal ICH with consequent porenchephaly, adult-onset ICH, microhemorrhages, lacunar strokes, and leukoaraiosis (Table 13.2) [58,60–63].

Genetic counseling and prognosis

Once again, professional genetic counseling is advisable prior to obtaining any genetic testing. Although discouraging neurological outcomes is the general rule for Mendelian ICH syndromes, relative unpredictability of each individual presentation (varying degrees of age of onset, development of cognitive decline, for example) is likely related to environmental and genetic modifiers. The apparent role of COL4A1 in cerebral vessels' tolerance of minor head trauma in humans raises the possibility that the rec-

ognition of *COL4A1* familial syndromes may offer immediate benefit to affected individuals. Pregnant mothers with carriers of a culprit *COL4A1* mutation might benefit from surgical delivery, while affected individuals may benefit from advice against contact sports and other activities that carry high risk of minor head injury.

Case 3: Young patient with stroke and no family history

In the absence of family history, genetic predisposition to stroke in a young patient is more difficult to prove. Stroke in young patients could be attributed to a constellation of modifiable vascular risk factors such as smoking, hypertension, diabetes, as well as less well-studied risk factors such as patent foramen ovale (PFO), cervical artery dissection, or lone atrial fibrillation [37]. Arguably, each of the mentioned disorders, particularly when they appear at an earlier age, may carry their own genetic vulnerability. In Case 3, dormant hypercoagulability due to factor V mutation has possibly been induced by smoking and use of oral contraceptive agents, causing thrombosis of cerebral veins [64,65]. Other hypercoagulable states as well as abnormalities of vessels and heart should be considered in young patients with sporadic stroke [65].

Case 3

A 19-year-old nursing student was evaluated in the emergency department for complaints of blurred vision and right facial numbness of sudden onset. Her medical history was only significant for a recent brief upper respiratory illness, 2-pack/year smoking history, and no family history of cardiovascular disease or stroke. She had used oral contraceptive pills since age 17 for birth control. On exam, she was fully alert and oriented, with evidence of right homonymous quadrantanopsia and hypesthesia in the upper-motor distribution of the right facial nerve. Noncontrast head CT showed a "delta" sign in the area of the superior saggital sinus. MRI with venous phase angiography confirmed an extensive area of obstructed blood flow in the superior saggital sinus, torcula, and left transverse and sigmoid sinuses, and demonstrated evidence of acute infarct with hemorrhagic transformation in the left temporo-occipital area. The patient was admitted for anticoagulation treatment. Further workup showed evidence of increased protein C resistance activity consistent with factor V (Leiden) mutation confirmed by genetic testing. The remaining hyprecoagulability panel was unremarkable. The patient was discharged on warfarin therapy and strong recommendations for smoking cessation with residual visual field defect. Her oral contraceptive was discontinued, and a follow-up with a gynecologist was arranged to discuss nonhormonal methods of contraception.

Differential diagnosis

Ischemic stroke in the young occurs as the result of the same general etiological factors involved in stroke in those who are older, although the cardio-embolic mechanism tends to be most common. Cardiomyopathies, dysrrhythmias, PFO with and without atrial septal aneurysm, cardiac tumors, and developmental abnormalities of the heart and great vessels account for a substantial proportion of cardioembolic strokes [66–68]. Hematological dyscrasias including hemoglobinopathies, polycythemia vera, and essential thrombocytosis, as well as dyslipidemias, are also frequently encountered underlying conditions in arterial ischemic strokes, whereas hypercoagulable states often make their impact via paradoxical mechanisms (such as using PFO as a hemodynamic conduit) to cross from the venous to the arterial side [69–71]. Vasculopathies (such as fibromuscular dysplasia [FMD] and Moyamoya disease) [72–74] are also more frequent in young patients with stroke and are not normally limited by a single syndrome or manifestation. Hemorrhagic strokes in young patients without family history should prompt an investigation into a vascular malformation (arteriovenous malformation, cavernous malformation, or aneurysm) [75,76], vasculopathy (Moyamoya disease, cocaine-induced vasculopathy, inflammatory or infectious vasculopathy) [77,78], or hematological dyscrasia with a hypocoagulable state (factor VII deficiency, idiopathic thrombocytopenic purpura, etc.) [79,80].

Diagnostic approach

In addition to a comprehensive clinical investigation that includes EKG, transthoracic and/or transesophageal echocardiogram, Holter monitoring, brain and vascular imaging (MRI for evidence of prior infarcts, MR/CT or catheter angiography, as well as T1-weighted fat-saturated images through the neck in suspected cases of dissection), a hypercoagulability screen should be obtained [81], including testing for factor V (Leiden), and prothrombin gene (G20210A) variants, anti-thrombin antibody levels, protein C and S levels, anticardiolipin antibody titer, and lupus anticoagulant, in addition to routine testing of platelet count and markers of coagulation (prothrombin time [PT], activated partial thromboplastin time [aPTT]) [82].

Role of genetic variation in disease risk, course, and biology

The genetic basis of stroke in patients without familial syndrome is most likely to be complex, or polygenic [15,34]. In patients with cervical vessel dissection, an effort to identify a heritable connective tissue syndrome should account for possible diagnoses of Marfan's syndrome, Ehlers–Danlos Type IV, osteogenesis imperfecta, homocystinuria, and pseudoxanthoma elasticum [34,83]. Although not a distinct single-gene disorder, FMD can lead to an arterial dissection [74]. Because in the majority of young-onset strokes, both stroke severity and risk of recurrent stroke can be highly variable, modifying the effects of known and unknown environmental and genetic factors involved in pathogenesis of each particular disorder should be considered [84].

Genetic counseling and prognosis

Careful review of the pedigree (family history of stroke, other cardiovascular disorders, or clotting, miscarriages, connective tissue disorders, etc.), thorough clinical investigation, and extensive laboratory considerations constitute a comprehensive approach to discover a specific genetic syndrome in patients with early-onset stroke. Genetic counseling preceding testing will address a broad spectrum of possibilities, with a special emphasis on sporadic occurrence of strokes in the young [85] and the role of modifiable risk factors in stroke prevention [37]. Smoking cessation [86] and discontinuation of oral contraceptive agents [87] are particularly important [88], in addition to blood pressure control, treatment of dyslipidemia and diabetes, and referral for counseling for drug abuse, as appropriate [89]. Although genetic testing may not identify a specific cause, or instead may bring an unexpected diagnosis, an up-front plan for testing and follow-up counseling is recommended. Prognosis for functional recovery is usually excellent [90,91], unless a particular diagnosis uncovers a high risk of recurrent stroke [92,93]. Decision making with regard to lifetime anticoagulation (for hypercoagulable syndromes), minimally invasive intervention (PFO closure), or surgical procedure (arteriovenous malformation resection, bypass surgery in Moyamoya syndrome, etc.) requires care, given the general lack of strong clinical evidence as guidance [94].

Case 4: Late-onset ischemic stroke

As with many common disorders, stroke (Case 4) can be considered to be a prototypical *complex* (*polygenic*) disorder [15,95], in which DNA sequence variation affecting multiple genes each with small effect can – through their cumulative effect – result in the development of a diseased state [96]. Potentially, multiple alleles with small effect size per allele (OR < 1.3) play a significant role on a population basis [97], given their prevalence, and thus, contribute substantially to the overall risk of stroke.

> **Case 4**
>
> A 67-year-old woman, former smoker with a history of hypertension, hyperlipidemia, and bilateral endarterectomies for severe asymptomatic carotid stenosis was in her usual state of health, when she collapsed at her desk at 10:30 AM on the day of admission. Emergency medical services (EMS) were activated, and she was brought to a local hospital where she remained unresponsive, with generalized jerking movements in all extremities. She was intubated for airway protection, and her initial noncontrast head CT showed hyperdense basilar artery. She arrived to our emergency department at 4 hours after her symptom onset, and even off sedation, she remained unresponsive, with down-beating nystagmus, small, hypotonic bilateral extremities without motor response, and bilateral lower extremity hypertonia with extensor posturing and upgoing toes. CT angiogram demonstrated extensive occlusion in mid-to-top of the basilar artery and also in the proximal left vertebral artery. MRI showed evidence of early acute ischemic changes in bilateral mid-to-lower pons in paramedian distribution, as well as a small infarct in the left medial thalamus. Following extensive discussion with the family, intra-arterial intervention was attempted with the use of mechanical clot disruption and urokinase. Blood flow was restored at 9 hours following the stroke onset, and the patient was transferred to the neuro-ICU for further management. First clinical examination following intervention demonstrated a patient who opened her eyes to command, followed commands in all extremities, with dysconjugate gaze, bifacial weakness, and bilateral upper more than lower extremity weakness.

Differential diagnosis and diagnostic approach

Stroke of late onset in a patient without significant family history should prompt an investigation including physical exam and neuroimaging, with comprehensive assessment of the cerebral vasculature, cardiac evaluation, and laboratory testing [98], unless particular clinical or neuroimaging features suggest a heritable cause [24,99,100]. Genetic counseling and testing are generally not indicated in the absence of strong suspicion of a genetic syndrome.

Role of genetic variation in disease risk, course, and biology

Late-onset stroke in a patient with no family history should be considered a complex genetic disorder [95], likely mediated by a large number of genetic variants with small effect size and brought on by the complex interaction of genes and environment. A number of risk alleles in nonfamilial stroke syndromes have historically been identified through use of candidate-gene association studies [101]. SNPs involved in homocysteine metabolism (*MTHFR*, C677T) [102,103], renin–angiotensin–aldosterone system (*ACE*, In/del) [104], coagulation cascade (*factor V* Leiden, *prothrombin*, *PAI-I*) [65,105], atherosclerotic (*PDE4D*-discovered through linkage analysis) [106,107], and inflammation (*ALOX5AP*-also discovered through linkage analysis) [108] have all been associated with greater risk of ischemic stroke in individual studies. Furthermore, a number of other candidate loci have been investigated including those involved in inflammatory response (IL-1, IL-6, C-reactive protein, TNF-alpha, toll-like receptor-4, P- and E-selectines, etc.), coagulation (fibrinogen), lipid metabolism (apolipoprotein E [APOE], paraoxonase), endothelial reactions (nitric oxide release), and integrity of extracellular matrix (MMP-9) [65,109]. Unfortunately, most of these discovered associations have not been consistently replicated in follow-up studies [12,107], a consequence most likely of the use of insufficiently stringent *P* value thresholds for significance and the application of sample sizes with inadequate power [110]. Recently, GWASs have identified and confirmed that variation on chromosome 9 is a risk factor for coronary artery disease [2–4], and investigators collaborating within the International Stroke Genetics Consortium (www.strokegenetics.org) have demonstrated that this chromosomal region is also involved in risk for large artery atherosclerotic ischemic stroke (unpublished data). If confirmed, further investigation of this region of the genome may shed light on the mechanisms of large artery stroke.

Genetic counseling and prognosis

Although genetic counseling is not indicated in a patient with late-onset stroke (unless a latent genetic syndrome is uncovered in the course of etiological investigation), a discussion of potential heredity and risk of stroke in proband's children may be helpful [111,112]. Understanding the concept of modifiable and nonmodifiable risk factors in stroke may improve individual future strategies for the primary and secondary prevention of stroke [113]. What is crucial, however, is not to lose focus on modifiable risk factors, such as hypertension, atrial fibrillation, smoking, hyperlipidemia, and diabetes mellitus, and their importance in reducing the risk of recurrent stroke [84]. Although accumulating evidence from meta-analyses suggests that *MTHFR* does play a role in the risk of stroke, there is currently no benefit to screening patients for polymorphisms in this gene.

Case 5: Spontaneous ICH in the elderly

This is the most severe subtype of stroke, causing death or severe disability in at least 60% of affected individuals (Case 5). Most often in the complication of chronic progressive cerebral small-vessel disease, there is evidence that genetic factors play a role in its pathogenesis. ICH can be more common within families, although not in a clear familial pattern, suggesting that either genetic or shared environmental exposures are at play. ICH is frequently categorized according to the location within the brain in which the hematoma arises (Figure 13.3). Hemorrhages centered in the basal ganglia, thalamus, brain stem, and cerebellum are frequently considered the manifestation of the so-called hypertensive vasculopathy, although factors other than hypertension contribute to their pathogenesis including advancing age, alcohol exposure, and a prior history of stroke. Hemorrhages arising at the cortical–subcortical junctions are termed "lobar" in location, and these are most often attributable to underlying CAA, a common small-vessel vasculopathy of the elderly. Chronic hypertension, as well as alcohol abuse and the presence of a prior stroke also play a role in lobar hemorrhage occurrence. Strikingly, the risk of both lobar and nonlobar hemorrhage is elevated in individuals with a history of ICH in a first-degree relative [114].

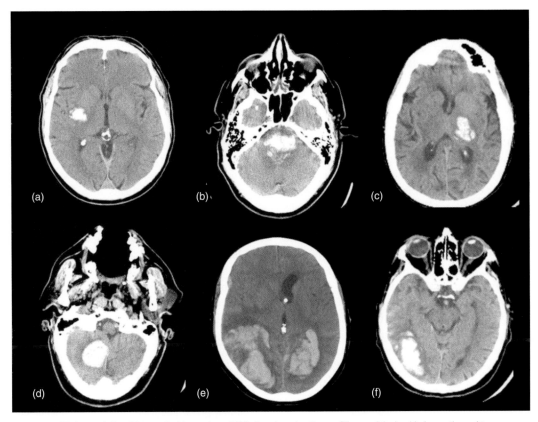

Fig. 13.3 CT characteristics of intracerebral hemorrhage (ICH). Hematoma location on CT scan of the head is frequently used to characterize location and suggest the etiology of ICH: (a) right basal ganglia; (b) pontine; (c) left thalamic; (d) cerebellar; (e) bilateral lobar; and (f) occipital lobar ICH.

Case 5

An 83-year-old man with a history of coronary artery disease, status post coronary artery bypass grafting, atrial fibrillation (on warfarin), hypertension, and hyperlipidemia was brought to the emergency ward (EW) by the EMS after being involved in a car accident. He was reportedly in his usual health until the morning of this admission, when he drove to a local mall with his wife. As per his wife's report, he showed no signs of illness until he drove onto the highway, where he initially acted "confused," looked around in distress, mumbled incomprehensibly, and then suddenly accelerated toward the shoulder, where he collided with the construction blocks left behind. A bystander called 911, and upon arrival, the patient was found to be confused and agitated, with incomprehensible speech, and not moving his right side well. In the

EW, he was found to have Wernicke aphasia, right homonymous hemianopsia, and right upper more than right lower extremity weakness. Urgent noncontrast head CT demonstrated left temporal hematoma, ~20 cc in size, without intraventricular extension or evidence of extensive edema or mass effect. Coagulation testing showed an international normalization ratio (INR) of 3.4, and the patient received an urgent reversal of anticoagulation with IV vitamin K administration followed by infusion of fresh frozen plasma. His repeat INR at 6 hours was 1.6, and head CT at 24 hours showed only slightly more of hematoma expansion (final volume of 25 cc). His clinical exam was stable and improved significantly with regard to motor function. He was discharged to a rehabilitation facility on day 5 with persistent hemianopsia and residual Wernicke-like aphasia.

Differential diagnosis and diagnostic approach

Although current standards of acute management of ICH do not require an intensive diagnostic evaluation other than to exclude underlying AVM, secondary prevention strategies may be informed by the distinction of lobar from nonlobar ICH, along with the confirmation of underlying CAA. Using the Boston Criteria, clinicians can make the diagnosis of probable CAA using clinical and neuroimaging criteria alone. These criteria are, in fact, sufficiently sensitive and specific for clinical decision making and have been validated in pathological case series. Lobar and nonlobar ICHs appear to differ markedly in their risks for recurrence. Up to 10% of lobar ICH survivors have recurrent lobar ICH per year, whereas the rate for nonlobar ICH is closer to 2–4% per year [115]. Accumulating evidence demonstrates that control of hypertension can substantially reduce the risk of recurrent nonlobar hemorrhages and may offer benefit for patients with lobar ICH. Warfarin may increase the risk of recurrent ICH in survivors of lobar and nonlobar ICH, and the decision to anticoagulate ICH survivors is therefore one that requires careful attention to risks and benefits [116].

Role of genetic variation in disease risk, course and biology

The gene for APOE, well-established as a risk factor for AD, is also a confirmed risk factor for CAA [117]. Of the three common alleles, e4 and e2 appear to be associated with risk of CAA-related ICH, in contrast to their relationship to AD risk, where e4 is the risk allele, but e2 is actually protective. Patients with pathologically confirmed CAA-related ICH have higher frequencies of e2 and e4, as do cohorts of individuals with *probable* CAA by clinical/neuroimaging criteria. Furthermore, in prospective cohort studies of lobar ICH survivors, the possession of e2 or e4 appears roughly to double the annual risk of recurrent lobar ICH [117].

Genetic counseling and prognosis

Currently, there is no role for genetic testing in bedside decision making for ICH survivors or those at risk for spontaneous ICH. Although *APOE* genotype is a risk factor for CAA-related ICH, it is neither sensitive nor specific for the diagnosis of CAA. The clinical/neuroimaging-based Boston Criteria are far

more useful in this regard. Although APOE may help differentiate those lobar ICH survivors who are at highest risk for recurrent ICH, the absence of any specific preventative strategies for lobar ICH recurrence makes this information of limited clinical utility. Furthermore, when deciding whether to offer anticoagulation to survivors of ICH who also have atrial fibrillation, currently identified genetic markers of bleeding risk do not appear to confer a risk of ICH sufficiently high to warrant routine genetic testing for patients at average risk of thromboembolism. Even if patients undergo screening with MRI as well as genotyping, currently available data on the role of MRI on risk of ICH and warfarin-ICH do not support the use of these tests for withholding anticoagulation in patients with atrial fibrillation [118].

Discoveries, prior to the GWASs era, that common DNA sequence variants in *CYP2C9* and *VKORC1* play a substantial role in determining an individual's warfarin dose requirement led to the initiation of randomized clinical trials and an update of the US Food and Drug Administration label for Coumadin™/warfarin, suggesting that clinicians consider genetic testing before initiating warfarin [119]. Although these discoveries represent a crucial first step toward the application of genetic information to make anticoagulation safer, it is clear that identifying an individual patient's risk for hemorrhage on anticoagulation, or thromboembolism in atrial fibrillation (and other diseases), will require many more genetic discoveries. Ongoing whole genome association studies of ICH currently being conducted by the International Stroke Genetics Consortium offer the promise of identifying additional genetic risk factors for ICH and bleeding on warfarin. Perhaps, combining novel genetic risk factors with *APOE* as well as those known to modulate bleeding risk on warfarin may become a helpful bedside approach for screening patients for anticoagulation, whether or not they have had an ICH.

Conclusion

Prevention and treatment of stroke remain among the major challenges in clinical medicine [91]. Although single-gene disorders associated with stroke have been well characterized, disease-specific therapies are still limited, and frequently, healthcare providers are left with little to offer our patients beyond genetic counseling and diagnosis [34]. In addition, single-gene disorders are associated with only a small proportion of all strokes, even those that occur predominantly in the young. The discovery of the genetic variants that contribute to the risk of multifactorial stroke, on the other hand, could offer a promise of tackling this problem on a much greater scale [15]. Sets of genetic markers are already being evaluated for risk prediction in cardiovascular disease [20] and prostate [120] and breast cancers [121]. In stroke, such clinical risk assessment could open doors to a new era of primary and secondary prevention, in which individualized risk prediction can clarify bedside decision making for primary and secondary prevention. Furthermore, a major lesson from the initial results of GWASs in other complex diseases is to expect the unexpected: associated genetic variants are generally outside of genes once considered "candidates" and frequently outside of any gene altogether. Unraveling the links between these new genetic risk factors may hold the greatest

hope for finally gaining control of the public health epidemic that cerebrovascular disease represents, because it is in these unexpected links that new mechanisms and, ultimately, new drug targets will be found. For now, clinicians are advised to continue to focus on rigorous treatment of all modifiable risk factors for stroke and to offer thoughtful, competent genetic counseling before obtaining genetic tests in their patients. Systematic genetic screening of individuals at risk for stroke will require further study.

Acknowledgements

The authors are grateful for the support of the Bugher Foundation – American Stroke Association, National Institutes of Neurological Disorders and Stroke (R01 NS04217), and the Deane Institute for Integrative Study of Atrial Fibrillation and Stroke.

References available online at www.wiley.com/go/strokeguidelines.

Surgical and Interventional Treatment for Carotid Disease

Kumar Rajamani and Seemant Chaturvedi

EXAMPLE CASE

A 66-year-old man presented to the emergency room with acute onset of expressive speech difficulty. The patient and his family did not notice weakness, loss of consciousness, or seizure activity. His past medical history was notable for diabetes mellitus and hypertension for 10 years each. There was no history of coronary artery disease or peripheral vascular disease.

On examination, the patient was in sinus rhythm with a blood pressure of 150/80 mm Hg. He had a moderate expressive aphasia, intact comprehension, mild right facial weakness, a pronator drift of the right upper extremity, and drift of the right lower extremity. His National Institutes of Health (NIH) Stroke Scale score was 6. ECG was normal.

Subsequent duplex ultrasonography revealed an 80–99% stenosis of the left internal carotid artery (ICA). This was confirmed as a severe stenosis on magnetic resonance angiography. Magnetic resonance imaging of the brain showed a 3-cm, cortically based left frontal infarct. Successful left carotid endarterectomy (CEA) was performed 7 days after the stroke.

MAJOR POINTS

- Carotid endarterectomy is proven effective for severe symptomatic stenosis.
- The benefit of carotid endarterectomy is reduced and less certain in patients with asymptomatic stenosis.
- Low-dose aspirin is recommended in the perioperative period for endarterectomy patients.
- Physicians should consider clinical and radiological variables in decision making.
- Carotid artery stenting is still investigational for the majority of patients with carotid stenosis.

Introduction

Patients with ischemic stroke or transient ischemic attack (TIA) are commonly screened for an ICA stenosis. Despite the frequent performance of carotid imaging studies, clinicians should keep in mind that large-vessel atherosclerosis accounts for no more than 20% of ischemic strokes [1]. Fewer than 10% of patients are candidates for carotid revascularization.

For patients who have had recent carotid territory symptoms, CEA can be very useful for decreasing the long-term stroke risk if there is moderate to severe stenosis. Many patients without recent carotid

---

A Primer on Stroke Prevention Treatment: An Overview Based on AHA/ASA Guidelines, 1st Edition. Edited by L Goldstein.
© 2009 American Heart Association, ISBN: 9781405186513

territory symptoms (asymptomatic stenosis) also undergo CEA, although the benefit is less certain. Some patients with carotid stenosis are not ideal candidates for surgery due to medical comorbidities (e.g., severe heart or lung disease) or anatomical factors (e.g., previous surgery or neck radiation). Carotid artery stenting (CAS) has been investigated for stroke prevention in these "high-risk" patients. CAS is also being evaluated in conventional risk patients as an alternative to CEA.

CEA for symptomatic carotid stenosis

Before 1990, CEA had been used as a tool for stroke prevention for many decades with uncertainty regarding its benefits. After two relatively unsuccessful attempts for a definitive answer to the clinical question of CEA's value [2,3], two large-scale randomized studies – the North American Symptomatic Carotid Endarterectomy Trial (NASCET) [4] and the European Carotid Surgery Trial (ECST) [5] – were launched in the 1980s. A third randomized study, the Veterans Affairs Cooperative Study [6], was stopped early after the NASCET and the ECST found a clear benefit of surgery.

High-grade symptomatic ICA stenosis

The NASCET and the ECST were pivotal studies that evaluated CEA in comparison with the best, prevalent medical therapy for the prevention of ischemic stroke in patients with symptomatic carotid stenosis. Patients with ICA stenosis determined by angiography, and an ipsilateral TIA, nondisabling ischemic stroke, or retinal ischemic symptoms were included in both randomized controlled trials. The two studies published interim reports in 1991 and a final report in 1998 [7], with each finding a benefit for CEA in patients with a high-grade stenosis (i.e., 70–99% occlusion). Pooled analysis combining the two studies and data from the Veterans Affairs trial (VA309) found that CEA was associated with an absolute risk reduction (ARR) of 16% over 5 years [8]. A meta-analysis of these studies reported a relative risk of 0.67 for the combined end point of nonfatal stroke, nonfatal myocardial infarction (MI), and death (95% confidence interval [CI] 0.54–0.83) [9]. The NASCET and the ECST findings emphasized the efficacy and durability of stroke prevention achieved with CEA in patients with high-grade stenosis, even after more than 8 years of follow-up.

Moderate-grade and low-grade symptomatic ICA stenosis

The NASCET study reported comparatively less impressive results for CEA versus medical therapy in patients with moderate carotid stenosis (30–69%) than in patients with high-grade stenosis [7]. Among patients with less than 50% stenosis, the risk of stroke after 5 years' follow-up did not differ significantly between the surgical arm and medical treatment arms (14.9% vs. 18.7%). In patients with stenosis in the range of 50–69% (high-moderate stenosis), however, the 5-year risk of ipsilateral stroke was 15.7% in the surgical group compared with 22.2% in the medical group (ARR 6.5%, $P = 0.045$). Notably, in this group, CEA did not confer a benefit to women, neither to patients with diabetes nor to patients with previous TIA. Women with 50–69% stenosis were found to have a low risk of stroke on medical therapy, and consequently benefited from surgery only if they met the criteria for additional risk factors such as age greater than 70 years, severe hypertension, history of MI, or a hemispheric (as opposed to a retinal) event [10]. Women also tended to have higher perioperative complication rates than men. The influence of gender on benefit with CEA is discussed in more detail later in this article.

With regard to patients with moderate stenosis, the ECST findings varied considerably from the NASCET study findings. Patients in the 30–49% and 50–69% stenosis groups, both categorized as moderate-grade stenosis, did not have a major benefit with surgery. This difference in outcome between the two major trials is partially related to differences in the methods used to estimate the degree of stenosis on carotid angiography. The method employed in the ECST tended to overestimate the degree of stenosis compared with the NASCET method [11]. Hence, many of the patients with moderate stenosis according to the NASCET criteria were classified as having high-grade stenosis in the ECST – many patients with 50–69% stenosis included in the moderate-grade stenosis group in the ECST would have been classified as having less than 50% stenosis in the NASCET.

Rothwell *et al.* reanalyzed the angiograms of patients studied in the ECST according to the

Table 14.1 Risk of ipsilateral stroke after carotid endarterectomy compared with best medical therapy in North American Symptomatic Carotid Endarterectomy Trial (NASCET) and European Carotid Surgery Trial (ECST) at 5 years

Stenosis (%)	Risk in NASCET (%)			Risk in ECST (%)		
	Medical	Surgical	ARR	Medical	Surgical	ARR
70–99	28.0	13.0	15.0	26.5	14.9	11.6
50–69	22.2	15.7	6.5	9.7	11.1	−1.4
<50	18.7	14.8	NS	6.2	11.8	−5.6

ARR, absolute risk reduction; NS, nonsignificant.

method of stenosis measurement used in the NASCET and found remarkable consistency in the results (Table 14.1) [12]. In the 30–49% stenosis group, surgery was not associated with a reduction in stroke or death compared with medical treatment (ARR 1.3%; $P = 0.6$). In the low-grade (<30%) stenosis group, surgical treatment was harmful, increasing the risk of stroke and death (ARR −3.6%; $P = 0.007$).

Accurate measurement of carotid stenosis is therefore critical for clinical decision making. In their final report, the ECST authors recommend that the NASCET method of measuring carotid stenosis be adopted as the standard [12]. In the NASCET method, the distal ICA, where the walls of the vessel are parallel, is used as the measurement reference.

In the combined analysis of the symptomatic trials by Rothwell *et al.*, data were included on 6,092 patients with 35,000 patient years of follow-up. As mentioned previously, the 5-year ARR was 16.0% for patients with 70–99% stenosis (number needed to treat [NNT] of 6.3). For subjects with 50–69% stenosis, the ARR was 4.6% (NNT of 22).

Timing of surgery

The issue of proper timing of CEA following TIA or stroke has been much debated. Some are concerned that carotid surgery after a major cerebral infarction could result in adverse outcomes caused by cerebral hemorrhage [13,14]. In the NASCET trial, however, postoperative intracranial hemorrhage occurred in only 0.2% of patients and was nonfatal in each case [15]. Altered autoregulation and hyperperfusion in the ischemic vascular bed distal to the endarterectomy might be responsible for these intracranial

hemorrhages. Others have suggested that the use of antithrombotic agents in the perioperative and postoperative periods could be the cause [16].

In the past, concerns about postoperative hemorrhage often led to a delay in surgery for a few months after the initial ischemic event. A delay in surgery, however, exposes the patient to an excess risk of recurrent stroke in the interim period. Lovett *et al.* have shown that the risk of stroke recurrence within the first month is high, especially in large-vessel disease [17]. Another study estimated the risk of subsequent stroke after TIA to be approximately 10.5% at 3 months, with the majority of recurrent strokes occurring in the first week [18].

In the pooled analysis of the symptomatic CEA trials, Rothwell *et al.* found that CEA was not only safe but was most beneficial when performed within 2 weeks of the index event [19]. Consequently, current treatment guidelines from the American Academy of Neurology as well as the American Stroke Association/American Heart Association (ASA/AHA) recommend that CEA for patients with nondisabling strokes should be performed without delay and preferably within 2 weeks of the primary stroke [20,21]. In the case presentation described at the outset, CEA was performed after 7 days without complications.

ASA/AHA guidelines indicate that CEA should be performed by a surgeon with a stroke/death rate of <6% for patients with severe (70–99%) stenosis and a stroke or TIA in the territory of the stenosed vessel within the preceding 6 months (Class I, Level A recommendation). For patients with recent symptoms and 50–69% stenosis, CEA is recommended depending on factors such as age, gender, severity of symptoms, and medical comorbidities (Class I,

Level A). For patients with <50% stenosis, there is no evidence that CEA is useful [21].

Which patients benefit most from CEA?

The multicenter CEA trials have led to several sub-group analyses of various clinical and radiological features and their relationship to benefit from surgery. Clinicians should recognize that even when performed by vetted surgeons, CEA is not a benign procedure. In randomized trials of symptomatic patients, the perioperative risk of stroke or death was approximately 7% [8]. In fact, if this benchmark of safety cannot be achieved, the benefit of CEA is lost. Hence, identifying the patients at greatest risk for recurrent events is clinically relevant. Subgroup analyses should, however, be viewed as exploratory because of potential group imbalances and limited statistical power. However, information from the pooled studies is more credible.

Men versus women

In addition to the degree of stenosis and the timing of surgery, age greater than 75 years and male sex were predictors of benefit in the pooled analysis of the endarterectomy trials [19]. It was observed that women on medical therapy had fewer recurrent events and higher operative risk, resulting in a worse surgical risk/benefit ratio compared with men. In a meta-analysis of all published studies between 1980 and 2004, women had a significantly higher risk of perioperative stroke and death than men (odds ratio 1.31; $P < 0.001$) [22]. The cause for this imbalance is unclear, but the smaller size of the carotid arteries in women is a possible explanation. Similar raised risks were described in another report combining data from the NASCET and the Aspirin and Carotid Endarterectomy (ACE) Study [10]. The benefit from CEA was similar in women and men with high-grade ICA stenosis (5-year ARR 15.1% vs. 17%, respectively), but women had higher risk of periop-erative stroke and death. Although men benefited from CEA in the moderate-stenosis group, there was no clear benefit in women with the same disease severity.

Age

Due to the aging of the population, clinicians increasingly encounter patients age 80 years and older with carotid stenosis. The NASCET initially excluded patients aged 80 years and older, and although the ECST studied patients of any age, it is not clear how many patients of this age group were actually included. In a review of more than 2,500 CEA procedures performed in octogenarians, the combined perioperative stroke and death rate was 3.45% [23]. Another pooled analysis of trials of CEA for symptomatic stenosis found that the benefit was higher in patients aged >75 years, as compared with younger patients [22]. Administrative database studies have shown an increased perioperative mortality with increasing age, and therefore, careful patient evaluation is mandatory when CEA is contemplated in octogenarians [24]. If an elderly symptomatic CEA candidate is medically fit, CEA should not be withheld. As benefit accrues over 1–2 years after surgery, these patients should ideally have life expectancy that exceeds this period.

Symptoms at presentation: ocular versus hemispheric stroke

Data suggest that risk of stroke recurrence can be stratified on the basis of symptoms at presentation. Retinal symptoms carry lower risk. In the NASCET, the risk of recurrent stroke among medically treated patients presenting with transient monocular blindness was lower than that in those presenting with hemispheric TIAs (10% vs. 20% over 3 years, adjusted hazard ratio of 0.53, 95%, confidence intervals 0.30–0.94) [25]. The risk of subsequent ischemic events was higher in individuals with transient monocular blindness treated medically if they had coexisting risk factors including age greater than 75 years, symptomatic peripheral vascular disease, and 80–94% stenosis of the ICA without adequate collateral circulation. Consequently, among patients with transient monocular blindness, CEA was beneficial only when ICA stenosis (>50%) was associated with these stroke risk factors. In the patient described at the outset, male gender and hemispheric stroke increased the likelihood of benefit from CEA.

Contralateral ICA occlusion

Another factor that requires consideration when treating a patient with symptomatic carotid stenosis is the presence of a contralateral ICA occlusion. Although some believe this condition does not impact prognosis after CEA [26,27], others have reported that it is associated with increased perioperative risk [28]. Gasecki et al. described 43 patients in the NASCET database with contralateral ICA occlusion [29]. They found the risk of perioperative stroke to be higher in these patients than in those who had significant contralateral stenosis but were not occluded (14% vs. 5%). The long-term outcome at 2 years, however, was better in the surgery group than in the medical group (22% vs. 69% risk of ipsilateral stroke, hazard ratio 2.15). The authors concluded that there is significant benefit from CEA performed for symptomatic high-grade stenosis, even in the presence of contralateral ICA occlusion.

Carotid plaque ulceration

The pathophysiological mechanisms of plaque ulceration and the potential for thrombosis and distal embolization have been studied extensively. After the inspection of more than 1,000 postoperative specimens following CEA, Park et al. concluded that plaque ulceration is associated with symptomatic rather than asymptomatic plaques [30]. Fisher et al. not only confirmed this finding after careful study of samples collected from the NASCET study and Asymptomatic Carotid Atherosclerosis Study (ACAS), but also showed that ulcerated plaques develop in the contralateral carotid artery as often as they develop in the ipsilateral symptomatic artery [31]. In the NASCET Study, although patients were not randomized prospectively on the basis of plaque ulceration, a post hoc analysis revealed that the presence of angiographically determined ulceration significantly increased the risk of stroke in medically treated patients with severe stenosis by up to three times [32]. These patients, however, are candidates for CEA because of the degree of stenosis alone. Moreover, the detection of carotid plaque ulceration both by carotid duplex and by angiography is currently unsatisfactory. In a study comparing surgical specimens with angiographic data in 500 patients from NASCET, angiography had a 45.9% sensitivity and 74% specificity with a positive predictive value of 71% for diagnosing plaque ulceration [33]. Future improvements in imaging technologies may allow a more accurate identification of plaque ulceration, which could result in a more efficient stroke prevention by CEA.

Carotid "near occlusion"

When using catheter angiography to assess severe carotid stenosis, the flow in the distal ICA beyond the stenosis is occasionally reduced and seems "collapsed." These patients are classified as having "near occlusion." The diagnosis of near occlusion is made by the delayed appearance of contrast in the ipsilateral intracranial ICA compared with the external carotid artery and a smaller diameter of the ICA compared with the external carotid artery. The contrast is diluted because of the collateral circulation. Morgenstern et al. identified 7.6% of the NASCET population as having carotid near occlusion, and observed that the risk of stroke recurrence in this group was significantly less than that in the 90–94% stenosis group (11% vs. 35%) [34]. The ARR of stroke in the CEA-treated group with near occlusion was 7.9% compared with the medically treated group. Using combined NASCET and ECST datasets, Fox and coworkers identified subsets of patients with near occlusion; the risk of stroke in the medically treated arm in this group was 15.1% compared with 10.9% in the surgical arm (ARR of 4.2%, $P = 0.33$) [35]. The reason for the low risk of stroke in this group is unclear but could be because of good collateral circulation from the opposite side or the ipsilateral external carotid artery. As acknowledged by the authors, however, the sample size and event rates were too small to make definitive conclusions. CEA can be considered in these patients, although the benefit is uncertain.

CEA for asymptomatic carotid stenosis

The role of CEA in asymptomatic individuals is much less certain and still debated. The largest trials are the ACAS [36] and the Asymptomatic Carotid Surgery Trial (ACST) [37].

In the ACAS, otherwise healthy patients with an asymptomatic stenosis (>60%) were randomized to receive either best medical treatment or best medical therapy in addition to endarterectomy [36]. The study was stopped early after 2.7 years of average follow-up. In the surgical arm, the recurrent combined event rate for ipsilateral stroke, any perioperative stroke, and death at 5 years was projected to be 5.1%, compared with 11% in the medical arm – a relative risk reduction of 55% (ARR of 5.9%, $P = 0.004$). The surgical benefit requires a very low perioperative risk (1.5% achieved in the trial). Whether this low perioperative stroke rate can be achieved in routine clinical practice is doubtful. For example, in a study of over 1,800 asymptomatic CEA cases from Ontario, the perioperative stroke and death rate was 4.7% [38].

Although it is frequently reported that the ASCT findings were similar to those of the ACAS, there were important differences between the studies. In the ACAS, the primary analysis compared strokes occurring in the territory of the operated carotid artery, while the ACST included strokes in any vascular territory. In addition, conventional angiography was not mandated for either group in ACST. After 5 years' follow-up, the risk of recurrent stroke for the surgical group in ACST was 6.4% and 11.8% for those on medical treatment [37]. The risk of perioperative stroke or death was 2.8%. Importantly, this study showed a significant reduction of fatal or disabling strokes in the surgical arm (3.5% vs. 6.1% in medically treated group, ARR 2.6%; $P < 0.004$). Approximately half of all ipsilateral strokes were fatal or disabling. The ACAS showed a trend toward reduction in fatal and disabling strokes with surgery but did not reach statistical significance (ARR 2.7%; $P = 0.26$). There was no clear benefit of CEA in those age 75 years and over in ACST.

A meta-analysis of data from 5,223 patients from the major trials of CEA for asymptomatic carotid stenosis found that surgery was associated with a reduction in the combined risk of any perioperative or subsequent stroke and all-cause perioperative mortality (relative risk 0.69, 95% CI 0.57–0.83) [39]. The overall risk of perioperative stroke or death was 2.9%. Subgroup analysis revealed men received more benefit from surgery than women, and younger patients benefited more than older patients. Unlike the symptomatic stenosis trials, stenosis severity did not correlate with surgical benefit. Despite these findings, some have argued against the routine use and widespread enthusiasm for CEA in asymptomatic patients. Barnett et al. highlighted that the absolute annual risk reduction of stroke in this asymptomatic group is about 1% with an NNT of 83 to prevent one stroke in 2 years [40]. Moreover, it has been estimated that approximately half the strokes in asymptomatic individuals are not related to the stenosed carotid artery but are rather lacunar strokes or caused by cardioembolic events [41].

As discussed earlier, the benefit of surgery in patients with carotid stenosis is highly dependent on perioperative stroke risk. A low perioperative stroke risk is especially critical for asymptomatic patients in whom the marginal benefit can be lost if the risk is not within the recommended limits. Practicing clinicians must, therefore, be aware of the local and institutional complication rates, in order to advise patients. In a study of 12 academic centers and 1,160 procedures, Goldstein et al. reported a perioperative risk of stroke or death of 2.8% [42]. Notably, the rate was higher in symptomatic than in asymptomatic individuals. Postoperative stroke and death were also significantly higher in women, older individuals (>75 years), those with associated congestive heart failure, and those undergoing simultaneous coronary artery bypass grafting surgery.

Guidelines from the ASA/AHA indicate that patients with asymptomatic stenosis should be screened for other treatable causes of stroke and that intensive treatment of stroke risk factors should be pursued (Class I, Level C) [43]. In addition, the use of aspirin is recommended in subjects with asymptomatic stenosis. CEA is recommended in highly selected patients with high-grade stenosis, and the surgeon should have a stroke/death rate of <3% (Class I, Level A). There should be a thorough understanding of the goals of the procedure, the patient's life expectancy and comorbidities, and patient preferences. The American Academy of Neurology guidelines recommend that CEA for asymptomatic stenosis be considered only for patients 40–75 years old with at least a 5-year life expectancy. In addition, the surgeon's complication rate should be reliably documented to be less than 3% [20].

Perioperative drug therapy

A retrospective analysis of data from the NASCET suggested that patients receiving low-dose aspirin (0–325 mg/day) in the perioperative period had higher risk of perioperative stroke and death than those on higher doses (650–1,300 mg/day). This observation led to the randomized ACE trial [44], which found that the perioperative stroke or vascular death risk in the low-dose aspirin (81–325 mg/day) arm was 6.2% compared with 8.4% in the high-dose arm (650–1,300 mg/day), pointing out the importance of conducting prospective trials to test hypotheses generated from exploratory analyses. A more recent systematic review of all trials has attempted to address the question of optimum anti-platelet therapy during CEA for symptomatic and asymptomatic carotid stenosis [45]. This study found that perioperative stroke risk among those receiving antiplatelet agents was reduced, but that the risk of perioperative death was not altered. The findings also indicated that antiplatelet agents could increase the risk of hemorrhage. The widespread belief that antiplatelet agents reduce the risk of native-vessel or graft thrombosis and MI after vas-cular surgery (including CEA), however, means that most patients should be given antiplatelet therapies in the perioperative period.

Evidence that statins [46] and beta-blockers [47] reduce morbidity and mortality when used during vascular surgery is mounting. A retrospective analy-sis found that the use of statins, compared with the absence of statin treatment, during CEA signifi-cantly reduced the risk of perioperative stroke (1.2% vs. 4.5%; $P < 0.01$) and death (0.3% vs. 2.1%; $P < 0.01$) [48]. These observations are intriguing, but more definitive studies are needed before broad rec-ommendations for routine use of these medications can be advocated in the perioperative period.

The risks associated with CEA

The risks of surgery should be carefully discussed with patients before CEA. Risks include periopera-tive ischemic stroke, hemorrhagic stroke, cranial nerve injury, MI, congestive heart failure, and neck hematoma with consequent airway compromise. Perioperative ischemic stroke occurs as a result of thrombotic occlusion of the operative site, distal thromboembolism of debris from the operative site, cross clamping of the ICA, or a combination of these factors. Ischemic stroke usually not only occurs within the first 12–24 hours after surgery but can also occur later in recovery. If a patient wakes up from anesthesia with a deficit or develops one soon thereafter, emergent exploration of the operative site for thrombosis or other correctable operative defects is usually undertaken. Cerebral angiography can be performed with a view to identifying occluded vessels. The benefit of reoperation, however, cannot be predicted. Of the 10 patients who underwent

reoperation in the NASCET, none had any benefit [15]. Furthermore, Findlay and Marchak reported that 13 of 24 patients had postoperative strokes fol-lowing CEA and underwent emergency reoperation [49]; yet only four of these patients were reported to show any benefit.

Severe carotid stenosis with limited collateral flow can result in postoperative hyperperfusion syn-drome. In addition to increased blood flow, which is associated with this syndrome, use of anticoagula-tion and occurrence of a perioperative ischemic event with subsequent hemorrhagic transformation might also be important. The prognosis is often grave and early recognition during surgery – by noting increase in the cerebral blood flow – is important. Hemorrhagic stroke is, fortunately, rare. Only 0.2% of the NASCET cohort had this compli-cation. A retrospective review of patients undergo-ing CEA found that hemorrhages occurred in 0.6% patients, mainly in patients with hypertension [14].

Wound complications such as infections and hematoma occurred in 9.3% of patients in the NASCET. Wound hematoma is a particular concern because in the NASCET, it was associated with higher perioperative stroke risk (14.5% vs. 5.9% in patients without hematoma) [15]. Large hematomas can also result in airway compromise, requiring immediate evacuation. Smaller hematomas can be managed conservatively. Cranial nerve injuries include those to the hypoglossal nerve, vagus nerve, or branches of the facial nerve and occur in 8.6% of patients but are commonly transient and mild.

Overall, the risk of complications with CEA is higher in symptomatic patients, patients with con-tralateral ICA occlusion, patients with hemispheric rather than retinal ischemic events, in patients aged 75 years or more, in women, and in patients undergoing reoperation [42,50,51]. Severe systemic illnesses such as congestive heart failure, severe respiratory insufficiency, uncontrolled hyperten-sion, and unstable angina are contraindications to CEA.

Carotid angioplasty and stenting (CAS)

Endovascular approaches are attractive because they are less invasive than traditional surgical procedures. Carotid angioplasty with or without the placement of a stent has been developed and studied as an alternative to CEA over the past 10–15 years. Risks and benefits as compared with CEA remain under investigation.

CAS in "high-risk" patients

Previously discussed trials of CEA such as the NASCET and the ACAS excluded patients who were at high risk for perioperative complications with these patients tending to have substantially poorer outcomes than reported in the trials [24,52]. Patients at "high risk" for CEA have been treated with CAS as part of industry-supported registries and randomized trials. Commonly used criteria for "high risk" CEA candidates are listed in Table 14.2.

The Study of Angioplasty with Protection in Patients at High Risk for Endarterectomy (SAPPHIRE) [53] included both symptomatic and asymptomatic patients (about 70% were asymptomatic) with an ICA stenosis who were considered to be high risk for CEA. Patients were randomly assigned to CEA or CAS. CAS with distal emboli protection was not inferior to CEA in these high-risk patients (30-day risk of stroke, death, or MI was 4.4% in the CAS group compared with 9.8% in the CEA group, $P = 0.09$). After 1 year, the combined rate of stroke, death, and MI was lower in those randomized to CAS (12% vs. 20% for CEA, $P = 0.004$ for noninferiority). Moreover, a second revascularization procedure was required less often in the

CAS group compared with the CEA group (0.6% vs. 4.3%, $P = 0.04$). Most of the difference in the composite end point was due to the lower risk of non-Q wave MI events with CAS.

Information on the 3-year outcome of patients in SAPPHIRE has been reported, although follow-up was incomplete (78% of patients had 3-year data) [54]. There was no difference in the combined rates of periprocedure (within 30 days) stroke, MI, or death, or ipsilateral stroke between 31 and 1,080 days, (26.2% for CAS vs. 30.3% for CEA at 3 years, $P = 0.71$). The relatively high 3-year death rate in both groups, averaging 22%, is troubling and raises questions about the value and necessity of either procedure in a high surgical risk cohort.

There have been numerous reports of CAS outcomes from single-center case series and multicenter registries. The 30-day risk of stroke, death, and MI ranges between 1% and 8% [55]. In industry-sponsored registries, the 30-day combined risk of stroke, death, and MI has varied from 3.8% to 8.6% [55].

The Food and Drug Administration has approved the use of specific stenting systems for limited applications in the treatment of carotid artery disease. The Centers for Medicare and Medicaid Services only reimburses for treatment with the approved devices for symptomatic high-risk patients with >70% stenosis. Symptomatic patients with 50–69% stenosis and asymptomatic patients with >80% stenosis are covered only if treated as part of an approved clinical trial or registry.

AHA/ASA guidelines indicate that CAS is not inferior to CEA and can be considered in patients with symptomatic stenosis of >70% in whom the stenosis is difficult to access surgically or who have significant medical comorbidities (Class IIb, Level B). CAS practitioners should have a periprocedural stroke/death rate of <4–6% (Class IIa, Level B) [21].

CAS in "average-risk" patients

Two recent randomized controlled trials of CAS compared with CEA in average-risk patients have been completed. The Stent-Supported Percutaneous Angioplasty of the Carotid Artery versus Endarterectomy trial [56] included 1183 symptomatic patients who were randomized to either CAS or CEA. The 30-day risk of ipsilateral stroke or death was 6.84% for the CAS group compared with 6.34%,

Table 14.2 Commonly cited criteria determining "high risk" for carotid endarterectomy

Medical	Surgical/anatomical
Left ventricular EF <30%	Contralateral carotid occlusion
Age ≥80 years	Prior radiation to neck
Recent MI (≤30 days)	Open tracheostomy
Class III/IV angina or CHF	High cervical bifurcation
Severe COPD	Low/thoracic bifurcation
Need for CABG in <30 days	Contralateral recurrent laryngeal nerve palsy
Significant renal failure	Prior ipsilateral carotid endarterectomy

CABG, coronary artery bypass grafting; CHF, congestive heart failure; COPD, chronic obstructive pulmonary disease; EF, ejection fraction; MI, myocardial infarction.

and the study failed to prove the noninferiority of the stenting procedure. A similar study, the Endarterectomy versus Angioplasty in Patients with Symptomatic Severe Stenosis [57], was stopped earlier than planned because of futility and safety concerns. The 30-day rate of stroke and death was 3.9% in the CEA group compared with 9.6% in the CAS group ($P = 0.01$). This discrepancy persisted after 6 months, leading to the conclusion that widespread use of CAS is not justified in this group of patients. There was criticism of the trials because of the limited training of the interventionalists, multiple device types used (some without embolic protection), and lack of standardized medical therapy [58].

There are still ongoing studies of CEA versus CAS in average risk patients. The NIH-supported Carotid Revascularization Endarterectomy versus Stent Trial aims to recruit 2,500 patients with either symptomatic (>70% stenosis by ultrasound or >50% by angiography) or asymptomatic (70–99%) stenosis. The Asymptomatic Carotid Trial I is a randomized study of CAS and CEA with a 3:1 randomization ratio and involves patients <80 years. This study aims to recruit over 1,600 subjects. Other CAS studies in conventional risk patients are ongoing in Europe. There is also a need to compare CEA and CAS with aggressive, modern medical therapy, although such a trial has not been organized as of yet [59]. An overview of current CAS recommendations can be found in Table 14.3.

Conclusions

CEA is of benefit in carefully selected patient populations for secondary and, to a lesser extent, primary stroke prevention. This procedure prevents stroke in carefully selected symptomatic patients with high-grade and moderate-grade ICA stenosis of more

Table 14.3 Status of carotid stenting according to patient profile

1 Symptomatic high-risk patients with 70–99% stenosis can be considered for CAS.
2 Symptomatic high-risk patients with 50–69% (moderate) stenosis should be offered CAS only in the setting of an approved clinical trial or registry.
3 Asymptomatic high-risk patients with >80% stenosis should be offered CAS only in the setting of an approved clinical trial or registry.
4 Conventional risk patients with symptomatic >50% stenosis and asymptomatic patients should be offered CAS only in the setting of an approved randomized clinical trial.

CAS, carotid artery stenting.

than 50%. The absolute benefit is less in asymptomatic patients with high-grade stenosis. The overall benefit of the operation is highly sensitive to the periprocedure stroke risk. "High-risk" patients such as those with comorbid medical conditions can be considered for CAS if they have high-grade symptomatic stenosis. Those high-risk patients with moderate-grade symptomatic or with asymptomatic stenosis >80% can be considered for CAS in the setting of an approved clinical trial or registry. It remains, however, unclear if any revascularization procedure is necessary in patients who are at high surgical risk because of comorbid conditions. Until high-quality data are available, CAS is not a recommended treatment for conventional risk patients with carotid stenosis. Documentation of the institutional complication rates for both CEA and CAS is important.

References available online at www.wiley.com/go/strokeguidelines.

Intracranial Atherosclerosis

Farhan Siddiq, Burhan Z. Chaudhry, and Adnan I. Qureshi

EXAMPLE CASE

A 55-year-old right-handed man with a past medical history of hypertension, hyperlipidemia, and carotid artery disease, developed acute left upper-extremity weakness after waking up in the morning. The patient was taking aspirin, metoprolol, and a statin. Neurological examination in the emergency department revealed mild dysarthria, left-sided central facial nerve palsy, and left upper-extremity drift. Left upper-extremity strength was 3/5 (the National Institutes of Health [NIH] Stroke Scale score was 4). The remainder of the examination was normal. He was not a candidate for intravenous (IV) recombinant tissue plasminogen activator therapy due to presentation 3 hours after the onset of symptoms. Magnetic resonance imaging (MRI) revealed a watershed distribution ischemic stroke in the right cerebral hemisphere (Figure 15.1). A four-vessel angiogram was obtained, which revealed a hemodynamically significant (estimated greater than 95%) 9-mm-long supraclinoid right internal carotid artery stenosis (Figure 15.2). No thrombus was visualized. A decision was made to perform angioplasty of this lesion (Figure 15.3). After revascularization with angioplasty (Figure 15.4), a Wingspan® stent was placed (Figure 15.5). The patient was started on clopidogrel, and aspirin was continued. The patient was symptom free at the time of a 4-month follow-up visit.

MAJOR POINTS

- Approximately 5–10% of ischemic strokes are related to high-grade intracranial stenosis.
- In one study, 22% had a recurrent stroke within 2 years.
- Medical therapy includes aspirin, clopidogrel, and aspirin-dipyridamole combination.
- There is no evidence that warfarin is superior to aspirin in this setting.
- Indications for endovascular therapy include high grade stenosis with recurrent ischemic symptoms.
- Because of a lack of definitive data from prospective controlled trials, recommendations for endovascular intervention are based primarily on expert opinion.

A Primer on Stroke Prevention Treatment: An Overview Based on AHA/ASA Guidelines, 1st Edition. Edited by L Goldstein.
© 2009 American Heart Association, ISBN: 9781405186513

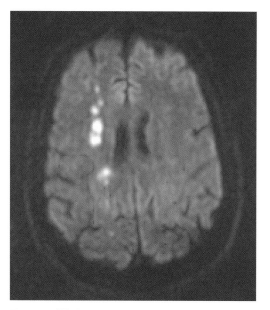

Fig. 15.1 Diffusion-weighted magnetic resonance imaging demonstrated hyperintense signal in the right middle cerebral artery distribution in the watershed region between the deep and superficial branches.

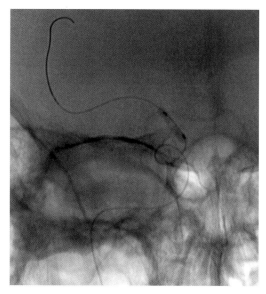

Fig. 15.3 The inflated balloon visualized in the anteroposterior projection during primary angioplasty of the right internal carotid artery (supraclinoid segment) stenosis.

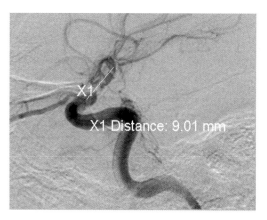

Fig. 15.2 A lateral projection of the right intracranial view after a right internal carotid artery injection demonstrating high-grade right internal carotid artery (supraclinoid segment) stenosis.

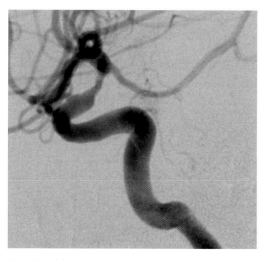

Fig. 15.4 A lateral projection of the right intracranial view after primary angioplasty subsequent to right internal carotid artery injection demonstrating significant resolution of the high-grade right internal carotid artery (supraclinoid segment) stenosis.

Introduction

This man presented with a symptomatic intracranial stenosis. He was initially started on aspirin for stroke prevention. His treatment failed, and he had a stroke in the vascular territory of the stenosed vessel. The magnitude of the stenosis was determined by the ratio of the diameter of the narrowest portion of the vessel within the stenosis to the proximal portion of the reference vessel. At that time, it was decided to perform an angiolasty and place a stent in the target vessel in an attempt to prevent further ischemic events.

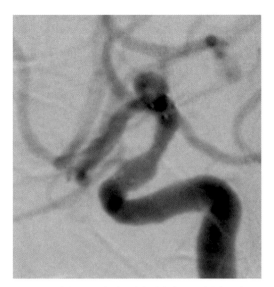

Fig. 15.5 A lateral projection of the right intracranial view after the self-expanding stent deployment subsequent to right internal carotid artery injection, demonstrating significant resolution of the high-grade right internal carotid artery (supraclinoid segment) stenosis.

Incidence of intracranial stenosis and atherosclerosis

Up to 47% of people by their fourth decade and 75–97% of people by their sixth decade show evidence of atherosclerosis in the circle of Willis [1–4]. Thirty percent of the population may have atherosclerotic changes in the intracranial vessels as early as in their second decade [1]. A study using transcranial Doppler (TCD) demonstrated that 12.6% of patients with one vascular risk factor had a stenosis of the middle cerebral artery (MCA). The prevalence quadrupled with increasing numbers of vascular risk factors [5]. Intracranial atherosclerotic disease may account for up to 8–10% of all strokes [6]. Segura *et al.* [7] reported that 5% of hospitalized acute stroke patients had a symptomatic intracranial atherosclerotic lesion. Another large hospital-based study [8] reported that 8% of acute strokes were caused by an intracranial stenosis. Recently, an NIH study group [9] reported that the first-year stroke rate was 11% in the territory of a stenosed intracranial vessel. The annual rate of recurrent stroke may be as high as 15% in patients with intracranial steno-occlusive disease [6,10–14].

Risk factors for intracranial stenosis and atherosclerosis

The extent of intracranial vessel atherosclerosis varies from one population series to another [1]. Intracranial stenosis may be significantly higher in Asian, African-Americans, and Hispanic populations [8,15,16]. The frequency and severity of atherosclerosis increases with advancing age among different populations [1]. Diabetes mellitus, hypertension, hypercholesterolemia, and duration of cigarette smoking; have also been implicated as independent risk factors for intracranial stenosis [6,17–20]. Elevated blood pressure and hyperlipidemia increase the risk of stroke and other major vascular events in symptomatic intracranial atherosclerosis patients [21]. Socioeconomic factors may also play a role. In an autopsy series, it was found that indigent women and urban men had higher prevalence of intracerebral atherosclerosis when compared with private women and rural men patients, respectively [22].

Mechanism of ischemic events associated with intracranial stenosis and atherosclerosis

Several mechanisms have been proposed for ischemic stroke caused by intracranial atherosclerotic disease. Hemodynamic restriction of cerebral blood flow (CBF) accounts for a large number of events [23,24]. Blood flow starts to decrease distal to stenosis of the MCA that is greater than 50% [25]. Maximum restriction of the CBF was observed in patients with more than 75% stenosis. Thrombotic occlusion at the site of stenosis due to plaque rupture and direct occlusion of adjacent penetrating vessels may be the cause of ischemic stroke in some cases [10,26,27]. Transcranial Doppler (TCD) scan performed in 387 stroke patients detected microembolic signals in 36% of those with symptomatic intracranial atherosclerotic disease during the acute phase, affecting areas that were distal to the site of the vascular lesion [7]. This effect dissipated in the chronic phase and was not seen in the setting of an asymptomatic intracranial stenosis. In situ thrombosis followed by acute artery-to-artery embolic phenomena may be a possible pathophysiological mechanism of the stroke caused by intracranial stenosis.

Risk of recurrent ischemic events associated with intracranial stenosis and atherosclerosis

Several studies have identified a high rate of recurrent stroke and death among medically treated patients with symptomatic intracranial stenosis. Among the 164 medically treated patients enrolled of patients in the Extracranial (EC)–Intracranial (IC) Bypass Study (EC-IC) 11.7% of patients per year had a recurrent ischemic episode during the 42-month follow-up period [28]. For patients with MCA stenosis, the ipsilateral recurrent stroke rate was 7.8% per year [7]. The retrospective Warfarin versus Aspirin Symptomatic Intracranial Disease (WASID) Study [14] reported an ipsilateral recurrent stroke rate of 8% per year for those treated with warfarin as compared with an 18% with aspirin. Outcome may be worse for the antithrombotic treatment failure group in another study [29]. In a retrospective study, 29 (56%) patients had a cerebral ischemic event while receiving either an antithrombotic (antiplatelet) agent, warfarin, or heparin. In the Cox regression model, older age was an independent factor associated with recurrent symptoms. Recurrent transient ischemic attacks (TIAs), nonfatal or fatal stroke, or death occurred in 15 of 29 (52%) of these treatment failure patients. In the prospective double-blind, multicenter WASID trial [6], 569 patients with 50–99% symptomatic stenosis of a major intracranial artery were randomized to receive warfarin or aspirin. Over a mean follow-up period of 1.8 years, the primary end point (ischemic stroke, brain hemorrhage, or vascular death) occurred in 22% of the patients in the aspirin group and 22% of those in the warfarin group. Among patients with intracranial stenosis of 70% or greater in the WASID Study [30], the risk of recurrent ipsilateral stroke was 23% and 25% for 1 and 2 years post-randomization, respectively. The stroke-free survival rate was 48% over 5 years among 102 patients with symptomatic stenosis in the vertebrobasilar circulation in another study [31]. Subsequent prospective studies have confirmed the high rates of stroke or death associated with intracranial stenosis. The results from a European, multicenter, prospectively maintained Groupe d'Etude des Sténoses Intra-Crâniennes Athéromateuses symptomatiques registry [32] evaluated the natural history of symptomatic intracranial stenosis.

During the 2-year follow-up, 38% of patients experienced an ipsilateral stroke or TIA. Among patients with a hemodynamic stenosis, 61% had a recurrent ischemic stroke or TIA in the territory of the stenotic artery, whereas only 32% of the patients without a hemodynamic stenosis had a recurrent event. The high recurrent stroke and death rates in medically treated patients highlight the importance of developing new treatment modalities such as endovascular treatment for intracranial stenosis.

Evaluation and detection of intracranial stenosis or atherosclerosis

Patients should ideally be evaluated by an experienced stroke neurologist prior to consideration of revascularization, in order to correlate the patient's symptoms and physical finding with the lesion and to exclude other potential causes of cerebral ischemic events. The usual evaluation includes a conventional catheter angiogram to demonstrate the extent of stenosis, MRI, magnetic resonance angiography (MRA), TCD, and CT angiography (CTA). A prospective multicenter trial [33] demonstrated that TCD and MRA can reliably exclude the presence of intrac-ranial stenosis. Confirmatory catheter angiography, however, is required for the identification and characterization of the lesion. Because MRA may overestimate the severity of intracranial stenosis, its use should be confined as a screening tool until further developments occur in this technology. With improvement in the three-dimensional CTA technique, there is a potential for a noninvasive test for identification and confirmation of intracranial steno-occlusive disease. The sensitivity and positive predictive value of CTA may be better as compared with MRA as a screening tool for intracranial stenosis (98%/93% and 70%/65%, respectively), especially in the presence of slow flow through the stenotic segment [34]. Classes II–III evidences suggest that TCD may provide important information about intracranial steno-occlusive disease [35], but there is currently no recommendation for population-based screening for intracranial stenosis for primary prevention strategy.

A functional CBF study may be obtained at the baseline and after an acetazolamide or carbon dioxide challenge test. Measurements of the cerebral mean transit time, cerebral blood volume, and

CBF can be obtained by various methods, including inhalation or IV injection of 133-xenon, single-photon emission CT, stable xenon CT, positron emission tomography, and CT and MRI perfusion studies after the injection of a contrast medium. The choice of the appropriate investigation depends on availability and experience of the treating physicians.

Intravascular ultrasonography (IVUS) is a safe and a useful technique for analyzing plaque morphology in coronary vasculature. There has been increasing interest for IVUS in intracranial atherosclerosis [36,37]. IVUS provides accurate real-time dynamic measurements of the artery morphology, histology of the plaque, and inflammation within the plaque [38]. This may be a useful adjunct for making the choice of revascularization device and assessing the extent of stent expansion. The use of IVUS in intracranial vasculature is limited due to difficulties in navigating the IVUS catheter to the target vessel through tortous intracranial anatomy.

Antiplatelet treatment of intracranial stenosis or atherosclerosis

In the EC-IC bypass trial [28], medical treatment included aggressive stroke risk factor management and 1,300 mg of daily aspirin. The annual mortality and stroke rate in the control group was 8–10%. Cilostazol, a phosphodiesterase III inhibitor, has been studied in a randomized, double-blinded, placebo-controlled trial in 135 patients with symptomatic intracranial atherosclerosis [39]. The primary outcome measure was increased degree of stenosis detected with MRA. Recurrent stroke and progression of intracranial stenosis on TCD were the secondary outcomes. Over the study's 6-month follow-up period, the rate of progression of intracranial stenosis in the cilostazol group was lower than that of the placebo group (3/67 [6.7%] cilostazol group vs. 15/68 [28.8%] placebo group, $P = 0.008$). The validity of this study still remains in question due to the false-positive and false-negative rates that are associated with both MRA and TCD. Relatively short follow-up period (6 months) was another criticism.

Other antiplatelet agents including clopidogrel, extended-release dipyridamole plus aspirin, and ticlodipine do not have sufficient data to support their use in primary or secondary stroke prevention as a specific measure for the patients with intracranial stenosis. The European Stroke Prevention Study 2 [40] and European/Australasian Stroke Prevention in Reversible Ischaemia Trial [41] demonstrated the benefit of aspirin in combination with dipyridamole for secondary stroke prevention over aspirin alone. Neither study performed any subgroup analyses comparing risk reduction between aspirin and aspirin–dipyridamole combination among patients with symptomatic intracranial stenosis. Therefore, we do not have any data supporting preferential use of aspirin–dipyridamole combination in patients with intracranial stenosis. Similarly, other acute stroke trials were not designed to evaluate the differential efficacy of antiplatelets as secondary prevention for symptomatic intracranial atherosclerosis [42,43].

Anticoagulation for intracranial stenosis or atherosclerosis

The use of anticoagulation for patients with atherosclerotic disease in the basilar artery was initially proposed in 1955 [44]. The effect of warfarin in comparison with aspirin was further studied in two large multicenter trials. The first trial was a retrospective study of 151 patients with symptomatic intracranial atherosclerosis [14]. Eighty-eight of these patients were treated with warfarin and 68 with aspirin. During the mean follow-up period of 14.7 months, the warfarin group had an 8.4% rate of stroke and death versus 18.1% stroke and death in the aspirin group (mean follow-up time: 19.3 months). A Kaplan–Meier analysis revealed a significantly higher rate of major vascular ischemic stroke in patients treated with aspirin compared with warfarin ($P = 0.01$).

Based on the results of the first retrospective trial, a second larger NIH-funded, multicenter, double-blinded, randomized trial was conducted between 1998 and 2003. The WASID trial [9] aimed to establish safety and efficacy of warfarin compared with aspirin in symptomatic intracranial disease (positive history of recent TIA or minor stroke). Patients with symptomatic intracranial stenosis of greater than 50% were randomized to receive either warfarin (international normalized ratio, 2.0–3.0) or aspirin (1,300 mg/d). The trial was halted early due to safety concerns with warfarin (higher incidence of hemorrhages) after 569 patients were randomized. The rates of ipsilateral ischemic stroke for the aspirin- and warfarin-treated groups were 12% and 11%, respectively, during a mean follow-up period of 1.8 years. The rates of death in the aspirin and warfarin groups were 4.3% and 9.7%, respectively ($P = 0.01$). The rates of major hemorrhagic complication in the aspirin and warfarin groups were 3.2% and 8.3%, respectively ($P = 0.02$). There was no difference between the two groups in terms of stroke prevention for patients with symptomatic intracranial stenosis, but the warfarin group had more morbidity and higher mortality.

Other medical therapies for intracranial stenosis or atherosclerosis

Aggressive medical management of hypertension (Class IIa, Level of Evidence B), diabetes mellitus (Class I, Level of Evidence A), and hyperlipidemia (Class IIa, Level of Evidence B) is recommended for the prevention of both recurrent stroke and other vascular events in patients who have had a stroke or TIA. The optimal management for hypertension is uncertain; however, the available data support the use of diuretics and the combination of diuretics and an angiotensin-converting enzyme inhibitor (Class I, Level of Evidence A) [45]. Lifestyle modifications along with blood pressure reductions should be included as part of a comprehensive medical therapy [45]. These modifications include the avoidance of heavy alcohol consumption (Class I, Level of Evidence A), light-to-moderate alcohol intake for both men and women (Class IIb, Level of Evidence C), weight reduction (Class IIb, Level of Evidence C), smoking cessation (Class I, Level of Evidence C), and at least 30 minutes of moderate-intensity physical exercise (Class IIb, Level of Evidence C). High-dose statins reduce the size of atherosclerotic plaque in coronary vasculature, but the use of statins has yet to be explored in patients with intracranial atherosclerotic disease [46,47].

Surgical treatment of intracranial stenosis or atherosclerosis

A surgical procedure involving the bypass from EC (superficial temporal artery) to IC (MCA) in an attempt to circumvent an occluded carotid artery or its branches was first described in 1967 [48]. Soon after, many reports were published describing the safety and feasibility of this innovation [49]. A large prospective, multicenter, randomized controlled trial was conducted to study the effect of EC–IC bypass in patients with internal carotid artery or MCA occlusion [28]. Patients with TIA, small hemispheric stroke, retinal infarction, and occlusive disease of the carotid artery or MCA were randomized to bypass surgery ($n = 663$) or best medical management ($n = 714$). At the mean follow-up of 55.8 months, fatal and nonfatal strokes occurred more frequently and earlier in the surgical group. The analyses of different angiographic lesion location failed to demonstrate any benefit of surgery. Patients with severe MCA stenosis and persistent ischemic symptoms after internal carotid artery occlusion had worse outcomes in the surgical group. Bypass surgery was largely abandoned for the treatment of intracranial stenosis after the publication of these results.

Despite the negative results of the EC–IC bypass study, several investigators have continued to evaluate the utility of this procedure in carefully selected patients with internal carotid artery (ICA) stenosis or occlusion who have continued hemodynamic compromise and cerebral hypoperfusion. Characteristically, these patients have a severely diminished cerebrovascular reserve capacity (CRC) owing to the occlusive disease and inadequate collateral circulation. During the last decade, there has been a revival of interest in cerebral revascularization with the introduction of newer surgical techniques. A report of 15 patients indicted that EC–IC bypass surgery may not have any effect on regionel CBF (rCBF) but may improve CRC in patients with intracranial stenosis and occlusion [50]. Another study found that EC–IC bypass surgery may be able to maintain cerebral blood oxygenation immediately after surgery or gradually within 1 year when the preoperative rCBF is below 24.5–25 mL/100 g/min [51]. A third study reported an increase in total brain blood supply and restoration of local perfusion in the hemodynamically compromised brain tissue in 25 patients with symptomatic ICA occlusion who had an EC–IC arterial bypass procedure [52].

Endovascular treatment of intracranial stenosis or atherosclerosis

At present, intracranial angioplasty with or without stent placement is reserved for medically refractory patients (symptomatic even with the "best medical management" including adequate antithrombotic treatment) and with adequate vessel diameter (2.5–4.5 mm diameter). The incidence of peri-procedural neurological events ranges from 5% to 33%. The technical success rates are increasing, and complications are decreasing over time with the advances in the endovascular technology [31,53–55]. Technical feasibility with success rates greater than 90% have been reported in numerous series. The rates of procedure-related complications, however, vary greatly among different studies, indicating that these procedures may be highly operator-dependent in terms of both success and complication (complication rates 0–20%) [56–69].

Examples of the criteria for selecting patients for endovascular treatment of intracranial stenosis in one study [30] include:

1 age greater than 18 years;
2 ischemic events referable to the artery with stenosis;
3 ischemic symptoms despite antiplatelet therapy, defined by regular use of aspirin 81 mg or higher daily (either alone or in combination with dipyridamole), clopidogrel 75 mg daily, or ticlopidine 250 mg twice daily, or anticoagulation defined by IV heparin (with an activated partial thromboplastin time >1.5 times control) or oral warfarin (with an international normalized ratio greater than 2.0);
4 intracranial stenosis, including the petrous and cavernous segments of the internal carotid artery and the intradural segment of the vertebral artery;
5 presence of an atherosclerotic lesion with angiographically visible reduction (greater than 50% stenosis) of the lumen of the affected artery. The magnitude of stenosis is determined by the ratio of the narrowest vessel diameter within the stenosis to the diameter of the proximal portion of the reference vessel. After the publication of the WASID trial, the eligibility criteria may be extended to include patients with angiographic stenosis of 70% or greater without medication failure, considering that such patients had a greater risk of ischemic events despite treatment with medication [30].

Summary of clinical studies evaluating primary angioplasty for intracranial stenosis

An early study reported a 25% restenosis rate 3 months after angioplasty in seven patients [61]. In an attempt to determine the ideal time for angiographic follow-up to detect restenosis, 35 patients had follow-up studies at 3 and 12 months [60]. The rate of restenosis was 29.6% at 3 months. Patients without restenosis at 3 months were also free of recurrent disease at 12 months. Lesions smaller than 5 mm in size with little or no calcification, and with smooth surface contours, had higher success rate with low morbidity and lower rate of restenosis.

In a series of 23 patients, the procedure success rate was 91.3% (one death after the procedure) with an annual rate of ipsilateral hemispheric stroke of 3.2% over a mean follow-up period of 35.4 months [55]. Another series included 120 patients with 124 intracranial stenoses who had primary angioplasty. Stenosis at the time of treatment varied from 50% to 95% (mean 82%). The combined peri-procedure (30-day post-procedure) stroke and death rate was 5.8% (three strokes and four deaths). During the follow-up period (mean 42 months), there were 11 strokes and 10 deaths. Six strokes were in the territory of the treated artery. The reported annual stroke and ipsilateral stroke rates were 4.4% and 3.2%, respectively. Long-term clinical follow-up suggests that stroke prevention rate following the procedure compares favorably with the expected rates among patients receiving medical therapy.

Subsequent revisions of the technique, using slow balloon inflation and undersized balloons in 50 patients, was associated with no abrupt vessel occlusions or strokes [57]. Forty-nine of the patients (98%) achieved good angiographic and short-term clinical outcomes, defined as stable or improved neurological status. The rate of asymptomatic restenosis at 3–12 months was 8% (4/49).

In 2006, Wojak et al. [62] reported 60 consecutive patients with 71 intracranial lesions (67 symptomatic and 4 asymptomatic) who were treated with a total of 84 primary angioplasty and angioplasty followed by stent placement (62 and 22, respectively).

A success rate of 90.5% was reported with a 4.8% rate of peri-procedural stroke and death. A total of 23 lesions had angiographic evidence of restenosis at the mean follow-up period of 4.6 months. Long-term clinical outcome was available for all 60 patients. Over a period of 224 patient years of follow-up, there were four strokes and no deaths due to neurological complications; four other patients died due to non-neurological causes. The annual stroke rate in treated vessel territory and annual stroke and death rate was 1.8%. The annual stroke and all-cause mortality was 3%.

Some authors have proposed theoretical advantages of stent placement over primary angioplasty by preventing early elastic recoil and negative remodeling [63,64].

Summary of clinical studies evaluating stent placement for intracranial stenosis

New coronary stents that have become available made placement in the cerebral circulation feasible. In one study, stent placement was attempted in 10 patients with 12 lesions [59]. The procedure was successful in eight patients (two lesions were inaccessible). Pretreatment vessel diameter of 80% was reduced to 7% in 10 lesions ($P < 0.001$), and no angiographic restenosis was seen at 3 months. No neurological events were reported at the mean follow-up of 11 months. After this successful deployment of stents in intracranial vasculature, many other reports followed describing the safety and potential effectiveness of intracranial stenting.

The Stenting in Symptomatic Atherosclerotic Lesions of Vertebral and Intracranial Arteries trial evaluated the safety and efficacy of a new balloon catheter and stenting device (Neurolink, Guidant, Advanced Cardiovascular Inc.) in 43 patients with intracranial stenosis and 18 with extracranial vertebral artery stenosis [12]. Peri-procedural stroke rate was 7% with a 95% success rate. Forty-two patients had a 12-month clinical follow-up. Four patients had a stroke after 30 days in the target lesion territory. Angiographic restenosis occurred in 35% of patients and was symptomatic in a third. Based on this finding, the Food and Drug Administration (FDA) granted a Humanitarian Device Exemption (HDE) approval for the Neurolink device [70].

A prospective study was conducted to evaluate the efficacy and feasibility of the another stent system comprising of a semicompliant balloon, a stainless steel stent, and a delivery catheter [71]. Peri-procedural stroke rate was 6.5%. Angiographic follow-up performed in 25 patients revealed seven restenoses (28%), one of which was symptomatic. The stroke rate was 4.3 per 100 patient years.

Stents eluting antiproliferative drugs have shown encouraging results in clinical trials for the prevention of restenosis after percutaneous coronary intervention [72]. Technical success rate (defined as the reduction of target lesion to stenosis <30%) of 100% and peri-procedure stroke rate of 5.5% (no deaths) were reported in 18 patients treated with these types of stents [73]. No major strokes or deaths occurred after 6 months. Estimated major stroke-free survival was 86% at 12 months following the procedure. Symptomatic angiographic restenosis rate was 5.5% (one lesion).

An HDE Safety Study was conducted at 12 sites in Europe and Asia for a self-expanding, nitinol stent sheathed in a delivery system [74]. Forty-five patients with medically refractory symptomatic intracranial atherosclerosis were enrolled, of whom 44 patients subsequently underwent stent placement. The procedural success rate was 98% with a 4.4% ($n = 2$) peri-procedural rate of death or ipsilateral stroke. Forty-three patients completed the 6-month follow-up with a 7.0% ($n = 3$) death and ipsilateral stroke incidence. Further lesion reduction was observed in 24 of the 40 patients (mean severity 28%) who had a 6-month angiographic follow-up. Based on the results of this study, the FDA granted an HDE approval for the Wingspan(TM) Stent System with Gateway(TM) PTA Balloon Catheter in 2007. US multicenter experience with the Wingspan Stent System study [75] reported a 98.8% success rate (one failure due to tortuous carotid artery). Five (6.1%) patients suffered major neurological complications in the peri-procedure period, four of which led to death. A recently published NIH registry on the use of the Wingspan stent [45] enrolled 129 patients with symptomatic intracranial stenoses (range 70–99%) from 16 medical centers and found a technical success rate of 96.7%. The frequency of stroke and death within the peri-procedural period was 14.0%. The rate of restenosis in 52 patients with angiographic follow-up was 25%.

Comparative role of primary angioplasty versus stent placement for intracranial stenosis

There is presently insufficient evidence to determine the relative efficacies of angioplasty, stent placement, or the combination of the two. Treatment paradigms are often based solely on operator preference and experience. Some investigators are recommending primary angioplasty as the preferred treatment for intracranial atherosclerosis, while others recommend stent placement whenever possible. Various factors play a role in deciding primary angioplasty versus stent placement for the treatment of medically refractory symptomatic intracranial stenosis. In general, primary angioplasty may be preferred for small vessels (<2 mm in diameter); long lesions which would require long or multiple stents (>12 mm); very tortuous proximal vessels (two or more acute curves requiring traversing as judged by experience); limited vessel length available distal to the lesion to allow the stable placement of microwire (basilar stenosis with hypoplastic or aplastic posterior cerebral arteries); lesions located in anterior cerebral or posterior cerebral artery or M2 segment of MCA; or if the guide catheter cannot be placed in the distal vertebral or internal carotid artery.

Whether angioplasty or stent placement is better for intracranial stenosis remains subject to great debate. One study reported the clinical and angiographic follow-up of 187 patients with symptomatic intracranial stenosis treated with angioplasty and stent placement in the target vessel (94 angioplasties, 96 stent placements) [76]. After adjusting for age, gender, and center, there was no difference in the rate of stroke and stroke and/or death between the groups. A randomized controlled trial is recommended to fully understand the effectiveness of angioplasty compared with stent placement in the intracranial circulation.

Recommended indications from professional organizations

American Heart Association/American Stroke Association guidelines indicate that the usefulness of endovascular therapy (angioplasty and/or stent placement) for patients with hemodynamically significant intracranial stenosis who have symptoms despite medical therapies (antithrombotics, statins, and other treatments for risk factors) is uncertain and is considered investigational (Class IIb, Level of Evidence C) [77].

The Brain Attack Coalition recognizes the lack of data from large, prospective randomized trials. Intracranial angioplasty and stent placement for cerebrovascular disease is considered an optional component for a comprehensive stroke center, although there are selected cases in which such techniques may be of value [78]. If a center does offer this procedure, it is recommended that cases be entered into a registry to track outcomes. It is further recommended that if a comprehensive stroke center does not offer extracranial and intracranial angioplasty/stent placement, it has an available referral arrangement to send selected patients to another facility that does offer these interventions.

It should be noted that the American Society of Interventional and Therapeutic Neuroradiology, the Society of Interventional Radiology, and the American Society of Neuroradiology [79] agree that sufficient evidence now exists to recommend intracranial angioplasty with or without stent placement for symptomatic patients with intracranial stenoses >50% demonstrated on catheter angiography, who have failed medical therapy. Patient benefit from revascularization for symptomatic intracranial arterial stenosis is critically dependent on a low peri-procedural stroke and death rate, and should therefore be performed by experienced endovascular centers. Patients with asymptomatic intracranial arterial stenosis should first be counseled regarding optimal medical therapy. Due to the lack of sufficient evidence, endovascular therapy is not recommended in asymptomatic patients with severe intracranial atherosclerosis. They should be counseled regarding the nature and extent of the disease, monitored for new neurological symptoms, and have periodic imaging at regular intervals of 6–12 months (MRA, CTA initially, and then cerebral angiography if warranted). Optimal prophylactic medical therapy should be instituted, which may include antiplatelet and/or statin therapy. These recommendations are summarized in Table 15.1.

Table 15.1 A summary of indications used for treating intracranial atherosclerosis in various studies, with quality of evidence

Treatment	Indications	Safety	Recommendations
Aspirin	Symptomatic intracranial atherosclerosis	Level I [6,23]	Grade C [77]
Warfarin	Symptomatic intracranial atherosclerosis refractory to initial medical management	Level II [6]	Grade C [77]
Surgery	Symptomatic intracranial atherosclerosis not amenable to endovascular therapy	Level II [23]	Grade C [77]
Angioplasty	Symptomatic intracranial atherosclerosis refractory to medical management	Level III [43,51,66,67,80]	Grade C [77]
Stent placement	Symptomatic intracranial atherosclerosis refractory to medical management	Levels II–III [12,58,60,65,66,68,70,72,74,81,82]	Grade C [77]

Level I – derived from multiple randomized controlled trials.

Level II – derived from a single randomized trial or nonrandomized studies.

Level III – consensus opinion of experts.

Table 15.2 Stents approved by the Food and Drug Administration for intracranial stent placements

Stent system		Year of approval	Recommended use
Neurolink Stent System (Guidant Corporation, Menlo Park, CA)	HDE	August 2002	Treatment of recurrent ischemic events attributable to atherosclerotic disease with >50% stenosis, refractory to medical therapy in intracranial vessels ranging from 2.5 to 4.5 mm in diameter accessible to the stent system
Wingspan Stent System with Gateway PTA Balloon Catheter (Boston Scientific Smart, Fremont, CA)	HDE	August 2005	Improving lumen diameter in patients with intracranial atherosclerotic disease ≥50%, refractory to medical therapy in intracranial vessels that are accessible to the system

HDE, Humanitarian Device Exemption.

Regulatory approvals, the FDA, and the Centers of Medicare and Medicaid Services (CMS)

Two stents are approved under the provision for humanitarian use devices by the FDA (see Table 15.2). Effective January 1, 2006, the American Medical Association issued specific CPT® Codes (61630 and 61635) for intracranial angioplasty and stent placement procedures (http://www.bostonscientific. com/Reimbursement.bsci/,,/navRelId/1000.1038/ seo.serve#Neurovascular%20Intervention). Effective November 6, 2006, the CMS decided to allow national Medicare coverage of intracranial angioplasty and stent placement as part of certain investigational device exemption clinical trials. Currently, however, procedures which involve the Wingspan Stent System and Gateway PTA Balloon Catheter for the HDE-approved indication remain a noncovered service under Medicare. Other health insurers who choose to cover intracranial angioplasty and stent placement cases will reimburse hospitals for inpatient care using a variety of mechanisms including per diems, diagnosis-related groups, case rates, or percentage of billed charges.

Future directions

Randomized controlled trials are warranted to clearly establish the role of intracranial angioplasty and stent placement for symptomatic intracranial artery disease. The best medical therapy is not established at this time for comparison. Various advances in stent delivery system are also anticipated to improve access to tortuous vessels. The NIH-funded, randomized, open-label, Stent Placement versus Aggressive Medical Management for the Prevention of Recurrent stroke in Intracranial Stenosis [83] trial will be able to answer some of the questions. This trial is designed to compare the intracranial stenting (Wingspan) and best medical therapy (management of blood pressure, lipids, and other risk factors for vascular events) for symptomatic intracranial atherosclerosis. The enrollment for this trial has started in February 2008, with publication of the results expected by February 2013.

References available online at www.wiley.com/go/strokeguidelines.

16   Patent Foramen Ovale

Marco R. Di Tullio and Shunichi Homma

EXAMPLE CASE

A 55-year-old right-handed man with no significant medical history and no history of neurological disease developed left-sided perioral tingling associated with significant dysarthria. The episode lasted for 2 minutes, resolved entirely, and then recurred 5 minutes later lasting for about an hour. Each episode was characterized by left perioral paresthesia (tingling and numbness) and dysarthria noted by the patient and his wife. The episodes were not associated with difficulty in understanding words or with word-finding difficulties, but rather an inability to form the words. There was no associated change in mental status, headache, visual changes, diplopia, or limb weakness or numbness. The patient had no history of similar episodes and no cardiovascular risk factors.

Physical and neurological examinations

In the emergency department, the patient was afebrile, blood pressure was 126/82 mm Hg, pulse was 58 and regular, and respiratory rate was 16 with oxygen saturation of 97% on room air. Cardiac auscultation revealed regular heart sounds with no murmurs or gallop. Lungs were clear to auscultation. The abdomen was soft and nontender. Peripheral pulses were normal. No peripheral edema was noted. Neurological examination was normal.

Laboratory studies

Complete blood count, electrolytes, renal function, and coagulation parameters were normal. An EKG showed normal sinus rhythm. A head CT scan without contrast was normal. Later, a magnetic resonance imaging (MRI) revealed a small lesion in the right frontal convexity consistent with ischemia. Magnetic resonance angiography of the neck and head showed no vascular stenoses. A transthoracic echocardiogram showed an atrial septal aneurysm (ASA) with evidence of a large shunt on contrast injection, consistent with the presence of an associated patent foramen ovale (PFO). Further laboratory testing, including a complete workup for hypercoagulability, was negative. The patient, completely recovered, was discharged from the hospital on aspirin treatment.

MAJOR POINTS

- The presence of a PFO is associated with increased risk of ischemic stroke, especially cryptogenic stroke, and with increased risk of recurrent events in patients with a first stroke.
- The association between PFO and stroke is present at all ages, although it is stronger in subjects younger than 55 years.
- Treatment with antiplatelet agents is recommended for secondary prevention in most stroke patients with a PFO; warfarin treatment is indicated in patients with associated deep venous thrombosis or hypercoagulable states.
- Until results of randomized treatment trials versus medical treatment are available, PFO closure should be reserved for patients who fail medical therapy or have contraindications to it.
- The incidental finding of a PFO in an otherwise asymptomatic subject does not represent an indication for preventive treatment.

A Primer on Stroke Prevention Treatment: An Overview Based on AHA/ASA Guidelines, 1st Edition. Edited by L Goldstein.
© 2009 American Heart Association, ISBN: 9781405186513

Introduction

The previous case is an example of a cerebrovascular episode, fortunately of mild severity, in a man with no risk factors or apparent embolic sources, but with a PFO and ASA revealed by echocardiography. In the past 20 years, the association between PFO and otherwise cryptogenic ischemic stroke has been recognized and has gained widespread acceptance. Since the first reports were published, this relationship has been confirmed and studied in different patient subgroups, possibly associated cofactors have been sought, and potential preventive strategies have been developed, although uncertainties remain. The present chapter will review the available evidence on the relationship between PFO and stroke, the main diagnostic techniques to detect a PFO, and the possible therapeutic options to decrease the stroke risk associated with its presence.

Frequency of PFO in the general population

A normal component of the fetal circulation, the foramen ovale usually closes after birth due to the fusion of the two components of the atrial septum: the septum primum and the septum secundum. In approximately one quarter of subjects, this fusion does not occur or is incomplete, resulting in small interatrial communication that persists into adult life. In a PFO, the septum primum and secundum overlap but do not fuse; in most cases, the PFO can only open when the pressure in the right atrium exceeds that of the left atrium, creating the conditions for a transient right-to-left shunt that resolves when the pressure gradient between the atria is reversed, as it happens during most of the cardiac cycle. A PFO has to be distinguished from an atrial septal defect (ASD), in which a segment of the septum is missing entirely, resulting in a fixed inter-atrial communication that allows a continuous and usually bidirectional shunt between the atria. The prevalence of PFO in the general population has been reported to be between 15% and 35% in autopsy studies [1–4]. The prevalence of PFO appears to decrease with age. In an autopsy study of 965 subjects of all ages, PFO prevalence was 34% in the first three decades of life, compared with 20% in

Table 16.1 Patent foramen ovale prevalence among patients with atrial septal aneurysm

Study	Method	Prevalence
Mügge et al. [7]	TE Echo.	54% (106/195)
Hanley et al. [12]	TT Echo.	49% (24/49)
Schneider et al. [13]	TE Echo.	77% (17/22)
Zabalgoitia-Reyes et al. [14]	TE Echo.	85% (17/20)
Pearson et al. [15]	TE Echo.	69% (20/29)
Silver and Dorsey [16]	Autopsy	50% (8/16)
Mattioli et al. [17]	TE Echo.	87% (39/44)
Burger et al. [18]	TE Echo.	56% (18/32)
Homma et al. [19]	TE Echo.	64% (44/69)
Total		59% (236/400)

TE Echo., transesophageal echocardiography; TT Echo., transthoracic echocardiography.

the ninth decade [3]. The size of the PFO increased with age, suggesting that some smaller foramina may close over time. The prevalence of PFO is similar in different race–ethnic groups [5,6].

An ASA is another abnormality of the interatrial septum that is often found in patients with a PFO, as was the case in our patient, and may also be associated with increased stroke risk. An ASA is a discrete protrusion of a redundant atrial septum into either atrial chamber. A protrusion of at least 10 mm is generally considered diagnostic of ASA [5,7]. An ASA is found in a much smaller proportion of the general population than a PFO (approximately 1–4%) [8–11]. A coexisting PFO is found in approximately 60% of patients in whom an ASA is present [7,12–19] (Table 16.1).

Detection of PFO

Transesophageal echocardiography (TEE) remains the most sensitive technique for the detection of a PFO in vivo. This test, which is semi-invasive and performed under conscious sedation, is generally well tolerated, and serious complications (laryngeal or gastroesophageal trauma, hypoxia, bronchospasm, cardiac arrhythmias, bleeding) are rare (estimated at 0.2% in a large series) [20]. The assessment for PFO is performed with the injection of contrast material, usually aerated saline solution, and the

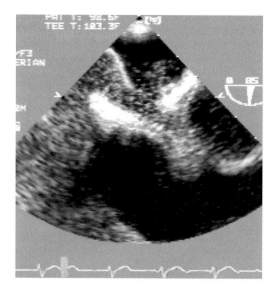

Fig. 16.1 Example of positive contrast study by transesophageal echocardiography with contrast injection. A separation is visible between septum primum and septum secundum, and microbubbles are seen shunting from the right atrium (bottom) to the left atrium (top).

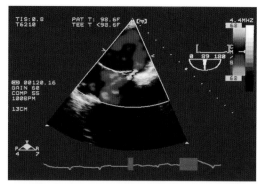

Fig. 16.2 Patent foramen ovale visualization by color Doppler during transesophageal echocardiography. An aliasing color flow jet is seen between the right atrium (bottom) and the left atrium (top).

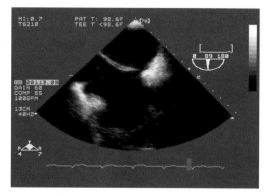

Fig. 16.3 Direct visualization of a patent foramen ovale by transesophageal echocardiography. The separation between septum secundum (left) and septum primum (right) is visible.

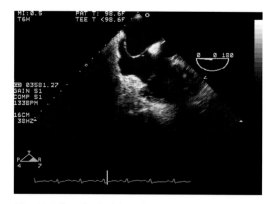

Fig. 16.4 Example of atrial septal aneurysm by transesophageal echocardiography.

appearance of microbubbles in the left atrium soon after the contrast material fills the right atrium is consistent with the presence of a PFO (Figure 16.1). The injection is then repeated during Valsalva maneuver and coughing, to increase the right atrial pressure and thus maximize the sensitivity of the test in visualizing any right-to-left shunt. Color flow Doppler can occasionally confirm the diagnosis (Figure 16.2), but its sensitivity is lower than that of contrast injection [21]. In many patients, the actual separation of septum primum and septum secundum can be visualized (Figure 16.3), which is a direct proof of the presence of a PFO, and may allow the direct measurement of the gap, a notion that can be used for risk stratification. The degree of shunting can also be inferred by the number of shunting microbubbles. TEE can also very accurately identify the presence of an ASA (Figure 16.4), with or without associated PFO. TEE also allows the differentiation of a PFO from an ASD, because in the latter it can directly visualize the fixed interatrial communication, its location, size, and prevalent shunt direction.

Transthoracic echocardiography (TTE) with contrast injection is a noninvasive, albeit less sensitive,

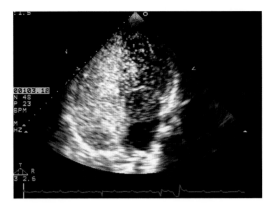

Fig. 16.5 Patent foramen ovale detection by transthoracic echocardiography with contrast injection. Microbubbles are visualized filling the right-sided chambers (displayed on the left in the picture) and shunting into the left atrium (bottom right) and from there into the left ventricle (top right).

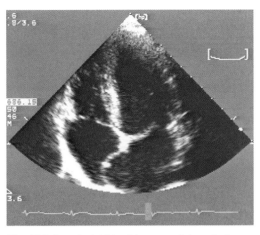

Fig. 16.6 Example of atrial septal aneurysm (between the two lower chambers in the picture) by transthoracic echocardiography.

imaging modality for diagnosing a PFO. An example of PFO detection by contrast TTE is provided in Figure 16.5. In studies that evaluated the accuracy of contrast TTE for PFO detection using TEE as the gold standard, TTE sensitivity was approximately 50–60% [22–29], but the PFOs that were missed were due to technically inadequate images, or were smaller and associated with lesser degree of shunt, therefore were possibly less relevant from a clinical standpoint [23]. When TTE is used, timing becomes important in differentiating an early shunt (within three cardiac cycles from the right atrial opacification), typical of a PFO, from a later shunt associated with transpulmonary circulation, a condition that can instead be evaluated directly by TEE through the visualization of microbubbles in the pulmonary veins. An ASA can also be visualized by TTE (Figure 16.6), although with less sensitivity than by TEE [7], especially for small aneurysms. In our patient, TTE with contrast was performed and was strongly positive both for a PFO and an ASA, making TEE unnecessary for the diagnosis. TEE may, however, be considered to better define the anatomy of the lesions if PFO closure is considered, as will be discussed later in the chapter.

Transcranial Doppler (TCD) imaging has also been used for detecting right-to-left shunts. Using TCD with contrast injection, shunting microbubbles appear as discrete spikes superimposed to the normal

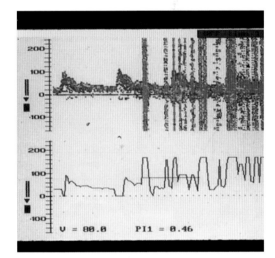

Fig. 16.7 Detection of microbubbles by transcranial Doppler in the middle cerebral artery of a patient with a patent foramen ovale. Microbubbles are displayed as vertical high-intensity signals superimposed to the normal blood flow.

blood flow detected in the middle cerebral artery (Figure 16.7). TCD sensitivity for PFO detection is intermediate between those of TEE and TTE, and as high as 91.3% in one study [27]. However, TCD is limited because it cannot assess the location of the shunt (e.g., intracradiac vs. transpulmonary). A comparison of the three diagnostic techniques in various published studies is provided in Table 16.2.

Table 16.2 Comparison of techniques for patent foramen ovale detection

Study	n	TTE	TCD	TEE
Teague and Sharma [22]	46	26% (12/46)	41% (19/46	–
Di Tullio et al. [28]	80	18% (14/80)	26% (21/80)	–
Jauss et al. [24]	50	–	28% (14/50)	30% (15/50)
Karnik et al. [25]	36	–	36% (13/36)	42% (15/36)
Job et al. [26]	137	–	42% (58/137)	47% (65/137)
Klötzsch et al. [27]	111	–	38% (42/111)	41% (46/111)
Nemec et al. [29]	32	23% (7/32)	41% (13/32)	41% (13/32)
Di Tullio et al. [23]	49	18% (9/49)	27% (13/49)	38% (19/49)
Total		20%(42/207)	36% (193/541)	42% (173/415)

TCD, transcranial Doppler; TEE, transesophageal echocardiography; TTE, transthoracic echocardiography.

Table 16.3 Relationship of cryptogenic stroke with patent foramen ovale (PFO) in younger patients

Study	n (patients)	Age	PFO (cryptogenic)	PFO (control)	P value
Lechat et al. [32]	26	<55	54% (14/26)	10% (10/100)	<0.001
Webster et al. [33]	34	<40	56% (19/34)	15% (6/40)	<0.001
Cabanes et al. [34]	64	<55	56% (36/64)	18% (9/50)	<0.001
de Belder et al. [35]*	39	<55	13% (5/39)	3% (1/39)	–
Di Tullio et al. [36]	21	<55	48% (10/21)	4% (1/24)**	<0.001
Hausmann et al. [37]	18	<40	50% (9/18)	11% (2/18)	<0.05
Handke et al. [41]	82	<55	44% (36/82)	14% (7/49)**	<0.001
Total			45% (129/284)	11% (36/320)	<0.001

*Includes different stroke subtypes.
**Controls were patients with stroke of known cause.

PFO, ASA, and risk of ischemic stroke

Although the first anecdotal report of a stroke associated with an interatrial shunt in a young woman dates back to Julius Cohnheim's description in 1877 [30], the association between PFO and ischemic stroke has been clearly recognized and studied only in the past 20 years. Approximately 40% of ischemic strokes do not have an apparent cause, and are therefore referred to as cryptogenic strokes [31]. Using contrast echocardiography, various case-control studies reported an association between PFO and cryptogenic stroke, especially in patients younger than 55 years [32–37]. Lechat and colleagues were the first to report a prevalence of PFO of 40% in young stroke patients (age <55) compared with 10% in controls; the prevalence was even higher (56%) in patients with cryptogenic stroke [32]. Almost at the same time, Webster and colleagues found a similar difference in young (age <40) stroke patients compared with controls (50% vs. 15%) [33]. Since then, several other studies have confirmed the association between PFO and stroke in younger stroke patients (Table 16.3). Stroke risk increases with age with only 3% of all strokes occurring before the age of 40 [38]. Therefore, the number of elderly patients with stroke and a PFO is much greater than the number of younger patients with stroke and PFO. The association between PFO and stroke in older patients has been controversial [35–

Table 16.4 Relationship of cryptogenic stroke with patent foramen ovale (PFO) in older patients

Study	n (patients)	Age	PFO (cryptogenic)	PFO (control)	P value
de Belder *et al.* [35]*	64	>55	20% (13/64)	5% (3/56)	<0.001
Di Tullio *et al.* [36]	24	>55	38% (9/24)	8% (6/77)**	<0.001
Hausmann *et al.* [37]	20	>40	15% (3/20)	23% (23/98)	NS
Jones *et al.* [39]	57	>50	18% (10/57)	16% (29/183)	NS
Handke *et al.* [41]	145	>55	28% (41/145)	12% (28/232)**	<0.001
Total			25% (76/310)	14% (89/646)	<0.001

*Includes different stroke subtypes.
**Controls were patients with stroke of known cause.
NS, not significant.

37,39]. In a group of 146 stroke patients, an increased prevalence of PFO was observed in patients with cryptogenic stroke in both individuals over 55 years (38% compared with 8% in patients with stroke of determined cause) and under 55 years (48% vs. 4%) [36]. Subsequent studies, however, reported conflicting results, confirming [35] or negating [37,39] the association between PFO and stroke risk in the elderly (Table 16.4). The association was also questioned in a meta-analysis that evaluated case-control studies published until 2000 [40]. A significant association between PFO and stroke was found in those under the age of 55 years (odds ratio 3.10, 95% confidence interval [CI] 2.29–4.21). There were also associations between ASA (odds ratio 6.14, 95% CI 2.47–15.22) and the combination of PFO and ASA (odds ratio 15.59, 95% CI 2.83–85.87) and stroke risk. In older patients, ASA (odds ratio 3.43, 95% CI 1.89–6.22) and PFO plus ASA (odds ratio 5.09, 95% CI 1.25–20.74) appeared to be associated with stroke, whereas PFO alone was not (odds ratio 1.27, 95% CI 0.80–2.01). Although these data were obtained from studies comparing stroke patients with normal controls, a similar trend was observed for PFO when comparing cryptogenic strokes with strokes of known cause, with a significant association with cryptogenic stroke observed in younger (odds ratio 6.00, 95% CI 3.72–9.68) but not in older (odds ratio 2.26, 95% CI 0.96–5.31) patients [40]. Insufficient data were available to allow an analysis for ASA alone and for PFO plus ASA.

More recently, the largest TEE study performed to date [41] reaffirmed the association between PFO and ischemic stroke even in patients over the age of 55. PFO was more frequent in cryptogenic stroke patients than in patients with stroke of determined cause in both the younger subgroup (43.9% vs. 14.3%; odds ratio 4.70, 95% CI 1.89–11.68; $P < 0.001$) and in the older subgroup (28.3% vs. 11.9%; odds ratio 2.92, 95% CI 1.70–5.01; $P < 0.001$). After adjustment for age, aortic plaque thickness, hypertension, and coronary artery disease, PFO remained strongly associated with cryptogenic stroke in both the younger (odds ratio 3.70, 95% CI 1.42–9.65; $P = 0.008$) and the older groups (odds ratio 3.00, 95% CI 1.73–5.23; $P < 0.001$) [41].

The role of an ASA as a risk factor for stroke has also been assessed in case-control echocardiographic studies. The prevalence of ASA is greater among patients with embolic events than among controls [14,36,42–44]. As mentioned previously, ASA is associated with PFO in approximately 60% of patients. In addition, the PFOs found in the presence of ASA tend to be larger compared with those without an associated ASA [19,45]. Thus, the association of ASA with embolic events may be based on the high prevalence of large PFOs. Although no TEE was performed in the patient described at the beginning of the chapter, the shunt was very large by TTE with contrast injection. However, the meta-analysis mentioned earlier in this section [40] suggested the existence of an increased stroke risk also in patients with isolated ASA, and the risk was higher in subjects with PFO plus ASA than in those with either condition alone. In situ thrombus formation could be responsible for stroke in patients with isolated

ASA, but this was an infrequent finding in a large series of patients [7]. Atrial arrhythmias have been hypothesized to play a role in the increased risk of stroke seen in patients with these right atrial abnormalities [46], but clear evidence to this regard is lacking [47].

The association between PFO and stroke has been established. The mechanism of stroke such as paradoxical embolization to the brain from a venous source often remains presumptive. Anecdotal cases of thrombotic material trapped in the PFO (Figures 16.8 and 16.9) represent proof that the mechanism indeed occurs, but in the vast majority of cases, the diagnosis of paradoxical embolization is an exclusion diagnosis, based on the combination of neuro-imaging findings compatible with embolism, the absence of other obvious stroke mechanisms, and the presence of cofactors that may increase the likelihood of a thrombus to form and embolize through the PFO.

Associated factors

Some anatomical characteristics of the atrial septum and of the right atrium can predispose to an increased propensity for paradoxical embolization through a PFO. The size of the septal separation seen by TEE, although a rough, two-dimensional representation of a three-dimensional structure, has been associated with increased stroke risk. In studies that have used contrast TTE [33], TEE [48–50], TCD [24,51], or cardiac catheterization [52], patients with presumed paradoxical embolization appeared to have larger PFOs compared with those seen in control groups. In the PFO in Cryptogenic Stroke Study (PICSS), large PFOs were significantly more prevalent among cryptogenic stroke patients compared with those with known cause of stroke [53]. Additionally, stroke patients with larger PFOs have been shown to have brain imaging findings suggestive of an embolic mechanism [54], and there is some evidence that PFO size may be an independent risk factor for recurrent cerebrovascular events [55].

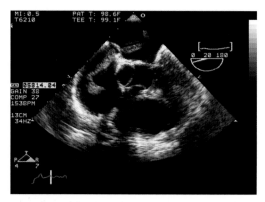

Fig. 16.8 Transesophageal echocardiography visualization of large thrombus crossing the patent foramen ovale and extending into the left atrium (top) and the right atrium (bottom).

Among atrial anatomical variants, a prominent Eustachian valve (the structure that directs the blood from the inferior vena cava toward the fossa ovalis region of the atrial septum) is more commonly seen in patients with suspected paradoxical embolism [56].

Hemodynamic conditions may also play a major role in determining the chances of paradoxical embolization. Although higher right atrial pressure can transiently occur during the normal cardiac cycle [57], cardiac lesions that more consistently elevate the right atrial pressure will increase the chance of right-to-left shunt. As a result, paradoxical embolization is often reported in patients with pulmonary embolism [58,59]. Similarly, patients with right ventricular infarction [60], severe tricuspid regurgitation [61], or those on a mechanical left ventricular assist device have an increased degree of right-to-left shunting through a PFO [62]. Although right-sided pressure elevation can increase the flow

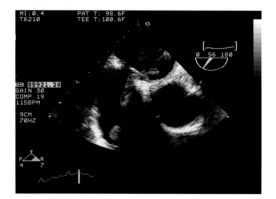

Fig. 16.9 Same case as in Figure 16.8. Changing the imaging angle has allowed a better visualization of the segment of thrombus trapped in the stretched patent foramen ovale.

across PFO, it will be decreased with left-sided pressure elevations [63].

Venous thrombi and hypercoagulable states, which predispose to thrombus formation, are associated with increased frequency of paradoxical embolization in patients with a PFO. A greater prevalence of deep venous thrombosis was observed in one study in patients with cryptogenic stroke compared with the control group [64]. Several other studies did not confirm this finding [65,66]. More recently, pelvic vein thrombi were found more frequently in young patients with cryptogenic stroke compared with those with defined causes of stroke [67]. Pelvic veins and abdominal veins are not routinely studied in patients with cryptogenic stroke and PFO, preventing an accurate assessment of the frequency of thrombosis in those locations and a better understanding of its importance in the stroke mechanism. Also, late performance of venous studies, early anticoagulation or thrombolysis after stroke, or both, may all decrease the rate of detection of a venous thrombus [64]. When a venous thrombus is found, however, the possibility that the PFO may indeed be implicated in the stroke mechanism becomes more real, and it affects the subsequent treatment, as will be discussed later in this chapter.

Several studies reported a higher frequency of prothrombotic states, such as G20210A and factor V Leiden mutations, in patients with cryptogenic stroke and PFO [68–71]. In addition, common risk factors for venous thromboembolism, such as recent surgery, trauma, or use of oral contraceptives, may all increase the likelihood of paradoxical embolization through a PFO [72].

Prevention of recurrent stroke

In stroke patients in whom paradoxical embolization through a PFO appears the likely stroke mechanism, several therapeutic options have been explored in an attempt to reduce the likelihood of recurrent events.

Medical treatment
Oral anticoagulation with warfarin or treatment with antiplatelet drugs has been considered in stroke patients with a PFO, under the assumption that these therapies would reduce the likelihood of thrombus formation, and therefore the potential for

paradoxical embolization. The annual rate of stroke recurrence in cryptogenic stroke patients with PFO has been reported to be anywhere between 1.5% and 12% [53,73–77]. The wide range probably reflects relevant differences in the composition of the study groups. In a pooled analysis of published studies on a total of 943 stroke patients, the combined rate of recurrent stroke, death, and transient ischemic attack (TIA) for medical treatments was 4.86 events/100 person-years [78]. The possible difference in efficacy between warfarin and aspirin has also been studied, although the results are not conclusive. In a retrospective study of 90 stroke patients younger than 60 years, 52% of whom had a PFO, warfarin was more effective than aspirin in reducing the risk of recurrent stroke [77]. However, the treatments in that study were not randomly assigned, and treatment crossover was frequent. A study mentioned earlier in this chapter, PICSS has been the only randomized, double-blinded study of warfarin and aspirin treatment in patients with noncardioembolic stroke and a PFO [53]. In 630 patients with stroke, PFO prevalence was 39% in patients with cryptogenic stroke and 29% in those with stroke of known cause ($P < 0.02$). PICSS was a substudy of the Warfarin Aspirin Recurrent Stroke Study, in which patients with noncardioembolic stroke were randomized to aspirin 325 mg or warfarin (target international normalization ratio 1.4–2.8) [79]. Over 2 years of follow-up, there were no significant differences in the rates of recurrent stroke or death among patients with or without PFO (14.8% vs. 15.4%; hazard ratio 0.96, 95% CI 0.62–1.48; $P = 0.84$), and this also applied to cryptogenic stroke (14.3% vs. 12.7%; hazard ratio 1.17, 95% CI 0.60–2.37; $P = 0.65$). There were no significant differences in the rates of recurrent stroke or death among cryptogenic stroke patients treated with warfarin (9.5%) or aspirin (17.9%; hazard ratio 0.52, 95% CI 0.16–1.67; $P = 0.28$). No significant excess in risk of recurrent stroke or death was seen in patients with both PFO and ASA [53]. In a study from France, however, the recurrent stroke rates in cryptogenic stroke patients below age 55 treated with aspirin were 4.2% in patients without PFO, 2.3% in patients with PFO alone, and 15.2% in patients with PFO and ASA [74]. This study generated the hypothesis that aspirin treatment may not be sufficient in protecting against recurrent stroke when both PFO and ASA are present. Current American Heart Association/ American Stroke Association (AHA/ASA) guidelines for the prevention of stroke in patients with ischemic stroke or TIA are based on the combined information obtained from the studies described earlier. Antiplatelet treatment is currently recommended in most stroke patients with a PFO [80]. Warfarin is considered a reasonable choice for high-risk patients with other indications for oral anticoagulation, such as a coexisting venous thrombosis or hypercoagulable state [80]. The role of PFO closure and its place in the AHA/ASA recommendations will be discussed in the following section.

Percutaneous PFO closure

In recent years, great attention has been paid to the transcatheter closure of PFO, which might arguably represent a cure for PFO-related embolic events. Several nonrandomized or case series studies have been published in the United States and in Europe, generally showing feasibility and providing preliminary information of efficacy of this type of PFO closure. A pooled analysis of studies published until 2004 reported on a total of 1430 stroke patients who underwent PFO closure with a variety of devices [78]. The mean age of the patients was 46 years, and the average duration of follow-up was 18 months. There was a variable use of warfarin or antiplatelet agents after the closure. The combined rate of recurrent stroke, death, or TIA for PFO closure was 2.95 events/100 person-years, which compares favorably with the results of medical therapy [78]. Complications from the device implantation have included major complications such as death, major hemorrhage, cardiac tamponade, and fatal pulmonary emboli, which, in a meta-analysis of 1355 patients, occurred in approximately 1.5% of the patients [81]. Other complications such as atrial arrhythmias, device arm fractures, device embolization, device thrombosis, EKG changes, and arterial-venous (AV) fistula formation were reported in 7.9% [81]. More recent studies have reported lower rates of recurrent embolic events and lower complication rates, likely reflecting improved design and construction of the closure devices and greater operator experience in their implantation. In 131 patients who underwent PFO closure with the Amplatzer ($n = 101$) or the Cardioseal ($n = 30$) devices, Slavin and colleagues reported no recurrent embolic events over a mean

follow-up of 30 months [82]. Temporary problems after device implantation, such as chest pain and palpitations, were reported by 23% of patients, and occurred more frequently in subjects with nickel hypersensitivity [82]. Spies and colleagues reported on 247 patients with presumed paradoxical embolization (mean age 53 years) who underwent PFO closure with the Intrasept occluder, a fourth generation device of the Cardia device family [83]. Acute complications from device placement occurred in four patients (1.6%). On an average follow-up of 14 months, seven recurrent strokes/TIAs occurred (2.8%) [84]. In a multicenter European study recently published, 430 patients (mean age approximately 51 years) underwent PFO closure with the Intrasept device [85]. Peri-procedural complications occurred in 11.5% of patients, 0.2% of which were defined as major. Over a relatively short follow-up (median 0.8 years), recurrent stroke rate was 0.5% and TIA rate was 2.5% [86].

The correct position of the PFO closing device, and the possibility of complications such as superimposed thrombus, fracture of the device arm, migration of the device or pericardial effusion can be monitored by TTE (Figure 16.10), but the monitoring for complications is more accurately performed by TEE because of the greater proximity of the transducer to the device and the consequent higher imaging resolution (Figure 16.11). Recently, three-dimensional transducers have become available, which may allow for further refinement of the imaging of the deployed device (Figure 16.12).

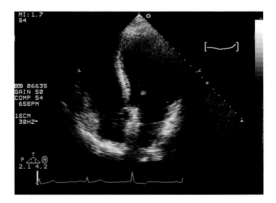

Fig. 16.10 Visualization by transthoracic echocardiography of a patent foramen ovale closing device deployed between the two atrial chambers (bottom).

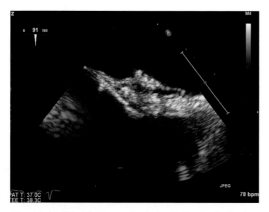

Fig. 16.11 Patent foramen ovale closing device visualization by transesophageal echocardiography. The two arms of the device are seen encasing the septum.

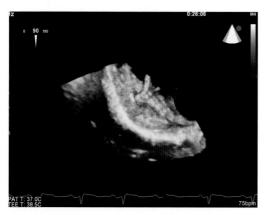

Fig. 16.12 Visualization of patent foramen ovale (PFO) closing device by three-dimensional transesophageal echocardiography. The device arm deployed on one side of the atrial septum is visualized. Also visible is the segment connecting the two arms, seated in the PFO opening.

Transcatheter PFO closure may also be associated with a risk of intra- or peri-procedural embolization to the brain. Transient microembolic signals were detected by TCD during the procedure in 28 of 29 subjects undergoing PFO closure [87]. Repeated MRI of the brain in 35 subjects with documented cerebral infarctions at baseline documented the appearance of new microembolic lesions after the PFO closure in three of them (8.6%) [88].

Scant data are available on the comparison of medical treatment and PFO closure in reducing the risk of recurrent thromboembolic events. In a meta-analysis including 1355 patients who underwent PFO closure (10 studies) and 895 patients treated medically (six studies), recurrent neurological thromboembolism at 1 year ranged from 0% to 4.9% of subjects with PFO closure (major and minor complications were 1.5% and 7.9%, respectively), and from 3.8% to 12% of subjects treated medically [81]. However, limitations arising from nonrandomized treatments, nonstandardized definitions, different assessment of outcomes, and baseline imbalances prevented an accurate efficacy comparison. Patients treated medically were older, were more frequently men, and had greater frequencies of diabetes mellitus and cigarette smoking, whereas patients undergoing PFO closure had more frequent history of repeated thromboembolic episodes at baseline [81]. In 308 patients with cryptogenic stroke and PFO, who were treated either medically (158 patients) or underwent percutaneous PFO closure (150 patients), Windecker and colleagues reported a trend toward a reduction at 4 years of combined death, stroke, or TIA (8.5% vs. 24.3%; $P = 0.05$; 95% CI 0.23–1.01), and of recurrent stroke or TIA (7.8% vs. 22.2%; $P = 0.08$; 95% CI 0.23–1.11) for PFO closure compared with medical treatment [89]. Patients with more than one cerebrovascular event at baseline and those with complete occlusion of PFO were at lower risk for recurrent stroke or TIA after percutaneous PFO closure compared with medically treated patients (7.3% vs. 33.2%, $P = 0.01$, and 95% CI 0.08–0.81, and 6.5% vs. 22.2%, $P = 0.04$, and 95% CI 0.14–0.99, respectively) [89]. The authors concluded that PFO closure may be at least as effective as medical therapy in preventing recurrent stroke, and possibly more effective in patients with repeated events [89]. However, treatment was not randomized, with patients with larger PFOs or multiple cerebrovascular events more frequently assigned to PFO closure.

No data from randomized trials are currently available on the comparison between medical therapy and PFO closure in preventing recurrent embolic events. In their absence, the current AHA/ASA guidelines for the prevention of stroke in patients with ischemic stroke or TIA considered the available data insufficient to make a recommendation for PFO closure in patients with a first stroke and a PFO [80]. PFO closure was recommended for consideration in patients with recurrent cryptogenic stroke despite medical therapy [80].

There are currently several industry-sponsored (AGA Medical – Plymouth MN, NMT Medical – Boston, MA) randomized clinical trials comparing medical regimen with device implantation in patients with ischemic neurological events. Results of these trials are likely to add important information in the management of patients with ischemic stroke and PFO.

In the patient described at the beginning of the chapter, aspirin treatment was chosen because of the data from PICSS, which showed no significant increase in risk of recurrent stroke in patients with PFO and ASA treated with aspirin [53]. The data from the French PFO/ASA study, which showed high risk of recurrent stroke in patients with PFO plus ASA below the age of 55 despite aspirin treatment [74], did not provide information on the relative efficacy of warfarin treatment or PFO closure in this patient group. Also, this patient had no evidence of hypercoagulability or history of deep venous thrombosis, which would have mandated the use of warfarin. Warfarin treatment or PFO closure would have to be considered in the case of recurrent symptoms despite the treatment with aspirin.

Surgical closure

Several small studies reported on the results of surgical PFO closure on the risk of recurrent cerebrovascular events [90–93]. A pooled analysis of the published studies yielded a total of 161 patients, with a mean age of 43 years and an average duration of follow-up of 22 months [78]. The annual rate of stroke was 0.34% (95% CI, 0.01–1.89%) and that of stroke or death was 0.85% (95% CI, 0.10–3.07%) [78]. Even with the use of a minimally invasive approach [94], surgical PFO closure is rarely performed, and its main indications appear to be in the rescue of failed transcatheter procedures, in the PFO closure in subjects with hypersensitivity to some device components (such as nickel hypersensitivity), and in patients undergoing cardiac surgery for other concomitant indications.

Newer PFO closing devices

Other modalities for closing a PFO are currently under investigation, which include the development of anatomically fitted devices more suitable to different PFO anatomical variants and other methods that do not entail surgery or even the deployment of a metal device. Among the latter techniques, radio-frequency thermal coaptation of the atrial septum has been successfully performed in experimental models, and there is preliminary experience with the technique in humans. In 30 subjects with PFO (average PFO size 8.5 ± 2.7 mm), Sievert and colleagues reported a 90% procedural success rate (27/30) [95]. Over a mean follow-up of 6 months, PFO closure persisted in 43% of subjects, and secondary closure with a repeat procedure was obtained in 63% of the remainder [95]. Bioabsorbable atrial septal repair implants are also being developed and tested, which have the theoretical advantage of a more physiological approach to the septal closure and, unlike the current devices, allows the possibility of transseptal access to the left atrium for future procedures. In a multicenter study on 58 patients with an ASD or a PFO, the reabsorbable device was successfully implanted in 57 patients (98%), with the only side effect being transient atrial arrhythmias in five patients (8.8%) [96]. Closure rates by contrast echocardiography at 30 days and 6 months were 92% and 96%, respectively [96].

PFO and risk of stroke in the general population

All the data on PFO and ischemic stroke risk presented earlier in this chapter have been obtained in case-control studies, in which the frequency of PFO was compared among stroke patients and stroke-free controls matched to cases by pertinent demographics and clinical variables. The risk of stroke estimated in those studies was affected by the obvious circumstance that enrolled patients had a stroke as the qualifying event and, therefore, were not necessarily representative of the general population. In other words, the PFO-related risk of ischemic stroke obtained in those studies may not be representative of the risk of stroke that an otherwise asymptomatic subject would face by virtue of merely having a PFO. Also, the reliability of the results of case-control studies depends on the assumption that cases and controls only differ for the variable under investigation (PFO), a circumstance that is unlikely and can never be entirely proven. In addition, case-control studies may point at an association between two variables (such as PFO and stroke), but they do not prove causation. Cause–effect relationship and temporal trends can only be examined in prospective studies. The PFO-related risk of stroke in the general population has been addressed in two prospective, population-based studies to date. In the Stroke Prevention Assessment of Risk in a Community (SPARC) Study, 577 volunteers underwent TEE to assess for cardiac embolic sources including a PFO, and the incidence in them of cerebrovascular events was evaluated over a median follow-up of 61 months [9]. The prevalence of PFO was 24.3%. After adjustment for other established stroke risk factors, PFO was not found to be independently associated with increased risk of cerebrovascular events (hazard ratio 1.46, 95% CI 0.74–2.88). In the Northern Manhattan Study (NOMAS), 1100 stroke-free subjects underwent contrast TTE for PFO detection [10]. PFO prevalence was 14.9%, reflecting the lower sensitivity of TTE compared with TEE for the detection of small shunts. Over a mean follow-up of approximately 80 months, PFO was not found to be independently associated with ischemic stroke risk (hazard ratio 1.64, 95% CI 0.87–3.09). Despite differences in the population samples (predominantly white and including prior strokes or TIAs in SPARC; tri-ethnic and stroke-free in NOMAS; Table 16.5) and in the techniques used for PFO detection, both studies obtained similar results. Both studies found a higher incidence of stroke in subjects with isolated ASA, but the numbers are too few to allow firm conclusions. Based on these studies, the risk of stroke in subjects with PFO in the general population appears low, at least within the follow-up duration examined by the two studies. No preventive measures should therefore be contemplated in asymptomatic subjects in whom a PFO is merely an incidental finding. The possibility exists that a subgroup of subjects with PFO may have an increased risk of stroke, but their effect on the overall stroke risk in the community is diluted because of the preponderance of subjects in whom a PFO is just an innocent bystander [10]. A better understanding of the associated cofactors of increased stroke risk that were discussed earlier in the chapter might help identify subjects with PFO at increased stroke risk among the larger group of subjects with a PFO.

Summary

The presence of a PFO is associated with increased risk of recurrent events in patients with ischemic stroke, especially those with cryptogenic stroke. The association of PFO and stroke has been demonstrated in patients younger than 55 years as well as

Table 16.5 Prospective studies on patent foramen ovale (PFO) and stroke risk in the general population

	SPARC [9]	NOMAS [10]
n of subjects	577	1,100
Male sex (%)	293 (50)	460 (42)
Age (mean ± SD)	66.9 ± 13.3	68.7 ± 10.0
Race–ethnicity	White	Black 26%, Hispanic 49%, white 25%
Previous stroke/TIA	6.3%	None
PFO detection	Contrast TEE	Contrast TTE
PFO prevalence	24.3%	14.9%
Follow-up (months)	61 (median)	79.7 ± 28.0
Adjusted hazard ratio for stroke		
PFO	1.46 (0.74–2.88)	1.64 (0.87–3.09)
PFO + ASA	0	1.04 (0.14–7.74)
Stroke incidence for isolated ASA	2/5 (40%)	2/8 (25%)
Adjusted hazard ratio for stroke	3.72 (0.88–15.71)	3.66 (0.88–15.30)

ASA, atrial septal aneurysm; NOMAS, Northern Manhattan Study; PFO, patent foramen ovale; SD, standard deviation; SPARC, Stroke Prevention Assessment of Risk in a Community; TEE, transesophageal echocardiography; TIA, transient ischemic attack; TTE, transthoracic echocardiography.

in those older than 55, in whom the association may be less strong, but who constitute the vast majority of patients with stroke. A better understanding of the factors that may increase the stroke risk in individual patients with a PFO may lead in the future to more rational and effective preventive strategies. At the current state of the knowledge, treatment with antiplatelet agents is recommended for secondary prevention in most stroke patients with a PFO, although warfarin treatment appears indicated in some patient subsets, such as those with associated deep venous thrombosis or hypercoagulable states. Insufficient data are available at this time on the comparison between medical treatment and percutaneous PFO closure. The latter is currently reserved for patients who fail medical therapy, although new evidence from randomized treatment trials and newer modalities for closing the PFO might change this approach in the future. The incidental finding of a PFO in an otherwise asymptomatic subject does not represent an indication for preventive treatment, given the high prevalence of this finding in the community and the weak association with stroke risk documented in population-based samples. The possibility that an ASA may be associated with high stroke risk needs to be verified in appropriately sized ad hoc studies.

References available online at www.wiley.com/go/ strokeguidelines.

Vascular Cognitive Impairment

José G. Merino and Vladimir Hachinski

EXAMPLE CASE

Mr. P is a 56-year-old man admitted to the hospital because his wife found him sitting on the toilet, with a blank stare, incessantly repeating the phrase "just one moment please." He had been well until 1 year ago when he was diagnosed with lacunar disease after he presented to the hospital with dysarthria and clumsiness and a CT scan showed bilateral centrum semiovale lacunes. Since then, his personality changed: he became morose, reclusive, and increasingly irritated. His job performance deteriorated, and he repeatedly became lost on the way to work. In the last 2 months, he became more apathetic and almost mute. His wife had to help him get dressed and go to the bathroom. He had a history of diabetes mellitus and was a heavy smoker.

The examination on the day of admission to the hospital revealed a quiet, heavyset man, with a blood pressure of 144/98 mm Hg. His general physical examination was unremarkable. He was alert but oriented only to name and date, and his attention was poor. He had a paucity of spontaneous speech and mild dysarthria. He was also aphasic (naming and repetition were mildly impaired, comprehension was normal, and he made frequent paraphasic errors). He was unable to do the Luria hand sequence or to copy a design. His recall of current events was poor, as was his short-term memory for objects presented verbally and visually; cueing helped recall. He did not have apraxia, alexia, or agraphia, but abstraction, constructional, and visuospatial

MAJOR POINTS

- Vascular cognitive impairment (VCI) refers to a heterogeneous group of conditions in which vascular factors are associated with or cause cognitive deficits.
- VCI is due to ischemic and hemorrhagic stroke, chronic hypoperfusion, global ischemia, and mixed primary neurodegenerative and cerebrovascular causes.
- No single clinical feature has a diagnostic value in an individual case and the diagnosis relies on a combination of clinical, radiological, and neuropsychological features. While there are several diagnostic schemes for vascular dementia, none exist for VCI.
- VCI leads to many different patterns of cognitive impairment that range from mild VCI no dementia to severe vascular or mixed dementia, and there is no pathognomonic pattern of cognitive deficits.
- Control of vascular risk factors may prevent the development of VCI. Cholinesterase inhibitors and memantine have a modest effect on advanced VCI.

A Primer on Stroke Prevention Treatment: An Overview Based on AHA/ASA Guidelines, 1st Edition. Edited by L Goldstein.
© 2009 American Heart Association, ISBN: 9781405186513

abilities were impaired. His thought processes, although slow, were goal directed, and he denied hallucinations. He described his mood as "good," but his affect was flat. His performance on the Mattis Dementia Rating Scale was below the first percentile for an age- and education-matched cohort, and he scored 17/30 in the Folstein Mini Mental State Examination. He had a right homonymous hemianopsia, impaired upward gaze, a decreased right nasolabial fold, as well as pronation of the right arm and mild bilateral dysmetria. Deep tendon reflexes were brisk, and plantar responses were extensor bilaterally. He walked with a stooped, slow gait with small steps and decreased right arm swing.

Laboratory investigations revealed normal chemistries, cell counts, coagulation and clotting, ammonia level, and liver and thyroid function. Venereal disease testing, Lyme titers, anti-nuclear antibody (ANA), and antiphospholipid antibodies were negative. A CT scan performed on the day of admission showed interval increase in the bilateral centrum semiovale ischemic lesions as well as left occipital and cerebellar infarcts. Less well-defined ischemic changes, possibly more recent, were noted in both thalami. A magnetic resonance imaging (MRI) confirmed these findings. His extra- and intracranial vessels were normal, as assessed by ultrasound. Transesophageal echocardiogram revealed a large, mobile, 2 × 4 cm mass attached to the left intra-atrial septum that was excised; pathological examination confirmed that it was an atrial myxoma. He was in sinus rhythm throughout his hospital stay. He was placed on antiplatelet drugs, and the management of his diabetes and hypertension were optimized. He was transferred to a nursing home for long-term care.

Introduction

The term vascular cognitive impairment (VCI) refers to a heterogeneous group of conditions in which vascular factors are associated with or cause cognitive deficits [1]. This concept replaces the more restricted one of "vascular dementia" (VaD) and applies to cognitive impairment of any severity caused by or associated with vascular factors. It includes patients with VCI–no dementia, VaD, and mixed vascular–neurodegenerative dementia (Figure 17.1) [2]. Because there is a strong interaction and synergism between cerebrovascular and Alzheimer-type pathology, and most elderly patients have some degree of both, vascular disease is probably the most common etiology of cognitive impairment [3–7].

The understanding of the role that vascular disease plays in the etiology of cognitive impairment has evolved over the past 50 years. In the first half of the 20th century, chronic cerebral ischemia due to atherosclerosis of the large arteries was considered the most common cause of dementia in the elderly. By the late 1960s, however, evidence from clinical, pathological, and imaging studies led to the idea that vascular disease affects cognition through discrete infarcts and not global hypoperfusion, and that most elderly patients with dementia had a neurode-generative rather than a vascular etiology. This idea led to the concept of multi-infarct dementia (MID) [8–11], which was replaced by VaD, because other vascular pathologies were associated with cognitive impairment. Several etiological subtypes have been described including MID, strategic infarct dementia, and dementia due to small-vessel disease, hypoper-fusion, and hemorrhage [10,12–17]. Over the last 10

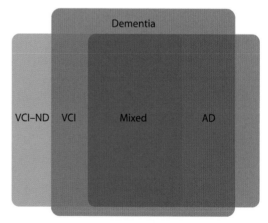

Fig. 17.1 Spectrum of vascular cognitive impairment (VCI) (taken from Moorhouse *et al.* [2]). Representation of the overlap and relative distribution of dementia syndromes. VCI-ND, vascular cognitive impairment-no dementia; AD, Alzheimer's disease.

years, VCI has replaced VaD as a paradigm to understand the association between vascular factors and cognitive decline because of the spectrum of cognitive impairments occurring in patients with cerebrovascular disease, from the brain-at-risk stage to severe dementia [3].

The concept of VCI is in flux. A lack of clear diagnostic criteria and an incomplete understanding of the interaction between vascular disease and neurodegenerative brain changes hamper the progress in understanding the pathophysiology of VCI, its clinical and neuropsychological features, and the development of new therapies. To address these shortcomings, the National Institute of Neurological Disorders and Stroke (NINDS) and the Canadian Stroke Network (CSN) convened a panel in 2007 to develop harmonization standards and define a set of data elements that should be collected in future studies aimed at defining VCI more fully, understanding its etiology, and identifying targets for treatment. These standards were not meant to become dogma; rather they are open to debate, study, and further validation [18]. Although developed to facilitate research, these harmonization standards can also be used to optimize the clinical evaluation and care of patients with VCI. In this chapter, we focus on some of these recommendations.

Etiology and pathophysiology

VCI may be due not only to "strokes, large, and small" [19], but also to chronic hypoperfusion, global ischemia, and mixed primary neurodegenerative and cerebrovascular causes [20]. An etiological classification of VCI includes several subgroups: large extra- and intracranial vessel disease, small-vessel disease, hypoperfusion, hemorrhage, and mixed vascular and neurodegenerative processes [2,21]. This distinction between subtypes is sometimes artificial in individual patients; for example, some have white-matter changes and lacunar and cortical infarcts. The initial cognitive impairment in Mr. P, described previously, may be due to small-vessel disease leading to lacunes and white-matter changes. He had a more rapid decline after having several cortical and subcortical infarcts that were likely due to emboli from the atrial myxoma.

Cognitive impairment is frequent after a stroke. In community-based series, the risk of dementia is four to six times higher among patients with a history of stroke than expected in the general population. In hospital-based studies, the prevalence of post-stroke dementia (PSD) at 3 months ranges from 5.9% to 32%; some of these patients may have had an underlying neurodegenerative process that preceded but was exacerbated by the stroke [22,23]. Cognitive impairment short of dementia is even more common, being found in 25–70% of patients 3 months after the stroke (the difference is due to the use of different definitions and neuropsychological tests) [24–26]. Age, educational level, pre-stroke cognitive status, temporal lobe atrophy, white-matter changes, cardiac comorbidities, and vascular risk factors (particularly when multiple) are all associated with the development of PSD [23,27]. PSD may be due to multiple cortical infarcts or to smaller strokes in strategic locations (e.g., angular gyrus, hippocampus, medial thalamus, caudate, right parietal cortex) that interrupt critical cortical–subcortical circuits and lead to well-defined cognitive syndromes [10,14].

Silent infarcts are more common than clinically apparent stroke and also have a deleterious effect on cognition. They occur in up to 20% of people in population-based epidemiological studies that use MRI and in 30–50% of patients with vascular risk factors, depression, or dementia [28–30]. By definition, these infarcts are not associated with stroke-like symptoms, but may occur with subtle neurological abnormalities, frailty, depression, and cognitive impairment [28]. The presence of silent infarcts increases the risk of subsequent stroke, independent of vascular risk factors, and doubles the risk of developing dementia (including Alzheimer's disease [AD]) and cognitive impairment among individuals with normal baseline cognition [31,32].

Small-vessel disease is associated with lacunar infarcts and white-matter disease, and studies using a variety of diagnostic criteria found that small-vessel disease is responsible for 40–70% of cases of VaD [33]. Lacunar infarcts may differentiate patients with VCI from those with stroke without dementia. Subcortical infarcts have been found to increase the risk of dementia substantially, after controlling for age and AD pathology [7,34,35]. Lacunes lead to psychomotor slowness due to loss of control of executive cognitive functioning, forgetfulness, changes in speech, affect and mood, urinary incontinence, and gait disturbance. These signs and symptoms, when found in conjunction with relevant imaging changes, constitute a homogenous subtype of VCI – subcortical ischemic VaD [33,36,37]. Although hypertension-induced lipohyalinosis of the small vessels is the main cause of lacunar infarcts, other vasculopathies, such as cerebral autosomal dominant arteriopathy with subcortical infarcts and leukoencephalopathy (CADASIL) and cerebral amyloid angiopathy (CAA), also cause small infarcts and are associated with the development of cognitive impairment. CADASIL (see also Chapter 13) is due to mutations in the *NOTCH3* gene on chromosome 19q12 that leads to the deposition of granular osmophilic material in, and destruction of, vascular smooth muscle cells, progressive thickening of the vessel wall and fibrosis, and luminal narrowing in small- and medium-sized penetrating arteries. It is characterized by migraine headaches, multiple strokes, white-matter lesions, seizures, vision problems, and personality changes [38,39]. CAA is due to the deposition of amyloid in the vessel wall, also leads to lacunar and hemorrhagic (micro- and macro-) strokes and white-matter lesions (Figure 17.2). CAA may lead to cognitive impairment even in the absence of hemorrhage, after controlling for age and AD pathology [38–40].

Changes in the white matter are commonly seen on CT and MRI scans in the elderly, and frequently occur in patients with lacunes and other vascular pathologies. Leukoaraiosis, a descriptive term that does not imply a specific etiology, occurs in 7% of patients with stroke, in 30–40% of unselected patients from memory clinics, and in over two-thirds of patients in clinical trials of VaD [41]. Confluent periventricular lesions are found in more than 10% of asymptomatic people 50–75 years old, and their prevalence increases with age [41,42]. Although patients with AD frequently have leukoaraiosis, these changes are more extensive and frequent when there is underlying vascular pathology [43,44]. Vascular risk factors (particularly hypertension, but also diabetes, smoking, hyperhomocysteinemia, and atherosclerosis of the large vessels) and increasing age are associated with the appearance of leukoaraiosis. The etiology of these lesions is not well understood, but small-vessel disease leading to hypoperfusion, ischemia and infarction, and, as a consequence, oligodendrocyte dysfunction, demyelination, and axonal damage is the presumed cause [45–47]. Deep subcortical white-matter lesions may represent a different entity from periventricular leukoaraiosis, as regions of confluent MRI-detected deep white-matter changes have myelin loss, gliosis, microinfarcts, and loss of nerve fibers, in contrast to periventricular halos that have a nonischemic appearance.

Extensive white-matter changes are associated with a syndrome characterized by cognitive impairment, personality change, gait disturbance, motor

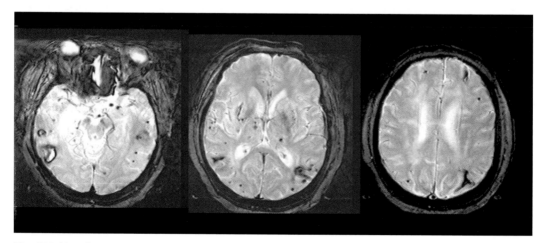

Fig. 17.2 Magnetic resonance imaging of a patient with probable cerebral amyloid angiopathy [96]. The patient has evidence of multiple lobar hemorrhages of varying ages as well as evidence of multiple microbleeds, most of them located on the gray-white matter junction.

deficits, and urinary incontinence, presumably because they disrupt white-matter tracts that interconnect distributed neural circuits, but sometimes they are asymptomatic [48]. Whereas these lesions are often found in asymptomatic individuals, in some patients even small amounts of white-matter abnormalities are associated with significant memory and language impairments. The extent and location of the changes in the white matter determine the neuropsychological profile among healthy community-dwelling individuals, stroke patients, and patients with mild cognitive impairment and dementia [21,43,49–53]. Leukoaraiosis of the deep white matter has been associated with executive impairment, slowed processing speed, and working memory and visuospatial abnormalities. There is a threshold effect; the more extensive the lesions, the more severe the cognitive impairment [43,49,50,52]. In addition, a rapid rate of progression of white-matter hyperintensities is associated with a greater risk of cognitive impairment [54].

Cortical and subcortical strokes and changes in the white matter may lead to cognitive impairment through several mechanisms. These lesions may affect cortical areas important for language, praxis, and self-awareness or, particularly when located in strategic locations (angular gyrus, hippocampus, medial thalamus, caudate, right parietal cortex), they may disrupt frontal–subcortical circuits and lead to specific cognitive syndromes (dorsolateral lesions cause executive dysfunction and impaired recall, orbitofrontal lesions lead to behavioral and emotional changes, and anterior cingulate lesions result in abulia and akinetic mutism) [10,14,43,53,55,56]. In addition, subcortical strokes may lead to thalamic cingulate gyrus and cortical gray-matter atrophy [53,56]. Brain atrophy, long associated with neurodegeneration, also plays a role in the genesis of dementia in patients with cerebrovascular disease. Medial temporal atrophy is an important correlate of cognitive dysfunction in stroke patients, and may have a stronger association with disease progression than white-matter changes [57,58]. Small-vessel disease and strategically placed infarcts contribute to global cognitive and functional impairments and to difficulties in mental flexibility, short-term memory and language, and short-term and working memory, over and above the effects of atrophy [53].

AD and vascular pathology have a complimentary and synergistic relationship, and there is a complex interaction between degenerative and vascular factors in the genesis of cognitive impairment [4,59]. Cerebral infarcts alter the clinical expression of a given load of AD pathology and increase the odds of having dementia among people with histopathological plaques and tangles [60]. Elderly patients often have coexisting Alzheimer and vascular pathology, and both processes may contribute to the development of cognitive impairment in most people with dementia [4,7]. AD and cerebrovascular disease have risk factors in common. The risk of AD is increased in people with diabetes mellitus, hypertension, atherosclerotic disease, and atrial fibrillation [4,60,61]. Vascular factors may play a role not only in the expression but also in the development of AD pathology. Microvascular damage is common in AD, and changes in the vascular endothelium increase the cleavage of amyloid precursor protein, promote tau phosphorylation, inhibit clearance of amyloid, and may lead to the development of plaques [2,62]. Mechanistically, there are many similarities between the molecular pathologies of AD and stroke, including neuroinflammatory events and antioxidant depletion. When combined, the two sets of processes may further neurodegeneration [6].

Genetic determinants of VCI include genes implicated in the development of vascular risk factors and stroke and its intermediate phenotypes, on the one hand, and genes that affect tissue response to ischemia (ischemic tolerance, neuroplasticity, etc.) on the other. In addition, there is an interaction with AD genes [18,63]. Monogenetic disorders associated with VCI include CADASIL, hereditary variants of CAA, sickle-cell disease, Fabry's disease, and homocystinuria. There are other inherited conditions that have VCI as part of their phenotypic spectrum but in which gene mutations have not been identified. Because they provide patient cohorts with a shared vascular pathology, the study of these conditions may lead to important insights into the pathophysiology and treatment of VCI [18,39].

Diagnosis

VCI is a complex nosological concept, and because there are no pathognomonic features – no single pathological feature is diagnostic in an individual case – the diagnosis relies on a combination of clinical, radiological, and neuropsychological features. Several diagnostic criteria were developed by consensus of experts and not by evidence in the 1980s that have been used in clinical trials (Table 17.1) [64–68]. These criteria, however, have several shortcomings. They identify patients in the later stages of the disease – the dementia phase – and are based on the AD paradigm, having memory loss as the most prominent clinical feature. Some include imaging criteria, but because of the requirement for a temporal relationship with stroke, they primarily identify patients with PSD. The criteria are not interchangeable and do not identify the same patients (Table 17.2) [69,70]. The NINDS–CSN harmonization standards aim to address these shortcomings. They focus on several key aspects of VCI that are important for diagnosis: clinical features, neuropsychology, neuroimaging, neuropathology, experimental models, genetics, biomarkers, and clinical trials. Rather than prescribe criteria, they provide screening questions to identify people with VCI, establish a minimum dataset for clinical practice or research studies, and develop an ideal dataset for VCI research. It is expected that their implementation will lead to data that, when integrated in a systematic fashion, will be used to develop diagnostic criteria and evaluate new treatments [2,18,71].

Clinical and epidemiological aspects

A detailed clinical evaluation is important to identify early cases of VCI, differentiate them from those with different etiologies, and identify modifiable risk factors. The clinical features of VCI are heterogeneous and depend on the location and extent of the cerebrovascular disease. Patients with VCI associated with multiple cortical strokes may have hemiparesis, sensory loss, corticospinal signs and visual field defects, whereas those with predominately subcortical disease and leukoaraiosis may have gait disturbance, urinary incontinence, and pseudobulbar features [48,72,73]. The NINDS–CSN harmonization criteria recommend the specific data points that should be sought and recorded in epidemiological studies and by clinicians caring for patients with potential VCI (Table 17.3).

Neuropsychology

VCI leads to many different patterns of cognitive impairment that range from mild VCI with no dementia to severe vascular or mixed dementia. There is no pathognomonic pattern of cognitive deficits [74–76]. Single strategic infarcts may lead to a discrete cognitive syndrome that depends on the location of the infarct, whereas subcortical lesions may affect all cognitive domains with a predominance of executive dysfunction: slowed motor, cognitive, and information processing speed, impairments in task shifting, and deficits in working memory [43,50,60,76–78]. Patients with mixed pathology, particularly later in the course of the disease, may have predominant memory loss and a pattern similar to AD [79]. Neuropsychological protocols must be sensitive to a wide range of abilities yet focus on the assessment of executive function [18]. The most frequently used screening test in clinical practice, the Mini Mental State Examination, is not sensitive for mild executive dysfunction, and its three-word recall may be insensitive to the subtle memory impairment often seen in VCI. The NINDS–CSN harmonization standards recommend three different test protocols that can be used in different settings: an extensive protocol (~60 minutes) that allows a detailed evaluation of patients with VCI, a shorter protocol (~30 minutes) for use as a clinical screening instrument for patients with suspected VCI, and a brief protocol (~5 minutes) that can be used by primary care physicians and in large epidemiological studies. The protocols include tests that met prespecified criteria and that could be used to differentiate VCI from AD (Table 17.4 and Figure 17.3).

Neuroimaging

VCI is a heterogeneous condition without pathognomonic radiological features. Neuroimaging studies, therefore, are not diagnostic but descriptive, and provide information about the presence of cerebrovascular disease, changes in the white matter, brain atrophy, and the coexistence of other pathologies (brain tumors, hydrocephalus). MRI is the ideal imaging tool, as different sequences can provide information about the anatomy and the presence of atrophy and other chronic pathologies (T1- and T2-weighted and fluid-attenuated inversion recovery [FLAIR]), acute infarction (diffusion weighted), integrity of white-matter fibers (diffusion tensor), and acute and chronic micro- and macrobleeds (gradient echo and T2*-weighted). Some conditions

Table 17.1 Diagnostic criteria for vascular dementia

Criteria		SCADDTC [66]*	NINDS–AIREN [67]*	ICD-10 (research) [68]	DSM-IV [65]
Dementia syndrome	Cognitive domains	Deterioration in more than one category of intellectual performance, independent of level of consciousness	Memory and two or more cognitive domains	Unequal distribution of deficits in higher cognitive functions (requires memory impairment [which must be present for 6 months] and executive dysfunction) and emotional control	Memory impairment *and* one or more of the following: aphasia, apraxia, agnosia, disturbance in executive function
	Severity	Deterioration from a known or estimated prior level of intellectual function sufficient to interfere broadly with the conduct of the patient's customary affairs of life	Decline from a previously higher level of functioning; deficits sufficiently severe to interfere with activities of daily living (ADLs) not due to physical effects of stroke alone	Impairments of ADL must result from cognitive deficits and not from physical dysfunction	The cognitive criteria cause significant impairment in social or occupational functioning and represent a significant decline from a previous level of functioning
	Documentation	Must be supported by historical evidence and documented by bedside mental status testing or neuropsychological examination	Clinical examination and neuropsychological testing	Must be objectively verifiable by history and neuropsychological testing	Not specified
CVD	Deficits on physical examination	Evidence of two or more ischemic strokes by history, neurological signs, and/or neuroimaging studies (CT or T1-weighted magnetic resonance imaging [MRI]) *or* occurrence of a single stroke with clearly documented temporal relationship to the onset of dementia	Focal signs on neurological examination consistent with stroke (with or without a history of stroke) and evidence of relevant CVD on brain imaging	Evidence of focal brain damage: unilateral spastic weakness of limbs, unilateral increased tendon reflexes, extensor plantar response, pseudobulbar palsy	Focal neurological signs and symptoms that are judged to be etiologically related to the disturbance
	Imaging	Required: evidence of at least one infarct outside the cerebellum by CT or MRI	Required: large-vessel infarcts, or a single strategically placed infarct as well as multiple basal ganglia and white-matter lacunes, or extensive periventricular white-matter lesions, or combinations thereof	Not required	Not required

225

Table 17.1 *Continued*

Criteria	SCADDTC [66]*	NINDS–AIREN [67]*	ICD-10 (research) [68]	DSM-IV [65]
Etiological relationship between CVD and dementia	Temporal relationship required if only a single stroke is documented	A relationship is inferred by onset of dementia within 3 months of stroke, abrupt deterioration or fluctuating, stepwise progression	Not specified clearly; a relationship must be "reasonably judged" to exist.	
Subtypes	Yes: cortical, subcortical, Binswanger's disease, thalamic dementia	Do not specify but recommend description of stroke features for research purposes	Allows subtypes-6 with only superficial clinical description: acute onset, multi-infarct dementia, subcortical, mixed cortical, and subcortical, other, unspecified	None
Levels of certainty WML	Yes. Also has mixed dementia category WML do not qualify as imaging evidence of CVD for probable diagnosis but may support possible IVD	Yes, probable, possible, definite		
Mixed dementia	Mixed dementia to be diagnosed in the presence of one or more systemic or brain disorders that are thought to be causally related to dementia.	Alzheimer's disease with CVD patients who fulfill the criteria for possible Alzheimer's disease and who also present clinical or imaging evidence of relevant vascular brain lesions. Include dementias due to hypoperfusion from cardiac dysrythmias and pump failure		

From Merino JG, Hachinski V. Diagnosis of vascular dementia-conceptual challenges. In: Paul RH, Cohen RA, Ott BR, Salloway S, eds. Vascular Dementia: Cerebrovascular Mechanisms and Clinical Management. Totowa, NJ. Humana Press, 2004: 57–71.

*This refers to probable vascular dementia.

CVD, cerebrovascular disease; DSM-IV, Diagnostic and Statistical Manual, 4th ed.; ICD-10, International Statistical Classification of Diseases and Related Health Problems, 10th Revision; NINDS-AIREN, National Institute of Neurological Disorders–Association Internationale pour la Recherché et l'Enseignement en Neurosciences; SCADDTC, State of California Alzheimer's Disease Diagnostic and Treatment Centers; WML, white matter lesions.

Table 17.2 Agreement in patient classification resulting from various criteria

Criteria	Chui *et al.* [70] $n = 25$	Pohjasvaara *et al.* [91] $n = 107$	Amar *et al.* [92]* $n = 20$	Amar *et al.* [92]† $n = 20$	Wetterling *et al.* [93] $n = 167$	Verhey *et al.* [94] $n = 124$
DSM-IV	25.7%	91.6%			27%	
SCADDTC probable	10.3%	86.9%	40%	20%	13%	12%
SCADDTC possible	14.3%		55%	35%		
SCADDTC probable and possible	20.6%		95%	55%		
NINDS–AIREN probable	5.1%	32.7%	40%	5%	7%	6%
NINDS–AIREN possible	6.3%		40%	20%		
NINDS–AIREN probable and possible	6.3%		80%	25%		
DSM-III		36.4%				
ICD-10		36.4%			13%	

From Merino JG, Hachinski V. Diagnosis of vascular dementia-conceptual challenges. In: Paul RH, Cohen RA, Ott BR, Salloway S, eds. Vascular Dementia: Cerebrovascular Mechanisms and Clinical Management. Totowa, NJ: Humana Press, 2004: 57–71.

*Hachinski Ischemic Score ≥7.

†Hachinski Ischemic Score = 4–6.

associated with VCI have suggestive imaging features (Figures 17.2 and 17.4). Although CT scans are widely available, they have limited utility in the evaluation of VCI because they measure only severe disease, the findings are difficult to quantify, and they are associated with radiation exposure. The harmonization standards detail the imaging features that should be recorded in research studies (Table 17.5).

Other considerations

The NINDS–CSN harmonization criteria include sections on neuropathology, biomarkers, experimental models, genetics, and clinical trials. Because these sections have limited clinical applicability outside a research context, they will not be discussed further in this chapter.

Mr. P has many of the characteristic features of VCI. He had several lacunar strokes and a rapidly progressive course characterized by personality change, executive dysfunction, and memory loss. The current admission was prompted by acute cognitive changes, and this was associated with acute strokes. The pattern of cognitive impairment, with prominent frontal dysfunction, mild language disturbance, memory deficits that improve with cueing, impaired abstraction and preserved praxis, reading and writing, is consistent with a subcortical pattern of decline, often seen in patients with VCI.

Treatment

Since vascular risk factors are treatable, it may be possible to prevent, postpone, or mitigate VCI [18]. Some trials of blood pressure-lowering agents suggest that this intervention may help delay cognitive decline in patients with stroke. In the Systolic Hypertension in Europe (Syst-Eur) study, for example, a reduction of 7/3.2 mm Hg for almost 4 years halved the risk of incident dementia. The effect, however, is modest. If 1,000 patients were treated with antihypertensive drugs for 5 years, 19 cases of dementia might be prevented [80]. In the Health Outcomes Prevention (HOPE) Study, fewer patients treated with ramipril (compared with placebo-treated patients) had a "change with cognition" [81]. Among individuals with cerebrovascular disease enrolled in the Perindopril Protection against Recurrent Stroke Study trial, the use of perindopril and indapamide significantly reduced the risk of cognitive impairment (from 11% to 9.1%). It also led to a nonsignificant reduction in the risk of dementia (from 7.1% to 6.3%, not significant). The effect was associated with a reduced risk of recurrent

Table 17.3 Recommended elements of the clinical evaluation

Variable	Clinical evaluation	Epidemiological studies
Demographics	Sex, birth date, race/ethnicity, education	Sex, birth date, race/ethnicity (including birth place and parents' place of origin), years in the current place of residence, primary language, number of years of education, occupation, literacy, living situation and level of independence, marital status, handedness, and a contact person
Informant	Demographics of informant should be collected	Source of informant, demographics, and amount and type of contact with the patient
Family history (first-degree relatives)	Stroke, vascular disease, dementia	Past strokes, vascular disease (myocardial infarction [MI], history of dementia and other neurological diseases), age at event and death
Health history	Cardiovascular or cerebrovascular conditions, hypertension, hyperlipidemia, diabetes mellitus (DM), alcohol use, tobacco use, physical inactivity, medications	Same. Use of specific questions to address al conditions. Surgery and cognitive impairment after surgery. MI, arrhythmia, angioplasty, stent, CABG or valve surgery, pacemaker, chronic heart failure, angina, pad, migraine, hypertension, hyperlipidemia, DM, sleep disorders, sickle-cell anemia, hypercoagulable states (including deep venous thrombosis, abortions, pulmonary embolism), chronic infections (including periodontal disease), autoimmune disorders, depression, substance use (including tobacco and alcohol), diet, lifestyle, renal disease, menopause, use of oral contraceptive pills, environmental exposure
Evaluation	Subjective impression: general health, changes in memory, speed of thinking, acting and mood over the past year, Activities of daily living Physical examination to include vital signs, waist circumference, timed gait Mental status examination (see Neuropsychology section) Laboratory studies may include ECG, echo, carotid ultrasound, urine studies, brain magnetic resonance imaging, C-reactive protein, lipids, homocysteine, glucose, HgA1C, insulin, clotting factors, fibrinogen	Objective symptoms and onset should be recorded Vital signs Neurological exam (including NIHSS) Mini Mental State Examination Behavioral assessment

CABG, coronary artery bypass grafting; NIHSS, National Institutes of Health Stroke Scale.

stroke [82]. On the other hand, a systematic review of blood pressure lowering among hypertensive individuals without cerebrovascular disease did not find evidence that blood pressure lowering prevents the development of dementia or cognitive impairment [83]. Some evidence suggests that improving metabolic control leads to cognitive impairment in patients with diabetes, but convincing data on the effect on cognition of controlling other vascular risk factors are not available [84].

After his first stroke, 1 year before the index hospitalization, Mr. P was started on an antiplatelet

Table 17.4 Neuropsychological batteries (modified from Hachinski V, *et al*. Stroke. 2006;37:2220–2241)

Sixty-minute protocol	Thirty-minute protocol	Five-minute protocol
Executive/activation	Executive/activation	Subtests of the Montreal Cognitive Assessment (MoCA) [98]
• Animal naming (from the CERAD neuropsychology assessment battery) • Controlled Oral Word • Association Test • WAIS III Digit Symbol-Coding • Trailmaking Test	• Animal naming (from the CERAD neuropsychology assessment battery) • Controlled Oral Word Association Test • WAIS III Digit Symbol-Coding	• 5-Word Memory Task (registration, recall, recognition) • 6-Item Orientation • 1-Letter Phonemic Fluency
Visuospatial • Rey-Osterreith Complex Figure		
Language • Short Form of the Boston Naming Test (2nd ed.)		
Memory/learning • Hopkins Verbal Learning Test (HVLT-R) or California Verbal Learning Test, second edition	Memory/learning • HVLT-R	
Neuropsychiatric/depressive symptoms • Neuropsychiatric inventory, Questionnaire Version • Center for Epidemiologic Studies-Depression Scale (CES-D)	Neuropsychiatric/depressive symptoms • Neuropsychiatric inventory, Questionnaire Version • CES-D	
Premorbid status • Informant Questionnaire for Cognitive Decline in the Elderly		
Supplemental • Simple and Choice Reaction Time tasks (future use once validated) • Complex Figure Memory • More detailed tests of semantics and syntax including the Pyramids and Palm Trees Test and the Token test • Boston Naming Test Recognition • Digit Symbol Coding Incidental Learning • Starkstein's Apathy Scale • Mini Mental State Examination (MMSE)	Supplemental • Trailmaking Tests A and B • MMSE	Supplemental • Remainder of the MoCA • MMSE • Animal Naming • Trailmaking Tests A and B

CERAD, Consortium to Establish a Registry for Alzheimer's Disease; WAIS III, Wechsler Adult Intelligence Scale III.

MONTREAL COGNITIVE ASSESSMENT (MOCA)

NAME :
Education :   Date of birth :
Sex :   DATE :

VISUOSPATIAL / EXECUTIVE			POINTS

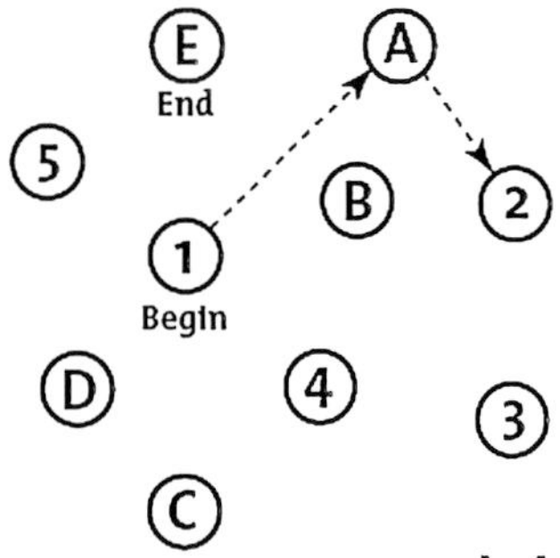

Copy cube

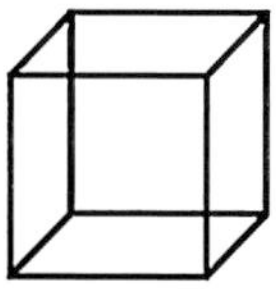

Draw CLOCK (Ten past eleven) (3 points)

[ ]   [ ]   [ ]   [ ]   [ ]   __/5
                                    Contour   Numbers   Hands

NAMING

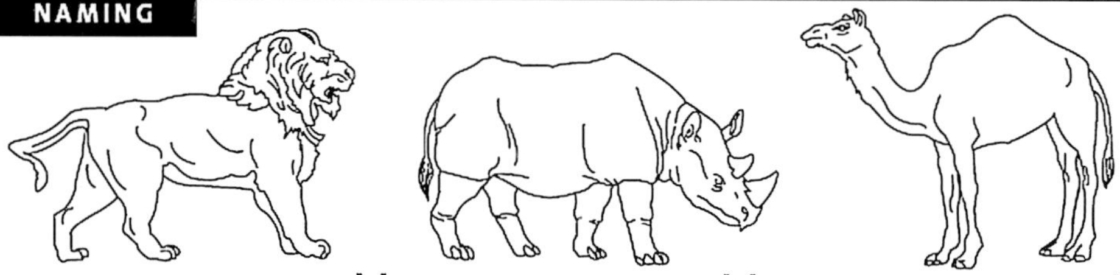

[ ]   [ ]   [ ]   __/3

MEMORY	Read list of words, subject must repeat them. Do 2 trials. Do a recall after 5 minutes.		FACE	VELVET	CHURCH	DAISY	RED	No points
		1st trial						
		2nd trial						

ATTENTION	Read list of digits (1 digit/ sec.). Subject has to repeat them in the forward order [ ] 2 1 8 5 4	
	Subject has to repeat them in the backward order [ ] 7 4 2	__/2

Read list of letters. The subject must tap with his hand at each letter A. No points if ≥ 2 errors
[ ] F B A C M N A A J K L B A F A K D E A A A J A M O F A A B   __/1

Serial 7 subtraction starting at 100   [ ] 93   [ ] 86   [ ] 79   [ ] 72   [ ] 65   __/3
4 or 5 correct subtractions: 3 pts, 2 or 3 correct: 2 pts, 1 correct: 1 pt, 0 correct: 0 pt

LANGUAGE	Repeat : I only know that John is the one to help today. [ ] The cat always hid under the couch when dogs were in the room. [ ]	__/2
	Fluency / Name maximum number of words in one minute that begin with the letter F [ ] _____ (N ≥ 11 words)	__/1

ABSTRACTION	Similarity between e.g. banana - orange = fruit [ ] train – bicycle [ ] watch - ruler	__/2

DELAYED RECALL	Has to recall words	FACE	VELVET	CHURCH	DAISY	RED	Points for UNCUED recall only	__/5
	WITH NO CUE	[ ]	[ ]	[ ]	[ ]	[ ]		
Optional	Category cue							
	Multiple choice cue							

ORIENTATION	[ ] Date	[ ] Month	[ ] Year	[ ] Day	[ ] Place	[ ] City	__/6

© Z.Nasreddine MD   Version 7.0   www.mocatest.org   Normal ≥ 26 / 30   TOTAL   __/30

Administered by:_____   Add 1 point if ≤ 12 yr edu

Fig. 17.3 Montreal Cognitive Assessment (downloaded from http://www.mocatest.org/ on July 14, 2008. Normative data and versions in other languages are also available on the website).

Table 17.5 Magnetic resonance imaging (MRI) imaging measures (adapted from Hachinski V, *et al*. Stroke. 2006;37:2220–2241)

Feature	Recommended MRI measure	Acceptable MRI measure
Brain atrophy	• Quantitative measurement of brain volume normalized for head size	• Estimates of Atrophy and Ventricular Size using the Cardiovascular Health Study (CHS) Scale • Estimates of Medial Temporal Lobe Atrophy using Scheltens Scale
White-matter hyperintensities (WMH)	• Quantitative measurement of WMH volume normalized for head size • Anatomical mapping also encouraged	• Preferred: ARWMC scale • Also acceptable: CHS WMH scale

Infarction	• All infarcts should be localized using a standard approach to generate quantitative measures of volume and location. Ideally, identified infarcts would also be mapped to a common stereotactic space [95]
	• All infarcts should be further differentiated from perivascular spaces by CHS criterion (see Table 17.2) independent of method to determine size and location
		1 Number and size at specified locations
		
		• Size (largest diameter):
		  a. Large >1.0 cm
		  b. Small 3–10 mm
		
		2 Location*:
		  • Anatomical locations
		    a. Supratentorial
		    b. Hemisphere
		    c. Cortical (may include subcortical)
		    d. Exclusively subcortical white matter
		    e. Exclusively subcortical gray matter
		  • Infratentorial

Hemorrhage	• All lesions should be localized using a standard approach to generate quantitative measures of volume and location. Ideally, identified lesions would also be mapped to a common stereotactic space [95]	**1** Number and size in each location
		  • Size (largest diameter)
		    a. Large hemorrhage >1 cm in diameter
		    b. Micro-hemorrhage†: <1 cm susceptibility on gradient echo
		  • Must report lower size limit cut-off, field strength
		  • Criterion in development and further work is necessary
		2 Location
		  • Same as infarcts

Other	Mass lesions, arteriovenous malformations, extra-axial fluid collections, malformations, dysplasia, or any other lesion that might complicate the assessment of cerebrovascular disease	

*Encourage the use of Talairach atlas [95] for precise anatomical localization.
ARWMC, Age-related white matter changes.

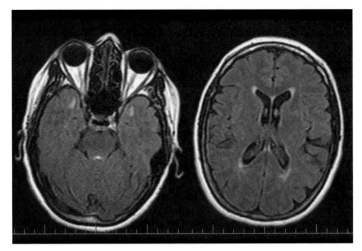

Fig. 17.4 Magnetic resonance imaging of a cerebral autosomal dominant arteriopathy with subcortical infarcts and leukoencephalopathy (CADASIL) patient. Note the confluent white-matter hyperintensities in the temporal poles, a characteristic finding in patients with CADASIL [97]. This relatively young patient has few periventricular white-matter hyperintensities.

agent and a statin, and his primary care physician tried several drugs to lower his blood pressure. These medications were continued, for stroke prophylaxis, after the removal of the atrial myxoma.

Cholinesterase inhibitors and memantine may have modest benefits for patients with VCI, but the results of clinical trials of these agents are difficult to interpret. As discussed earlier, the diagnosis of VCI is dependent on operational definitions, and the clinical trials of AD agents in VaD used the NINDS–AIREN criteria, and thus include patients with moderately severe dementia who probably have AD. Therefore, the findings may not be applicable to many patients with milder forms of VCI, or with primarily pure vascular pathology. They also include patients with a variety of cerebrovascular conditions and risk factors. The choice of end point influences the results of clinical trials. To date, most studies have focused on measures used in AD, but the use of tests that evaluate executive function may better capture the effect of different medications [39].

A meta-analysis of three donepezil, two galantamine, one rivastigmine, and two memantine trials found that these agents have a small benefit in cognition of uncertain clinical significance in patients with mild-to-moderate VaD; the authors postulate that the heterogeneity of the patients enrolled in the studies may explain the lack of noticeable effect [85].

On the other hand, the combined analysis of two large trials of donepezil for VaD showed some benefits in cognition, global function, and activities of daily living [86]. Memantine and galantamine had a modest benefit on cognition and behavior scales but not in clinical global measures [87,88]. Other promising agents that are undergoing trials include nimodopine and citicoline [89,90]. The use of one of these drugs might be considered in an attempt to improve Mr. P's cognitive outcome.

Conclusion

The concept of VCI is in flux, and a greater understanding of the relationship between vascular factors and cognition is evolving. Progress in VCI has been hindered by the lack of satisfactory diagnostic criteria, and a focus on the most severe extreme of the syndrome. The implementation (and continuous review as data becomes available) of the NINDS–CSN harmonization standards in research and clinical practice settings will lead to the development of criteria based on facts, and will deepen our understanding of this very frequent condition.

References available online at www.wiley.com/go/ strokeguidelines.

18 Stroke Outcome Assessments

Linda Williams

EXAMPLE CASE

A 54-year-old divorced man with hypertension and hyperlipidemia developed a sudden onset of difficulty in speaking and right-sided weakness while at work. He was brought by ambulance to the emergency department and was given tissue-type plasminogen activator (tPA). His deficits on admission included:

1 inability to follow commands;
2 inability to speak except for some garbled phonations;
3 near-total lower facial paralysis;
4 right arm proximal power 2/5;
5 right hand grip 0/5;
6 right leg proximal power 3/5;

7 right leg distal power 3/5;
8 diminished response to painful sensation in the right arm and leg.

He received 3 weeks of inpatient rehabilitation therapy and was discharged to his parents' home. At 3 months post-stroke, he was able to follow simple but not complex right/left commands, had minimal speech output with frequent paraphasic errors and neologisms, was unable to write spontaneously, and was unable to do simple mathematical operations. He walked with a mild hemiparetic gait and used a four-prong cane. He could lift his right arm above his head but could not grip with his right hand. He could feed and groom himself using his left hand. He

---

MAJOR POINTS

- Stroke outcomes should be conceptualized along a framework that includes impairments, disabilities, and handicap.
- In the most current World Health Organization paradigm, impairments equate to symptoms, disabilities to functional abilities, and handicap to participation.
- Stroke impairments may be most related to the underlying biology of stroke but are usually less important to the patient than functional ability and participation outcomes.

- Consideration of the content, the response format, and prior validation are paramount to selecting a tool that will adequately assess stroke outcome in a given population of patients.
- Global endpoint analysis, shift analysis, and prognosis-adjusted end points are examples of analysis strategies that may improve the sensitivity of existing stroke outcome measures to detect meaningful effect sizes in clinical trials.

A Primer on Stroke Prevention Treatment: An Overview Based on AHA/ASA Guidelines, 1st Edition. Edited by L Goldstein.

was able to dress himself and to get in and out of bed by himself, and was continent. He could go up 10 steps slowly using the handrail.

At 6 months post-stroke, he had some slight improvement in his right hand grasp but little improvement in expressive speech. He was able to follow complex commands and was better at monitoring and attempting to correct his paraphasic errors. He appeared frustrated by his difficulty in expressing himself. Due to his continuing language problems, he was unable to return to work. He required assistance from his parents for financial management. Since he was unable to work, he sold his home and was living with his parents. His parents relayed that he was having trouble sleeping and spent most of the day sitting by himself. He resisted their attempts to take him out shopping, or to go see a friend as he had done in the past.

Introduction

Precise measurement of stroke outcomes is critical because (a) stroke can be associated with considerable morbidity and cost, from both the personal and societal perspectives; (b) stroke incidence and prevalence is expected to increase as the population ages; and (c) efficient drug development and evaluation of nonpharmacological interventions rely on accurate and sensitive measures of stroke outcome. However, the methodology, conceptualization, and measurement of stroke outcomes are complex. This complexity exists because of the heterogeneity of the functional effects of stroke and because of the difficulty in assessing other critical variables that modify stroke outcomes.

This chapter will review the major types of stroke outcome measures frequently used in clinical trials, briefly discuss the use of surrogate outcome measures, and summarize the current debate about the most effective analysis strategies for outcome measures in stroke trials. The chapter concludes with a section on considerations when choosing an outcome measure for clinical stroke research and serves as a reference when interpreting the results of clinical trials.

Types of stroke outcome measures

Due to the heterogeneity of stroke symptoms and severity, there are many possible categories of outcome measures in stroke. Based on the original World Health Organization (WHO) classification of disease sequelae (Table 18.1), outcome scales have long been characterized as measuring impairments, disabilities, or handicaps [1]. *Impairments* are physi-cal consequences of dysfunction of a specific organ, *disabilities* are difficulties patients experience in normal activities because of their impairments, and *handicap* refers to the societal view of the disability, or how disease affects the individual's social, professional, or family roles. In stroke, impairments are usually summarized with ordinal scales (e.g., the National Institutes of Health Stroke Scale [NIHSS]). Disabilities are usually conceptualized as functional status and assessed by basic or instrumental activi-

Table 18.1 Content of commonly used stroke impairment scales

	CNS	NIHSS	SSS
Level of consciousness	+	+	+
Orientation		+	+
Commands		+	
Speech	+	+	+
Motor			
Face	+	+	+
Arm, proximal	+	+	+
Arm, distal	+		+
Leg, proximal	+	+	+
Leg, distal	+		+
Eye movements		+	+
Dysarthria		+	
Sensation		+	
Ataxia		+	
Neglect		+	
Limb tone			+
Gait			+

CNS, Canadian Neurologic Scale; NIHSS, National Institutes of Health Stroke Scale; SSS, Scandinavian Stroke Scale.

ties of daily living (IADLs) scales such as the Barthel Index (BI). Handicap, although less frequently assessed in stroke clinical trials, is typically measured by health-related quality of life (HRQL) scales.

It is important to note that this WHO classification has undergone modification from a focus on disease sequelae to a focus on the interaction between biological and societal aspects of human functioning [2]. This International Classification of Functioning (ICF) model considers body function and structure (rather than impairments), activities (rather that disability), and participation (rather than handicap) in relation to disease condition as well as to the contextual factors of existing personal and environmental characteristics. This model has been accepted by the World Health Assembly as the preferred method for classifying function related to health and so is likely to have an increasing influence on the conceptual framework for the measurement of health outcomes. Nonetheless, since the outcome measures currently used in stroke trials were developed prior to this classification, the review of these measures follows the earlier designation of measures of impairment, disability, and handicap (as measured by HRQL).

Impairment scales

Impairment scales are designed to measure the symptoms caused by stroke. As such, they are the most concrete or proximal outcomes to consider when assessing stroke outcome. This has the theoretical advantage of clarity and strength in relationship of the outcome to the stroke event. In reality, however, impairment scales have the challenges of symptom assignment, depth of measurement, and importance to the patient. First, the symptoms of stroke can be difficult to assign to the stroke itself versus some other cause. Any stroke impairment scale should have clear instructions about the assignment of symptoms that could be related to stroke but have some other specific cause (e.g., loss of sensation caused by radiculopathy or neuropathy vs. stroke). Because stroke can cause a variety of symptoms, some common and some rare, a stroke impairment scale is most relevant when it includes many symptoms, but can in turn suffer from the addition of unusual symptoms that often introduce measurement error in the scale. For example, this type of error has been demonstrated with the ataxia neglect

items of the NIHSS [3,4]. Some impairment scales were developed for or tend to measure outcome more fully in a specific stroke type (e.g., middle cerebral artery strokes or posterior circulation strokes). Finally, as is demonstrated by the construct of the ICF model, symptoms are the least important outcome to the patient, compared with the ability to function in daily life in the patient's unique environment.

Despite these theoretical limitations, impairment scales are commonly used in stroke trials and have fundamental importance in their ability to predict a wide range of eventual outcomes including function, quality of life, healthcare utilization, and mortality.

Many impairment scales have been developed, often regionally or nationally (e.g., Scandinavian [5] and Canadian Stroke Scales [6]; see the section on Neurologic deficit stroke scales in Herndon's *Handbook of Neurologic Rating Scales* for other examples [7]). Despite some limitations and a lack of demonstration of superiority over other impairment scales, the NIHSS has emerged as being the most commonly used in North American ischemic stroke trials and is also frequently used in studies of intracerebral hemorrhage. Emergency personnel, nurses, and other healthcare providers increasingly use the NIHSS as a uniform tool for communicating the status of stroke patients. The elements assessed in several commonly used impairment scales are given in Table 18.1.

NIHSS

The NIHSS assesses 11 items from a standardized neurological examination, focusing on findings common in acute stroke (e.g., assessment of hemisensory loss rather than distal peripheral neuropathic sensory loss). Items have a range of scores from 0 (normal) to 4, with some items having a maximal score of 2 or 3. Item scores are summed to create an overall score. Inter-rater reliability is enhanced with the use of formal training tapes [8,9], although at least a 4-point difference in score was demonstrated in multiple vignettes in a large sample of NIHSS certification tests [10]. Retrospective scoring of the NIHSS using the written physical examination has been validated [11–13].

Although various methods for modifying the NIHSS in content or scoring have been proposed

[14–16], the scale primarily used a simple summed measure. It is important to recognize that in many cohorts or populations, the NIHSS is not normally distributed. This observation in an individual study should underlie the statistical descriptions and tests used to assess the NIHSS (e.g., the use of a mean NIHSS score vs. a median score and parametric vs. nonparametric statistical tests). In addition to comparing group scores, several investigators have suggested methods of assessing and comparing change in intra-individual NIHSS scores over time [17].

The NIHSS has also been used in several other ways that are relevant to outcomes in clinical trials. Clinical differences in patients are apparent with the NIHSS, as those with left hemisphere strokes score significantly poorer (approximately 4 points higher) than those with right hemisphere strokes, due to the opportunity for language deficits to affect multiple scale items including language, dysarthria, and level of consciousness [14]. Although there is relatively little empirical comparison of the various uses of the NIHSS, the scale is sometimes dichotomized at 0 or 1 versus 2 and higher to indicate very favorable outcome. Other investigators have used change in NIHSS from 3 to as many as 11 points to indicate clinical worsening, or have suggested using change in NIHSS stratified by baseline NIHSS score as a stroke outcome measure [17–20]. A better understanding of the measurement properties of these many uses of the NIHSS compared with other measurements of patient outcome would be helpful in furthering this aspect of stroke outcome assessment.

Other impairment scales

Two other neurological impairment scales are frequently used in stroke research: the Canadian Neurologic Scale (CNS) and the Scandinavian Stroke Scale (SSS) [5,6]. The CNS includes eight items measuring the level of consciousness, orientation, speech, and motor function (face, distal and proximal arm, distal and proximal leg). Scores range from 0 to 10 (10 indicating no impairments). Scoring differs in patients with comprehension deficit. The SSS is a nine-item scale encompassing consciousness, orientation, speech, eye movements, facial palsy, motor (arm, hand, and leg), and gait. Scores range from 0 to 48 (48 indicates no impairments). Compared with the NIHSS, these two scales are

somewhat shorter but are more oriented toward middle cerebral artery stroke, with no assessment of ataxia or dysarthria. In addition, the CNS does not include an assessment of eye movements, making it unsuitable for posterior circulation stroke assessment.

> **Example Case, cont'd.**
> The clinical presentation of this patient underscores the observation that the commonly used impairment scales record different deficits. The NIHSS captures the patient's language dysfunction in three separate items (following commands, best language, and dysarthria) but does not capture the hand weakness. The CNS records speech abnormality in one item only but does account for the distal limb weakness.

Disability scales

Scales that measure functional status arguably represent the most diverse category of stroke outcome assessments. Scales have been developed to measure specific functions (e.g., upper extremity use, mobility, or balance) and to measure specific categories of functions (e.g., activities of daily living [ADLs] or IADLs). Because a discussion of these many types of scales is beyond the scope of this chapter, the focus will instead be on the more general functional outcome scales most commonly used in stroke studies. Since the ADL/IADL distinction is clinically important and relevant to patients, this distinction in scale focus is retained. However, most stroke clinical trials use ADL scales to measure functional outcomes since these are theoretically more closely related to the effects of stroke and are less likely to be impacted by other physical, social, or environmental variables than IADLs.

ADL scales

ADL scales refer to those activities necessary for the basic functions of everyday living. Typically, these include dressing, eating, toileting, mobility, and bathing.

The Barthel Index

Although its initial use was to measure the amount of assistive care an individual required, the BI has been one of the most commonly used ADL scales in stroke research [21].

It is comprised of 10 items that are each ranked on a 3-point scale (Table 18.2). The score is a simple sum of the 10 items with a possible total score of either 20 (if the 3-point scale is scored 0, 1, 2 or 3) or 100 (if the 3-point scale is scored 0, 5, 10, or 15). Items are weighted, in that transfers and ambulation have a maximal score of 15, bathing and grooming have a maximal score of 5, and all other items have a maximal score of 10.

The BI has been shown to have high reliability and validity in stroke patients [22], but due to its measurement of the most elemental aspects of function, it has a ceiling effect in many stroke cohorts, especially those that include patients with mild stroke [23]. It does not assess the cognitive effects of stroke (e.g., language or executive function) and so is unable to discriminate between patients with and without these important stroke-related deficits. This concern has limited its use as the primary outcome measure in acute stroke trials, but it remains a commonly used measure especially in stroke rehabilitation studies [24].

The Functional Independence Measure (FIM)

The FIM is a widely used measure of function in stroke patients and has become a standard measure of the effectiveness of inpatient rehabilitation for patients with stroke and other neurological conditions [25,26]. The FIM is a copyrighted scale with use and scoring manuals regulated by the Uniform Data Systems/Research Foundation of the State University of New York.

The FIM includes 18 items that are organized into six dimensions and two subscales (motor and cognitive). Each item is scored on a 7-point scale ranging from complete dependence to complete independence. Gradations between scale ratings can be subtle; hence, the use of the official scoring manual and training of any personnel conducting the FIM is essential for reliable score generation.

Although the FIM is a primary measure of rehabilitation efficiency and is clinically useful in setting and tracking individual patient goals, some studies have shown that it is not significantly more responsive as an outcome measure in stroke studies than the simpler BI [27,28]. These findings as well as the greater time to conduct and score the FIM have

Table 18.2 Barthel Index

Item	Definition
Feeding	10 = independent, able to apply any necessary device. Feeds in reasonable time
	5 = needs help, i.e., for cutting
	0 = inferior performance
Bathing	5 = performs without assistance
	0 = inferior performance
Grooming	5 = washes face, combs hair, brushes teeth, shaves
	0 = inferior performance
Dressing	10 = independent, ties shoes, fastens fasteners, applies braces
	5 = needs help but does at least half of task within reasonable time
	0 = inferior performance
Bowel control	10 = no accidents, able to use enema or suppository if needed
	5 = occasional accidents or needs help with enema or suppository
	0 = inferior performance
Bladder control	10 = no accidents, able to care for collecting device if used
	5 = occasional accidents or needs help with device
	0 = inferior performance
Toilet transfer	10 = independent with toilet or bedpan. Handles clothes, wipes, flushes, or cleans pan
	5 = needs help for balance, handling clothes or toilet paper
	0 = inferior performance
Chair/bed transfer	15 = independent, including locks of wheelchair and lifting footrests
	10 = minimum assistance or supervision
	5 = able to sit but needs maximum assistance to transfer
	0 = inferior performance
Ambulation	15 = independent for 50 yards. May use assistive devices, except for rolling walker
	10 = with help for 50 yards
	5 = independent with wheelchair for 50 yards, only if unable to walk
	0 = inferior performance
Stairs	10 = independent. May use assistive devices
	5 = needs help or supervision
	0 = inferior performance

limited its use in stroke trial, although it remains a frequent outcome measure in rehabilitation studies.

Example Case, cont'd.

Despite having significant remaining impairments, the patient is functionally independent in activities of daily living by 3 months post-stroke. Thus, his BI score is 100 (perfect). If a functional scale, especially one assessing less difficult items, is used as the sole outcome measure, the resulting ceiling effect can make it difficult to demonstrate a difference among treatment groups in a clinical trial.

IADL scales

IADL scales refer to the more complex, executive functions necessary for living independently and thus complement measures of ADLs. IADLs typically include procuring food and other necessities, cooking, and managing finances. Although of vital importance to patients, IADLs are not frequently used in outcome measures in pharmacological stroke clinical trials, although they may play a larger role in trials of rehabilitation interventions and in cohort studies. IADL scales that have been developed and validated in stroke patients include the Frenchay Activities Index, the Nottingham Extended ADL scale, and the Rivermead ADL Assessment [29,30].

HRQL scales

Although impairments and functional status are undoubtedly important stroke outcomes, they do not fully describe the impact of stroke on the person as a whole. For example, patients typically care more about what they can do with their hand (function) than whether their arm has a drift (impairment). Functional status is thus a more patient-centered outcome than impairment, but still focuses on one aspect of a person's life – physical performance of basic tasks, rather than considering the effects of stroke on the person as a whole.

Because of this limitation, there has been a gradual shift in outcomes assessment to incorporate the patient's perception of his own overall health status.

Consequently, HRQL is increasingly measured as a stroke outcome. Since the construct of HRQL typically encompasses the physical, psychological, and social aspects of life that may be influenced by changes in health states [31], HRQL scales can reflect a composite of impairments, disabilities, and handicaps after stroke.

HRQL can be measured with generic or disease-specific scales. Generic measures are designed to compare HRQL across populations or different diseases; disease-specific measures are designed to assess HRQL using questions and scales that are specific to a disease or condition. Generic HRQL measures are prevalent, well validated, and appropriate for the purpose of comparing HRQL changes after stroke to HRQL changes in patients with different conditions. Because they are designed to measure HRQL in diverse populations, the meaning of generic HRQL scores in stroke patients, the capacity of these scores to discriminate among patients with important clinical differences, and the capacity to measure change over time may be less than with stroke-specific HRQL scales [32,33].

Generic HRQL measures in stroke

Several generic HRQL measures have been and continue to be used for stroke outcome assessment (Table 18.3). The Medical Outcomes Study Short Form 36 (SF-36), the Sickness Impact Profile (SIP), and the EuroQoL have all been validated in stroke cohorts and continue to be used with some frequency.

The SF-36

The SF-36 is a 36-item scale that was developed for the assessment of health status in populations and has been used extensively in clinical and population-based research [34]. It is most often used descriptively to monitor patients or compare patients to the general population rather than as a primary outcome measure in clinical trials. Its strengths include its excellent measurement properties, the breadth of its measurement with relatively few questions, and the existence of national normative values [35]. Items are scored using a weighted algorithm to develop eight separate subscale (dimension) scores (Table 18.3).

The SF-36 has been used frequently to describe patients with stroke [33,36,37]. Although it does

Table 18.3 Generic health-related quality of life scales: domains and items

Scale	Domain	Number of items
Short Form 36	Physical functioning	10
	Physical role	4
	Bodily pain	2
	Emotional role	3
	Social functioning	2
	Vitality	4
	Mental health	5
	General health perceptions	5
	(Change in health status in the past year)	1 (not counted in scoring)
Stroke-Adapted Sickness Impact Profile-30	Alertness behavior	3
	Ambulation	3
	Body care and movement	5
	Mobility	3
	Communication	3
	Emotional behavior	4
	Social interaction	5
	Home management	4
EuroQoL	Anxiety/depression	1
	Mobility	1
	Pain/discomfort	1
	Self-care	1
	Usual activities	1

discriminate HRQL between stroke and non-stroke elderly, there are floor effects in some domains, especially those related to physical functioning.

In the interest of measurement efficiency, summary physical and mental composite scores have been developed from the SF-36 [38]. The SF-12 has gained popularity as a shortened version that can generate these two composite scales. Although efficiency improves when a scale is shortened, measurement accuracy may suffer. Thus, it is imperative to revalidate the shortened scale relative to the parent scale in the population of interest. When this was done in a stroke cohort, the scaling assumptions that go into the development of the SF-12 from the SF-36 were not fulfilled, suggesting that the calculation of SF-12 subscale scores in stroke patients may not be valid [32].

The SIP

The SIP is a well-validated generic HRQL measure comprised of 136 yes/no questions [39,40]. It has

been adapted and reduced to 30 items for stroke patients as the Stroke-Adapted SIP-30 (Table 18.3), with favorable comparison to the longer SIP despite primarily representing the domain of physical functioning [41,42]. The shortened version explained 91% of the variation in the original SIP score, but due to the exclusion of patients with aphasia, this does not include items relevant to communication.

The EuroQoL

The EuroQoL was designed to provide a single index score representing generic health status. It was developed collaboratively with input from researchers representing multiple countries to define a core set of HRQL items relevant across different cultures and individual characteristics [43–45]. The EuroQoL includes an additional item, a visual analog scale, representing the patient's health at the time of completion of the scale. This item is not included in the overall score, which uses weights developed for each item. The five-item scale (without the visual analog scale) is also known as the EQ-5D. These culturally specific utility weightings, derived separately for various countries, are then used to develop an overall utility score ranging from 0.0 to 1.0.

Although comprised of only five items each pertaining to a different domain of quality of life (thus susceptible to measurement error) and graded on a 3-point Likert scale (resulting in decreased discriminatory power), the EuroQoL is reliable and has discriminant and construct validity comparable to the SF-36 in stroke patients [46–48].

Stroke-specific HRQL measures
As the potential drawbacks of generic HRQL scales became apparent in stroke and in other conditions, the development of disease-specific HRQL scales proliferated. In addition to scales developed specifically for patients with hemorrhagic stroke [49] and scales developed from other stroke-specific scales [50], there have been three stroke-specific scales developed in the past decade (Table 18.4). These scales continue to be used in cohort studies and clinical trials, where work to further refine the scales and study their performance in different populations and in different study designs is ongoing.

Burden of Stroke Scale (BOSS)
The BOSS is the most recently developed stroke-specific scale [51].

Derived from focus groups of patients and caregivers, as well as literature and expert panel review, the BOSS includes 64 items reflecting 12 domains. These domains can be summarized in three composite scales (physical limitations, psychological distress, and cognitive limitations) or in an overall summary scale score. Lower scores (0 is normal) represent better functioning. This scale was validated in stroke patients and in healthy controls and included patients with communication difficulty in its initial development.

Stroke Impact Scale (SIS)
The SIS is a robust stroke-specific HRQL scale, developed from interviews with stroke survivors and caregivers. It includes 64 items in eight domains [52]. The SIS has been validated in multiple cohorts and for telephone and mail assessment [53,54]. Response sets for items are on a 5-point Likert scale, with scores calculated using a weighted algorithm

Table 18.4 Stroke-specific health-related quality of life scales: domains and items

Scale	Domain	Number of items
Burden of Stroke Scale	Mobility	5
	Self-care	5
	Communication	7
	Cognition	5
	Swallowing	3
	Social relations	5
	Energy and sleep	4
	Negative mood	4
	Positive mood	4
	Domain mood	7
	Domain satisfaction	7
	Domain restriction	8
Stroke Impact Scale	Strength	4
	Hand function	5
	Mobility	10
	ADL/IADL	12
	Memory	8
	Communication	7
	Emotion	9
	Participation	9
Stroke-Specific Quality of Life Scale	Energy	3
	Family role	3
	Language	5
	Mobility	6
	Mood	5
	Personality	3
	Self-care	5
	Social role	5
	Thinking	3
	Upper-extremity function	5
	Vision	3
	Work	3

ADL, activity of daily living; IADL, instrumental activity of daily living.

generating domain scores from 0 to 100. A shortened version, the SIS-16, reflects physical functioning [55]. The SIS is being used in several ongoing stroke and rehabilitation clinical trials.

Stroke-Specific Quality of Life (SS-QOL) Scale
The SS-QOL was developed from focused interviews with stroke survivors and caregivers and includes 49

items in 12 stroke-specific domains [56]. This scale has also been shortened to 35 items in eight domains [57]. Items are scored on a 5-point Likert scale, with domain scores representing the average score of items in that domain and the overall score the unweighted average of domain scores. It is more sensitive to stroke-related impairments than the SF-36 [33], and has been adapted for aphasic stroke survivors [50]; it has also been translated into Danish [58]. The SS-QOL is being used in several ongoing stroke clinical trials.

Example Case, cont'd.

Although the patient's language deficits would make completing an HRQL scale challenging, a proxy report by his parents revealed scores below the median for other similar stroke patients at 6 months post-stroke in the domains of work, role function, language, upper-extremity function, and mood. He had been able to convey to his parents that if he could get back to some kind of paid work, he would feel that he was again making a contribution to his family. In this patient, with relatively good large motor function, a generic scale might not be sensitive enough to capture remaining mobility problems. A primary component of his outcome at this point appears to be depression, highlighting the importance of using scales that capture changes in mood post-stroke. Referral to a vocational rehabilitation program might also be another potentially effective intervention identified by the HRQL scale assessment.

Global outcome scales

Global outcome scales are designed to summarize outcome in a single, meaningful paradigm. Whereas the use of a global outcome scale can have great face validity (e.g., is the person independent or not), the use of a single question to evaluate outcome can be problematic from a measurement standpoint. In the framework of classical test theory, the use of a single question does not allow the examiner to distinguish variability in the characteristic of interest (e.g., patient's true outcomes) from variability in measurement. Nonetheless, global outcome scales that

employ specifically defined categories or descriptions of outcomes are among the most commonly used and well-understood stroke outcome measures.

Simple questions

Simple self-reported questions have the advantage of efficiency and face validity, and several studies have investigated the use of various simple questions compared with other standard outcome scales. The consideration in deciding to use a simple question versus a scale usually depends on weighing time and cost efficiency against precision, realizing that the simple questions may be faster to collect but may necessitate increased sample size to demonstrate a given effect. Examples of simple questions that have been compared with other outcome scales include a two-item questionnaire that measures dependency ("In the last 2 weeks, did you require help from another person for everyday activities?") and recovery ("Do you feel that you have made a complete recovery from your stroke?") [59–61], and a five-item subset of a longer questionnaire [62].

The Glasgow Outcome Scale (GOS)

The GOS (Table 18.5) was originally developed as a companion to the Glasgow Coma Scale; its intent was thus first to describe outcomes in patients who

Table 18.5 Glasgow Outcome Scale

Grade	Description
1	Dead.
2	Persistent vegetative state. Patient exhibits no obvious cortical function.
3	Severe disability (conscious but disabled). Patient depends on others for daily support due to mental or physical disability or both.
4	Moderate disability (disabled but independent). Patient is independent as far as daily life is concerned. The disabilities found include varying degrees of dysphasia, hemiparesis, or ataxia, as well as intellectual and memory deficits and personality changes.
5	Good recovery. Resumption of normal activities even thought there may be minor neurological or psychological deficits.

presented in coma [63,64]. Although it has been used in clinical stroke studies, it has most often been used in studies of traumatic brain injury and non-traumatic coma. The categorizations are so broad as to reduce the distribution in ischemic stroke survivors, and thus, this scale is less commonly used than other global outcome scales in stroke, specifically the modified Rankin Scale (mRS).

mRS

The mRS may be the most frequently used outcome measure in clinical stroke research. Its popularity derives both from its face validity, its relative efficiency, and its generally well-accepted dichotomization categorizing dependent from independent stroke survivors. As is evident from observing the language in the descriptive statements (Table 18.6), the mRS considers impairments, functional ability, and role outcomes and thus attempts to assess outcomes across the range of meaning as described in the ICF model. As has been suggested, it should thus be considered a global functional health index with strong emphasis on physical disability [65] rather than a pure handicap measure.

The mRS includes six categories of outcome ranging from no symptoms at all (entirely normal) to complete dependence. Some versions of the mRS have also included a category for death. Commonly, the mRS is dichotomized at scores of 0–2 versus 3–5,

as this cut-point has been reported to reliably distinguish independence (scores 0–2) from dependence (scores 3–5). Some studies have also dichotomized the mRS at a score of 0 or 1 versus others, to indicate a very favorable outcome. Although choosing to define stroke outcome by Rankin as "good" (Rankin 0–1 vs. others) or "poor" (mRS 3–6 vs. others) may seem esoteric, the analysis of thrombolysis trials demonstrate that the overall effect of treatment remains consistent with either definition; individual trial successes and failures, however, can vary by choice of cut-point [66]. This variability likely has its roots in the underlying reliability characteristics of the mRS and has stimulated the evaluation of shift in mRS score rather than dichotomized analyses (see section on the Analysis of stroke outcome measures in clinical trials).

Despite the fairly detailed description of the categories, it is evident that there is still a significant possibility for subjective assessment in the mRS. This variability is because it is clinically possible to have a factual description of a patient's outcome in more than one category and because the information required to assign an mRS category can come from questioning the patient, a caregiver, and/or observation. This important characteristic of the mRS has been demonstrated by multiple studies showing lower than desirable inter-rater reliability [67]. However, reliability can be improved with the use of a structured interview to assign an mRS score that will in turn improve the precision of measurement and thus decrease the sample size needed to show a given effect [67,68]. Recently, a training program for mRS assessment has been demonstrated to be successful; this type of training and the use of a structured interview should become a standard procedure when using the mRS in any clinical research study [69].

Table 18.6 Modified Rankin Scale

Grade	Description
0	No symptoms at all.
1	No significant disability despite symptoms; able to carry out all usual duties and activities.
2	Slight disability; unable to carry out all previous activities, but able to look after own affairs without assistance.
3	Moderate disability; requiring some help, but able to walk without assistance.
4	Moderately severe disability; unable to walk without assistance, and unable to attend to own bodily needs without assistance.
5	Severe disability; bedridden, incontinent, and requiring constant nursing care and attention.

Example Case, cont'd.
The patient has remaining deficits, walks independently, but still requires help with IADLs (e.g., financial management); thus his Rankin score was 3.

Analysis of stroke outcome measures in clinical trials

From the preceding review, it is clear that there are many types of stroke outcome measures and no universally agreed upon "best" measure to use in clinical research. How common scales are used to define good or bad outcome varies from trial to trial [70]. Further, some trials have been controversial because of differences between several outcome measures. For these reasons, considerable effort has been put toward evaluating the best methods for analyzing outcome measures in the context of stroke clinical trials [71].

One approach that has been used to address the problem of multiple outcomes measured within a trial is to use a global endpoint analysis to simultaneously assess improvement in multiple scales [72]. This approach, which requires the selection of a cut-point defining good outcome for each measure, was used in the National Institute of Neurological Disorder and Stroke (NINDS) tPA trial, in which improvement favoring the intervention group was found in all four of the trial's outcome measures (tPA trial). As demonstrated by the retrospective analysis of the European Cooperative Acute Stroke Study (ECASS), however, the use of the global test statistic may result in a positive global outcome even if one of the individual outcome measures does not indicate a significant treatment effect [19]. This can lead to uncertainty over the interpretation of trial results.

Another approach that has been suggested is the shift analysis for mRS scores. This has both clinical appeal, in that it considers each individual subject's change across the full range of observed outcomes, and also has analytical appeal as it may be statistically more sensitive in detecting a treatment effect than a dichotomized outcome. Reanalysis of the NINDS-rtPA and the ECASS trials showed that although the use of this analysis strategy would have resulted in ECASS-II being a positive trial (favoring tPA treatment), the shift analysis was not necessarily more sensitive than the dichotomized Rankin score. A recent survey indicated that the shift analysis strategy is viewed favorably among stroke specialists [73].

Although the shift approach may be viewed favorably by some trialists, most still use a dichotomized stroke outcome scale to assess the effects of an intervention. How this dichotomized outcome is analyzed has critical effects on the difference in outcome the trial will be powered to detect. The Optimising Analysis of Stroke Trials collaborative group compared analysis strategies for dichotomized outcomes using data from more than 50,000 individual patients in 55 stroke and rehabilitation trials [74]. They found that across different trial types and sizes, analysis strategies that retained the scale scores as ordered categorical data (e.g., ordinal logistic regression, t-tests, robust ranks test) performed better than tests that dichotomize the data into favorable versus unfavorable outcome (e.g., chi-square or analysis of variance). This advantage has similarly been demonstrated for stroke prevention studies [75], and results in an approximate 25% reduction in needed sample size for acute stroke trials employing a functional primary outcome measure [74].

Because stroke patients vary widely in their type of deficits, severity of deficits, and probability of achieving good outcome, another approach has been to use prognosis-adjusted end points. This strategy can theoretically increase the statistical power of a trial while considering the individual improvements among all patients enrolled [76].

An additional consideration in analyzing stroke outcome measures deserves mention: the use of risk adjustment in the analysis of outcome data. Risk adjustment has been suggested as a means to account for unmeasured imbalance in stroke severity and prognosis, and may increase the odds of detecting a favorable outcome while reducing necessary sample sizes [77]. Other investigators have suggested using baseline variables to select study subjects most likely to benefit from an intervention, thus increasing the efficiency of the study at the cost of decreasing generalizability [78]. Arriving at a universal set of risk adjustment variables that apply broadly to stroke trials with different entry criteria and are accepted widely remains a challenge, but this general strategy deserves further investigation as a means to improve the design of clinical trials.

> **Example Case, cont'd.**
> The difference between the functional assessment (e.g., Barthel of 100) and the global assessment (Rankin of 3) underscores the potential uncertainty that can arise when using multiple types of outcome assessments in clinical trials. A comprehensive understanding of the scales, their prior performance in the specific population, and a thoughtful planned analytic strategy are needed to employ multiple scales successfully in clinical trials.

Conclusion

Stroke outcome assessments are complicated because of heterogeneity in stroke symptoms and severity.

Consideration of the population enrollment criteria (to ensure that full range of expected stroke impacts is assessed) and of the study design (to maximize efficiency and power) should guide the choice of stroke outcome assessment in a given study. Some authors have suggested that ideally, primary outcome measures would capture activities, since these are more patient centric, and have supported the use of shift or ordinal analysis over dichotomization due to the loss of clinical information and sensitivity [70]. For studies evaluating stroke recovery over a longer period of time, outcome measures that assess a specific deficit more sensitively may be more appropriate [79].

References available online at www.wiley.com/go/strokeguidelines.

Other Statements Published in 2008

During the production of this book the following relevant AHA/ASA statements and guidelines were published.

<u>Stroke Specific</u>

Update to the AHA/ASA Recommendations for the Prevention of Stroke in Patients With Stroke and Transient Ischemic Attack Publ March 2008 Stroke 2008:39;1647–1652. Robert J. Adams, Greg Albers, Mark J. Alberts, Oscar Benevente, Karen Furie, Larry B. Goldstein, Philip Gorelick, Jonathan Halperin, Robert Harbaugh, S. Claiborne Johnston, Irene Katzan, Margaret Kelly-Hayes, Edgar J. Kenton, Michael Marks, Ralph L. Sacco, and Lee J. Schwamm. http://stroke.ahajournals.org/cgi/reprint/STROKEAHA. 107.189063

Management of Stroke in Infants and Children Publ July 2008. Stroke 2008:39;2644–2691. E. Steve Roach, Meredith R. Golomb, Robert Adams, Jose Biller, Stephen Daniels, Gabrielle deVeber, Donna Ferriero, Blaise V. Jones, Fenella J. Kirkham, R. Michael Scott and Edward R. Smith. http://stroke.ahajournals.org/cgi/reprint/STROKEAHA. 108.189696

Bederson JB, Connolly ES Jr, Batjer HH, Dacey RG, Dion JE, Diringer MN, Duldner JE Jr, Harbaugh RE, Patel AB, Rosenwasser RH. Guidelines for the management of aneurysmal subarachnoid hemorrhage: a statement for healthcare professionals from a special writing group of the Stroke Council, American Heart Association. *Stroke* 2009: published online before print January 22, 2009, 10.1161/STROKEAHA. 108.191395.

Definition and Diagnostic Evaluation of Transient Ischemic Attack – This one has been to SACC, it had some comments (minor) and has gone back to the lead author. No pub date yet. – If SACC approved by press time LIST THIS ONE AS IN PRESS

<u>General Relevance</u>

Resistant Hypertension: Diagnosis, Evaluation, and Treatment Publ April 2008. Hypertension 2008:51;1403–1419.

David A. Calhoun, Daniel Jones, Stephen Textor, David C. Goff, Timothy P. Murphy, Robert D. Toto, Anthony White, William C. Cushman, William White, Domenic Sica, Keith Ferdinand, Thomas G. Giles, Bonita Falkner and Robert M. Carey. http://hyper.ahajournals.org/cgi/reprint/ HYPERTENSIONAHA.108.189141

Population-Based Prevention of Obesity: The Need for Comprehensive Promotion of Healthful Eating, Physical Activity, and Energy Balance Publ June 2008. Circulation 2008:118;428–464. Shiriki K. Kumanyika, Eva Obarzanek, Nicolas Stettler, Ronny Bell, Alison E. Field, Stephen P. Fortmann, Barry A. Franklin, Matthew W. Gillman, Cora E. Lewis, Walter Carlos Poston II, June Stevens and Yuling Hong. http://circ.ahajournals.org/cgi/reprint/ CIRCULATIONAHA.108.189702

Contribution of Metabolic and Anthropometric Abnormalities to Cardiovascular Disease Risk Factors Publ June 2008 Conf Proceedings. Circulation 2008:118;e20–e28. Carl Grunfeld, Donald P. Kotler, Donna K. Arnett, Julian M. Falutz, Steven M. Haffner, Paul Hruz, Henry Masur, James M. Meigs, Kathleen Mulligan, Peter Reiss, Katherine Samaras and for Working Group 1. http://circ.ahajournals.org/cgi/ reprint/CIRCULATIONAHA.107.189623

Translating Research Into Practice for Healthcare Providers: The American Heart Association's Strategy for Building Healthier Lives, Free of Cardiovascular Diseases and Stroke Publ July 2008. Circulation 2008:118;687–696. Daniel W. Jones, Eric D. Peterson, Robert O. Bonow, Frederick A. Masoudi, Gregg C. Fonarrow, Sidney C. Smith, Jr, Penelope Solis, Meighan Girgus, Patricia C. Hinton, Anne Leonard and Raymond J. Gibbons. http://circ.ahajournals.org/ cgi/reprint/CIRCULATIONAHA.108.189934

The Impact of Prevention on Reducing the Burden of Cardiovascular Disease Publ July 2008. Circulation 2008:118;576–585. Richard Kahn, Rose Marie Robertson, Robert Smith and David Eddy. http://circ.ahajournals.org/cgi/reprint/ CIRCULATIONAHA.108.190186

ACCF/ACG/AHA 2008 Expert Consensus Document on Reducing the Gastrointestinal Risks of Antiplatelet Therapy and NSAID Use. Circulation 2008:118;1894–1909. Deepak L. Bhatt, James Scheiman, Neena S. Abraham, Elliott M. Antman, Francis K.L Chan, Curt D. Furberg, David A. Johnson, Kenneth W. Mahaffey and Eamonn M. Quigley. http://circ.ahajournals.org/cgi/reprint/CIRCULATIONAHA.108.191087

AHA/ACCF Sleep Apnea and Cardiovascular Disease. Circulation 2008:118;1080–1111. Virend K. Somers, David P. White, Raouf Amin, William T. Abraham, Fernando Costa, Antonio Culebras, Stephen Daniels, John S. Floras, Carl E. Hunt, Lyle J. Olson, Thomas G. Pickering, Richard Russell, Mary Woo and Terry Young. http://circ.ahajournals.org/cgi/reprint/CIRCULATIONAHA.107.189420

ACC/AHA/Physician Consortium 2008 Clinical Performance Measures for Adults With Nonvalvular Atrial Fibrillation or Atrial Flutter. Circulation 2008:117;1101–1120. N.A. Mark Estes, III, Jonathan L. Haperin, Hugh Calkins, Michael D. Ezekowitz, Paul Gitman, Alan S. Go, Robert L. McNamara, Joseph V. Messer, James L. Ritchie, Sam J.W. Romeo, Albert L. Waldo and D. George Wyse. http://circ.ahajournals.org/cgi/reprint/117/8/1101

Skyler JS, Bergenstal R, Bonow RO, Buse J, Deedwania P, Gale EAM, Howard BV, Kirkman MS, Kosiborod M, Reaven P, Sherwin RS. Intensive glycemic control and the prevention of cardiovascular events: implications of the ACCORD, ADVANCE, and VA Diabetes Trials: a position statement of the American Diabetes Association and a scientific statement of the American College of Cardiology Foundation and the American Heart Association. Circulation 2008: published online before print December 17, 2008, 10.1161/CIRCULATIONAHA.108.191305. Available at: http://circ.ahajournals.org/cgi/reprint/CIRCULATIONAHA.108.191305

Alberts MJ, Felberg RA, Guterman LR, Levine SR, for Writing Group 4. Atherosclerotic Peripheral Vascular Disease Symposium II: stroke intervention: state of the art. Circulation. 2008;118:2845–2851. Available at: http://circ.ahajournals.org/cgi/reprint/CIRCULATIONAHA.108.191174.

White CJ, Beckman JA, Cambria RP, Comerota AJ, Gray WA, Hobson RW 2nd, Iyer SS, for Writing Group 5. Atherosclerotic Peripheral Vascular Disease Symposium II: controversies in carotid artery revascularization. Circulation. 2008;118:2852–2859. Available at: http://circ.ahajournals.org/cgi/reprint/CIRCULATIONAHA.108.191175.

Index

Author Disclosure Table

Working group member	Employment	Research grant	Other research support	Speakers bureau/honoraria	Expert witness	Ownership interest	Consultant/advisory board	Other
Adams	NONE	NONE	NONE	*Genentech Boehringer-Inselbeim/*for speaking	NONE	NONE	B6B	NONE
Adeoye	NONE	NONE	NONE	NONE	NONE	NONE	NONE	NONE
Beckett	NONE	NONE	NONE	NONE	NONE	NONE	NONE	NONE
Brisman	NONE	NONE	NONE	*Given several talks at hospitals . . . grand rounds etc. in which I discussed cerebral aneurysms among other topics and was given small honoraria for some, probably totaling $1,000 or so.	*Legal case about a woman with a ruptured cerebral aneurysm	NONE	NONE	NONE
Broderick				Boehringer Ingelheim			+Steering committee at Novo Nordisk	
Bushnell	NONE	+(BMS/Sanofi, co-PI for AVAIL registry, NIH K02NS058760)	NONE	NONE	NONE	NONE	*(Boehringer Ingelheim Data Safety Monitoring Committee for flibanserin)	NONE
Chaturvedi	NONE	+(Boehringer-Ingelheim Schering J&J)	NONE	NONE	NONE	NONE	+(BMS/Sanofi Partnership Boehringer-Ingelheim) and *(Abbott Vascular Prize)	NONE
Deal	NONE	NONE	NONE	NONE	NONE	NONE	NONE	NONE
deVeber	NONE	NONE	NONE	NONE	NONE	NONE	NONE	NONE
Giromano	NONE	+Site PI of NIH funded SPS3 study	NONE	Boeringer Ingelheim	NONE	NONE	NONE	NONE

Continued

Working group member	Employment	Research grant	Other research support	Speakers bureau/honoraria	Expert witness	Ownership interest	Consultant/advisory board	Other
Goldstein	NONE	+NIH, AHA, VA	*AGA (RESPECT), Schering Plough (TIMI 50)	*Pfizer	NONE	NONE	*Pfizer, Johnson & Johnson, AGA, Novartis, TAP, Daiichi Sankyo, Stroke Group	NONE
Gorelick	NONE	NONE	NONE	NONE	NONE	NONE	NONE	NONE
Hachinski	NONE	NONE	NONE	*Mitsubi Tanaba Pharma Corporation Honorarium and Ferrer Group Honorarium	NONE	NONE	NONE	NONE
Homma	NONE	NONE	NONE	NONE	NONE	NONE	NONE	+AGA Medical OSMB Money
Howard	NONE	NONE	NONE	NONE	NONE	NONE	+(Bayer executive board for ARRIVE study)	NONE
Levine	NONE	+NIH	*Gaisman Foundation	+NCME/*Medlink	NONE	NONE	*Photothera	NONE
Mayberg	NONE	*(NINDS)	*(Federal government)	NONE	NONE	NONE	NONE	NONE
Merino	NONE	NONE	NONE	NONE	NONE	NONE	NONE	NONE
Papamitzakis	NONE	NONE	NONE	NONE	NONE	NONE	NONE	NONE
Park	NONE	NONE	NONE	NONE	NONE	NONE	NONE	NONE
Qureshi	NONE	AHA; NIH; MMF	NONE	NONE	NONE	NONE	NONE	NONE

Romano	NONE	+(Site PH of NIH funded SPS3 Study)	NONE	Boeringer Ingelheim	NONE	NONE	NONE
Rosand	NONE	+American Heart Association National Institute of Health Deane Institutte	NONE	NONE	NONE	NONE	NONE
Rost	NONE	+AHA/ASA Bugher Foundation	NONE	NONE	NONE	NONE	NONE
Sacco	NONE	NONE	NONE	NONE	NONE	+Boehringer Ingelheim *Glaxo SmithKline, Sanofi	NONE
Testai	NONE	NONE	NONE	NONE	NONE	NONE	NONE
Tullio	NONE	NONE	NONE	NONE	NONE	NONE	NONE
Williams	NONE	NONE	*VA HSR&D grants, none directly relevant to the chapter	NONE	NONE	NONE	NONE
Woods Duncan	NONE – Duke University	NONE – LEAPS NIH Funded	NONE	NONE	NONE	NONE – AHA Consultant	NONE

*Modest.

+Significant.

This table represents the relationships of writing group members that may be perceived as actual or reasonably perceived conflicts of interest as reported on the Disclosure Questionnaire which all writing group members are required to complete and submit. A relationship is considered to be "Significant" if (a) the person receives $10,000 or more during any 12 month period, or 5% or more of the person's gross income; or (b) the person owns 5% or more of the voting stock or share of the entity, or owns $10,000 or more of the fair market value of the entity. A relationship is considered to be "Modest" if it is less than "Significant" under the preceding definition.